Animal Welfare
A Cool Eye Towards Eden

John Webster

Professor of Animal Husbandry, Department of Veterinary Science,
The University of Bristol

A constructive approach to the problem
of man's dominion over the animals

D0230132

b

Blackwell
Science

© 1994 by
Blackwell Science Ltd
Editorial Offices:
Osney Mead, Oxford OX2 0EL
25 John Street, London WC1N 2BL
23 Ainslie Place, Edinburgh EH3 6AJ
238 Main Street, Cambridge,
  Massachusetts, 02142, USA
54 University Street, Carlton,
  Victoria 3053, Australia

Other Editorial Offices:
Arnette Blackwell SA
  224, Boulevard Saint Germain
  75007 Paris, France

Blackwell Wissenschafts-Verlag GmbH
  Kurfürstendamm 57
  10707 Berlin, Germany

Zehetnergasse 6
A-1140 Wien
Austria

All rights reserved. No part of this
publication may be reproduced, stored
in a retrieval system, or transmitted,
in any form or by any means,
electronic, mechanical, photocopying,
recording or otherwise, except as
permitted by the UK Copyright, Designs
and Patents Act 1988, without the
prior permission of the publisher.

First published 1995
Reprinted 1997

Set in 10/12 Times
by DP Photosetting, Aylesbury, Bucks
Printed and bound in Great Britain by
Hartnolls Ltd, Bodmin, Cornwall

DISTRIBUTORS

Marston Book Services Ltd
PO Box 269
Abingdon
Oxford OX14 4YN
(*Orders*: Tel: 01235 465500
         Fax: 01235 465555)

USA
Blackwell Science, Inc.
238 Main Street
Cambridge, MA 02142
(*Orders*: Tel: 800 215-1000
              617 876-7000
         Fax: 617 492-5263)

Canada
Copp Clark Professional
200 Adelaide Street, West, 3rd Floor
Toronto, Ontario M5H 1W7
(*Orders*: Tel: 416 597-1616
              800 815-9417
         Fax: 416 597-1617)

Australia
Blackwell Science Pty Ltd
54 University Street
Carlton, Victoria 3053
(*Orders*: Tel: 03 9347 0300
         Fax: 03 9347 5001)

A catalogue record for this book is
available from the British Library

ISBN 0–632–03928–0

Library of Congress
Cataloging in Publication Data
is available for this book

To Cordelia

Contents

Preface   viii

Part I: Introduction: Man's Dominion Over the Animals   1

1 Introduction: Man's Dominion   3
   Assessment of animal welfare: the five freedoms   10
   Life, liberty and the pursuit of happiness   14

Part II: Analysis: How Is It For Them?   17

2 Animal Mind and Animal Suffering   19
   Feeling and doing   19
   Do animals have minds?   23
   The evolution of mind   24
   Feelings, moods and cognition   27
   Measurement of 'behavioural needs'   31
   The nature of stress and suffering   35
   Conclusions   38

3 Hunger and Thirst   39
   Definitions   39
   Metabolic hunger and conscious appetite   41
   The allure of domestication   45
   Hunger for specific nutrients   47
   Thirst   54
   Oral satisfaction and oral stereotypies   55

4 Housing and Habitat   62
   Environmental requirements   62
   Thermal comfort   65
   Adaptation and acclimatization to heat and cold   70
   Comfort, hygiene and security at rest   74
   The need for space   78
   The problem of barren environments   81
   Environmental enrichment   84

5   **Pain, Sickness and Death**   **87**
    Unnecessary suffering   87
    What is pain?   89
    Indices of pain in animals   91
    Acute and chronic pain   95
    What is pain for?   98
    Sickness   99
    Relief of sickness   100
    Death and dying   104

6   **Friends, Foes, Fears and Stress**   **107**
    Animal conflict   108
    The nature of fear   112
    Stress and the general adaptation syndrome   116
    The company of their kind   121

Part III: Advocacy: What We Can Do For Them   **125**

7   **The Workers: Farm Animals**   **127**
    Food animals as a commodity   128
    Costs and benefits in livestock production   130
    The impetus for intensification   134
    Intensification and sustainability of livestock production 136
    How hard do animals work?   140
    The acceptable limits to productivity   142

8   **Pigs and Poultry**   **146**
    The welfare of pigs   **146**
    Accommodation for dry sows   147
    Farrowing and nursery accommodation   150
    Growing pigs   152
    Handling, transport and slaughter   153
    The welfare of poultry   **155**
    Broiler chickens and turkeys   155
    The laying hen   157
    Handling, transport and slaughter   158
    Priorities for change   160

9   **Cattle and Other Ruminants**   **167**
    Welfare of the dairy cow   **169**
    Metabolic hunger   171
    Lameness   172
    Milking and mastitis   175
    Metabolic diseases and exhaustion   177

The dairy cow and her calf 178
New techniques in cattle breeding 180
Beef cattle 183
Veal production 186
Sheep production **191**
Transport and slaughter 194

10 Horses and Pets **199**
What it is to be a pet 199
Boredom 202
Oral satisfaction in horses and dogs 202
Sex and social intercourse 205
Breeding and welfare 210
Euthanasia 213

11 Wild Animals **216**
Hunting and shooting 218
Fishing and whaling 222
Wildlife parks, zoos and circuses 225

12 Animals and Science **228**
'Scientific procedures' and 'cruelty to animals' 229
Costs and benefits 233
Assessment of costs 235
Refinement and replacement 238
Animal welfare research 240
Tinkering: biotechnology and genetic engineering 242

13 Right Thought and Right Action **247**
The middle way 247
Where do we stand? 248
Animal mind, animal welfare and suffering 249
Sources of suffering and pleasure 251
Right action 256
Compassion and anger 256
Research 257
Legislation 259
Education 263

Further Reading **266**
Index **269**

Preface

The main aim of this book is to offer constructive solutions to the problem of man's dominion over the animals. It is intended for anyone who feels it essential not only to the dignity of mankind but also to the quality of our own life to extend to other animal species the concept of man's humanity to man. Although the aim may be moral, the approach is strictly pragmatic. Animals are not affected by how we feel but by what we do.

Part II – *How is it for them?* – is an analysis of the nature of animal mind, animal welfare and suffering. It follows the logic of the *Five Freedoms* and considers hunger and thirst, housing and habitat, pain, sickness and death, friends, foes, fears and stress. In addressing these questions I draw much of my information from the biological sciences, especially physiology, ethology and psychology and attempt to place this knowledge within a framework of compassion and common sense. In Part II I am writing as a scientist while acknowledging the fact that science is an incomplete discipline for the resolution of problems of animal suffering and animal welfare. Not only does it not have all the answers, it cannot even address all the questions.

The book is not written as an academic treatise but addressed to anyone who wishes to improve the quality of life for animals. Some people with a passionate concern for animal welfare will find parts of it too technical or too conciliatory for their liking. To you I say I admire your passion but suggest that passion is most effective when allied to a cool head. Whenever we discuss problems of animal welfare we are discussing the quality of an animal's life and, because sentient animals are complex creatures, these problems are usually too complex to be reduced to slogans. Indeed, simplistic solutions to welfare problems, however well intended, can often do more harm than good. One of the reasons why the animal welfare movement has achieved so little is that it has demanded too much. If we are to convert a proper concern for animal welfare into effective action our approach must necessarily be pragmatic, utilitarian and circumspect.

Scientists working in animal welfare will undoubtedly find some of my arguments simplistic and most of them unsubstantiated by reference to what they call 'the literature'. However, if I were to support all my arguments with statistics and scientific references the book would be twice as long and half as readable. Within each subject area I cite a few references mostly to recent reviews or textbooks on which I have drawn for substantial parts of my argument. References to original scientific communications are normally only given when the work is very new, contentious or when I wish to illustrate a general argument from my own personal experience. This means that a lot of my assertions are not substantiated in the text by reference to others.

Those seeking more detailed evidence in support of these assertions can, at least, begin with the list of suggestions for further reading which appears at the end of the book.

Part III – *What we can do for them* – proceeds from analysis to advocacy. It considers the major welfare problems faced by animals on the farm and in the wild, in laboratories or as pets in the home. It also reviews new welfare problems that may emerge from developments in biotechnology and genetic engineering. In all cases it then proceeds to specific suggestions for action to improve welfare, where necessary, by research to improve our understanding of animals, education to bring human perceptions of animal welfare rather closer to the way that the animals themselves perceive the quality of their own lives and, finally, legislation to improve animal welfare in circumstances where this cannot be achieved through the operation of consumer choice and the free market.

This book deals with aspects of animal behaviour and aspects of the law. Both disciplines tend to encourage tortuous exercises in semantics designed to create definitions that will offend no shade of scientific or legal opinion. I have made no attempt to write as if for committees since it is the death of style. From time to time I create (and explain) 'Humpty Dumpty' definitions which mean exactly what I choose them to mean. However, I should at the outset explain three words which I use rather a lot. These are 'problem', 'I', and 'man'. The word problem is used in the scientific and rational sense as a situation that calls for a solution and is therefore a source of extreme interest rather than outrage. The word 'I' is intended to indicate caution rather than arrogance. If, when dealing with matters of science, I write 'The optimal air temperature for a caged hen is 21°C' I am stating a proven fact, although I am unlikely to quote the original source of that information. If I write 'I suggest that the threshold to pain in a sheep may be similar to that in man', I am expressing a personal opinion or belief, based on the best available evidence, but one I am always prepared to modify. Similarly, when dealing with matters of advocacy, I use the personal pronoun to avoid delusions of grandeur. I may write 'I believe hunting with hounds is cruel' but I shall not write 'Hunting with hounds should be abolished!' Finally my use of the word 'man' is gender-neutral; it refers to mankind. Any person who believes I should substitute person throughout should turn at once to the lines of Robert Burns which preface Chapter 1 and provide a philosophical basis for the whole book.

'I'm truly sorry Man's dominion
   has broken Nature's social union.'

I shall not mess around with the poetry of Burns for anybody.

My aim, I repeat, is to offer constructive solutions to the problem of man's dominion over the animals. These solutions will not be achieved by self-indulgent moralizing on the nature of animal rights but by practical approaches designed to reconcile our aspirations for those animals within our dominion with a proper concern for their welfare. I do not expect to achieve paradise but I do my best to be fair.

Acknowledgements

Thanks first to The Universities Federation for Animal Welfare (UFAW) for the award of the Hume Fellowship which nearly bought me the time to write this book and (which is much more important) gave me the strength of will to begin it. The main aim of UFAW is to improve the welfare of animals by improving our ability to understand them. This is my aim too and half the profits from the sale of this book will go to promote the further work of UFAW.

I thank Mike Baxter, RhapRh Owen and Joanne Webster for Figs. 3.3, 2.4 and 1.1 respectively. Figure 9.2 is reproduced by kind permission of Silsoe Research Institute. For all other photographs and illustrations I am indebted to John Conybear and Malcolm Parsons.

I am especially grateful to my readers and reviewers: Mike Baxter, Manuel Berdoy, Steve Kestin, Bob Macpherson, Kathy Meyer, Bevis Miller, Christine Nicol and Paul Watkins, whose balance of comments and criticisms has, I hope, kept me close to the 'Middle Way'.

John Webster

Part I
Introduction:
Man's Dominion Over the Animals

1 Introduction: Man's Dominion

'I'm truly sorry Man's dominion
has broken Nature's Social Union,
An' justifies that ill opinion,
                   which makes thee startle,
At me, thy poor earth bound companion,
                   an' fellow mortal!

I doubt na, whyles, but thou may thieve,
What then, poor beastie, thou maun live!

Robert Burns (1785)

Man has dominion over the animals whether we like it or not. Wherever we share space on the planet, and this includes all but the most inaccessible regions of land, sea and air, it is we, not they that determine where and how they will live. We may elect to put hens in a battery cage or establish a game reserve to preserve the tiger but in each case the decision is ours, not theirs. We make a pet of the hamster but poison the rat. These are very human decisions but they have much in common with decisions taken by other animals, since they reflect our own will to survive, preserve our genetic inheritance and enrich the quality of our lives. We need good food and battery eggs are nutritious and cheap. We need good hygiene, and fear that rats carry germs. Pets enrich our lives and those of our children. We admire the tiger not only for its fearful symmetry but as a symbol of freedom itself, so we offer it rather more freedom than we would think fit for the chicken. It is impossible, however, to avoid the issue that both the chicken and the tiger are living on our terms.

It was not ever thus. Primitive man shared with other animal species the absolute imperative to ensure his own survival at the expense of all species other than his own. Though less swift and strong than the lion and less well equipped to digest vegetables than the ox, man not only survived but prospered through his ability to communicate and so acquire an education, initially horizontally within the pack or tribe, and later, vertically from generation to generation. All this is common knowledge. It is perhaps less obvious that man, for all his intelligence, did not seriously begin to threaten the habitat and survival of other animal species until he acquired access to sources of power (rather than intelligence) greater than himself; not only gunpowder to kill animals at a distance, but also fossil

3

fuels to drive the invasion of habitat by trains, automobiles, earthmovers and concrete mixers.

Having acquired this power, man has recognized (imperfectly) the need to use it responsibly and with respect to other life forms. We may like to call this morality but it is as essential to our long-term interests as was the need of primitive man to fashion a spear. The North American Indian is greatly admired by those for whom ecology is largely an emotional issue because, unlike the white man, he lived in harmony with the buffalo. However, given his limited power base, he had neither the scope, nor the motivation to do otherwise. This, of course, made nobility so much easier.

Nobody knows what primitive man thought about the beasts he hunted. We do know that the North American Indian and Eskimo (or Inuit) cultures recognize the spirits of the slain buffalo or seal, which implies a reverence for life, or, at the very least, a fear of death. It suggests also that those who created the spirit legends acknowledged that the animals they hunted could experience sensations similar to their own, in particular the intense sensations of fear and pain. At some early stage this would have begun to arouse compassion in some people.

In time, man began to get to know animals as individuals and so to develop favourites: animals that acquired lasting value by virtue of their lasting utility, or their companionship, or both. The dogs that scavenged around the edges of the camp became, at first, tolerated, then a source of amusement, then uniquely loyal friends and hunting companions. Eventually, the real favourites escaped being eaten altogether. In India, the cow became sacred; in England, the horse. (That highly intelligent animal, the pig, has persuaded four of the world's great religions not to eat it but for rather different reasons.) Even the killing of meat animals raised by man acquired its own dignity. We may today criticize Shechita and Halal slaughter as primitive ritual but (as with the Inuit) these rituals do imply a respect for the life being taken. However, as it is unnecessary to invoke morality in the decision of the North American Indian to cohabit with rather than exterminate the buffalo, so also one does not have to presume too much altruism in early man to conclude that his care and concern for the animals he domesticated would have been related to their importance to him as individuals; for example, the cow, a lasting source of milk, fuel and traction, was more important than the chicken. As hunter-gatherer communities became progressively agricultural, meat would have become a luxury since, when crops are hard won, they are too valuable to feed to animals that contribute nothing more efficient than meat. Horses and cattle, subsisting largely on grasses we cannot digest ourselves, were far more valuable alive than dead. Pigs and chickens, with digestions more similar to ours, were gleaning and scavenging any food that was overlooked, dropped or thrown away. Ruminants that grazed and browsed the huge expanses of uncultivated land away from the villages were hunted as wild animals, primitive man making no arbitrary distinction between cattle and game.

In these early village communities we may assume that some men and women developed a degree of reverence for life itself and a degree of compassion (i.e. desire to avoid unnecessary suffering) for selected species of other animals – those which, when I was a schoolboy, were still called 'the friends of man' (or the farmer or the gardener). This list included the dog, the robin and the earthworm but excluded the fox, the jay and the slug. It is difficult to escape the conclusion that the philosophical basis for the treatment of animals in the English middle-class environment of my youth was much the same as that for primitive man; i.e. we made decisions as to the quality of an animal's life, indeed its very existence, almost entirely according to our view of its utility, its beauty, its entertainment value or its value as a friend.

I think, to be fair to my family, that they were more compassionate than primitive man, even if they were basing their concern for animals on the same premises. Man's humanity or inhumanity to man and other animals tends to vary in direct proportion to his own comfort, wealth and security. It is easier to care for others when one's own survival is not under threat. Moreover, animal welfare, like conservation of the environment and other civilized concerns, costs money. A scientist (as distinct from a moral philosopher) studying the evolutionary basis of animal and human behaviour would argue that a 'human' trait like altruism only becomes functional in a stable and reasonably egalitarian society. 'Do as you would be done by' only works if it's mutual.

To summarize the argument so far, man has, to date, cared for animals in direct proportion to their value to him, i.e. their ability to create wealth or enhance his own quality of life. In primitive times, this did not matter too much to the survival of other species because of the limited extent of man's dominion over the shared environment. With domestication, however, man has progressively taken away from animals and into his own hands the decisions he, not they, considers to be necessary for survival and good welfare. Most of this book is concerned with the impact of human decisions on the quality of life for domestic animals. At this stage it is necessary only to point out that the species that have allowed themselves to become domesticated have tended to ensure their survival, as a species, rather better than those that stayed in the wild (the chicken is more likely to survive the next hundred years than the tiger).

Today we have complete dominion – sufficient power to destroy the majority of species of 'higher' animals (birds and mammals) but sufficient wealth to allow us to behave towards them with responsibility and altruism. However, given such awesome power, it is not sufficient simply to feel compassion. If we wish to convert our compassion and reverence for life into practical benefit for the survival and quality of life in other species, we need more than right thought, we need right action.

During the last twenty years there has been a small boom in books on animal welfare, sometimes (but not often enough) considered within the wider context of conservation and human aspirations. The seminal work on farm animal welfare was *Animal Machines* by Ruth Harrison. I admire this work greatly mainly because it is both realistic and constructive, having made allowances for the degree of polemic necessary to get such arguments off the ground. The vogue in more recent years has been to concentrate on the morality of animal rights and human attitudes. Examples of this genre include *Animal Rights* by Andrew Linzey (1976) and *Animal Liberation: A new ethics for our treatment of animals* by Peter Singer. I admire and share the concern of these authors for animal welfare but I do not find their counsel particularly helpful. It does not matter to an animal how we think but what we do. Peter Singer attacks humans for the practice of 'speciesism', namely the exploitation of other species for our benefit but without their consent. He has developed this philosophy as an extension of utilitarianism, based on Jeremy Bentham's (1748–1832) classic dictum 'The question is not, Can they reason? Can they talk? but can they *suffer?*' It will become clear that I find utilitarianism can be a great help to those trying to do their best for animal welfare in a practical way. However, most philosophical arguments which involve the concept of animal rights or animal consent are fundamentally flawed because the individuals whose rights and whose consent are under discussion are not allowed to contribute to the argument. To turn Singer's argument on its head, I would suggest that he is guilty of (benign) speciesism by presuming to speak for animals without first pausing (at considerable length) to ask them what they think and feel.

My approach throughout this book will be first, to address, by use of scientific method, the nature of animal mind and animal suffering; to ask them first how they feel, and then try to build this understanding into practical recommendations for animal care and animal welfare that are fair to all parties, animals and man. I shall, throughout, pay due heed to the moral basis for our treatment of animals but I shall try to avoid getting bogged down by it.

In recent years, a new generation of ethologists (such as Marian Dawkins, 1980, 1993) and cognitive psychologists (such as Toates, 1986) have developed methods for the study of animal mind that are infinitely more subtle than those based on simplistic, outdated, Pavlovian-type stimulus-response theory. This approach poses subtle questions to animals set in a form which they can understand (and when they cannot one should always try to rephrase the question before assuming that the animal is stupid). The slow, patient but hugely important objective of this scientific work is to understand the minds of the animals whose lives we control; for example, their powers of perception, decision making, self-awareness, or capacity to learn from others. No amount of moral philosophy can possibly judge *a priori* such things as the extent to which the genotype and experience (or education) of an animal may affect its strength of motivation to achieve a specific source of satisfaction, avoid a specific source of suffering, or simply make an active, constructive contribution to the quality of its own life. Nor can it predict the frustration the animal may feel if it is thwarted in these devices and desires. If we believe, on moral grounds, that we need to understand chickens because we control their lives, then we need to study what matters to chickens; if we want to understand cows, we should study cows. Since it is neither moral, nor practical to control the life of a tiger, we should, if we understand them at all, learn to leave them alone.

The moral philosophy approach to animal welfare – i.e. that based upon our thoughts and values, not theirs – tends to generate broad, bold (and careless) conclusions such as 'Man has no right to cause any other animal to suffer'. Phrases like this tend to become debased into the slogans of the Animal Rights and Animal Liberation movements and used to justify abuse to and assaults on anyone who *uses* animals (scientists, farmers, butchers, etc.). I have a great deal of empathy with the most passionate advocates for animal welfare, otherwise I would not be writing this book. I do, however, often find it difficult to discuss welfare issues with them on a rational basis, which is also why I am writing this book. I only ask that bold, brave clarion call to arms like the one which begins this paragraph be given a little thought. Taken at face value, it can only mean 'man has no right to cause any animal to suffer to any degree for any reason whatsoever'. When expressed in full, this statement begs many questions. At this stage I offer only three:

● *Do all animal species actually experience suffering? If so, how?* If, for example, I wash my face (with an ethically acceptable soap) and, in so doing destroy a few thousand mites living in my eyebrows, have I caused them to suffer? I think almost everyone would say 'no' to this specific question but would have greater difficulty with others in the same set, such as, 'Do fish feel pain?' or 'Does a chicken miss being out of doors?'

● *Does the sin of causing an animal to suffer apply equally to sins of commission and omission?* Do we have any more right to subject a herd of elephants (or a flock of sheep) to mass starvation by doing nothing, than to control numbers by selective culling and so maintain the population in good health?

● *Does the end never justify the means?* If a sheep, say, were to be injected with a genetically-engineered vaccine, and then made to give a small amount of blood at two-week intervals, and if the only source of distress to the sheep was the procedure for blood sampling, and if that blood could keep five children alive, would we still have no right to proceed? Once again this is an extreme case, but it illustrates (I hope) the point that it is difficult to con-demn, out of hand, all scientific procedures with animals.

The most crucial limitation to the moral philosophy approach to animal welfare is the fact that what matters to the animal is not what we think or feel but what we do. When I first began to write on animal welfare some fifteen years ago, I illustrated my approach by describing a rabbit without food, in isolation, in a cold box, on dirty, wet litter. This rabbit would clearly be suffering from hunger, cold, poor hygiene and lack of companions, and the extent of its suffering would be the same whether our intentions for this particular rabbit were to love it as a pet, kill it for food, experiment on it to find a cure for cancer or to test a new cosmetic. A central feature of my entire argument is that, at this stage, our motivation would be of no concern to the rabbit. Its perception of its own welfare is determined entirely by its own view of the world. If we are to do our best for the welfare of the rabbit, whatever our ultimate intention may be and however good or bad that may make us feel, we have no option but to do our best to understand how the rabbit perceives and interprets its world and adjust our actions accordingly.

Having challenged some of the more simplistic assumptions of the animal welfare activists and so, I hope, provoked them to read on, I offer an equally unsettling image to the reader who can live quite comfortably within the *status quo*, who finds our current classification of other animals as pets, farm animals, game, vermin etc. perfectly satisfactory. Glance briefly at Fig. 1.1, a photograph taken by flashlight of a brown rat in a larder. A normal reaction to the brief glimpse of a rat in one's larder would be horror or, at least, a cold resolve to destroy the rat as quickly as possible, together with any others that happened to be around. Now study the picture more carefully. The rat is not only sleek to the point of being chubby but clearly quite unalarmed by flash photography. Her name is Cordelia. She is not only the pet rat of my daughter but featured in her doctoral thesis on behaviour and disease transmisssion in wild rats, demonstrating rat behaviour for photographers and even appearing on live television. Indeed, she is something of a minor celebrity, totally at ease in human company and altogether charming.

This image further illustrates two of the central pillars of my argument. In

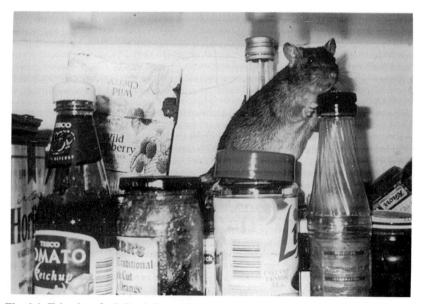

Fig. 1.1 Friend or foe? Cordelia at play.

the first analysis, a rat is a rat whether we define it as vermin or as a pet. We could not, however, describe Cordelia as a typical brown rat, even one bred, as she was, from a laboratory strain. Her character, intelligence and response to people have developed through being raised in a greatly enriched environment with loving human contact. If she had been reared in a natural, satisfactory environment with other rats, she would have adapted equally well to that and, eminently sensibly, become fearful and dangerous in the presence of man. If she had been reared in total isolation in a barren laboratory cage she would have been relatively ignorant and less able to handle complex decisions (like how to reconcile curiosity and fear in a novel situation). She may also have developed disturbed, pointless behaviour patterns called stereotypies. Later, I shall discuss all these issues in much greater detail. At this stage, I present the image of Fig. 1.1 simply to re-emphasize the point that the mind of an animal, and thus its perception of its own welfare, is determined by its genotype (species and breeding) and its education (experience and interpretation of that experience).

Having set up a series of questions and images designed to cast some doubts in the minds of anyone who thinks about animals at all from any set of preconceptions, I should now outline the set of preconceptions that leads me to write a book subtitled 'A Cool Eye towards Eden'. I do not wish to preach philosophy, religion or morals. If you find this book interesting and of practical help in your dealings with animals, that is enough. The moral state to which I aspire is (to quote Albert Schweitzer) 'to extend the circle of my compassion to all living things'. This does not absolutely preclude me (nor him) from killing another animal, for reasons of necessity, as humanely as possible, and in circumstances where that death does not cause distress to others (e.g. dependent offspring). My interpretation of necessity is considerably less austere than Schweitzer's. Although I do not hunt, shoot or fish for pleasure, I do eat most meat. On the basis that what matters to the animal is not what we think or feel but what we do I eat pheasant that have been shot for fun by somebody else in the woods but I do not eat broiler chicken that have been reared for strictly business reasons in the most intensive production systems.

I prefaced this introductory chapter with lines from the first and best of all animal welfare poems – Robert Burns' *To a mouse, on turning up her nest with the plough*, November 1785. I quote them again:

> 'I'm truly sorry Man's dominion
> has broken Nature's Social Union,
> An' justifies that ill opinion,
>   which makes thee startle,
> At me, thy poor earth bound companion,
>   an' fellow mortal!
>
> I doubt na, whyles, but thou may thieve,
> What then, poor beastie, thou maun live!'

I do believe that man has evolved beyond the stage where his treatment of his fellow mortals (as defined by Burns) needs to be determined by strict Darwinian principles of genetic survival at Malthusian limits of environmental exploitation. Man cannot create the Garden of Eden upon this earth but I see many good reasons for aiming in that general direction. My vision of such an Eden is not, however, one in which 'the wolf shall also dwell with the lamb and the leopard shall lie down with the kid . . . and the lion shall eat straw with the ox.' (Isaiah 11,v. 6–7). The lion would not survive long on a diet of straw. The leopard that lay down with the kid would not only become a very unsuccessful (and therefore distressed) leopard but it and the kid would now be competing for the same food source and so both become more vulnerable to starvation and extinction as a species. Similarly the ploughman will continue to destroy the nests of mice but he must continue to plough.

This book is intended for anyone who feels it essential not only to the dignity of mankind but also to the quality of our own life to extend to other animal species the concept of man's humanity to man. This does not and can not mean waiving our rights over all other species and setting them free, not least because most of them have nowhere to go. I am less interested in animal rights than in human responsibilities. Andrew Paton (1993) wrote that the answer to the accusation of speciesism is simply humanism. If this humanistic approach is to succeed in practice, rather than simply make us feel good, it must necessarily be pragmatic, utilitarian and circumspect. One of the reasons the animal welfare movement has achieved so little is that it has demanded too much.

I turn therefore a cool eye towards Eden, first to ask 'What do animals want? How is it for them? How do they perceive their own quality of life?' In addressing these questions I draw much of my information from the biological sciences, especially physiology, ethology and psychology and attempt to place this knowledge within a framework of compassion and common sense. I then turn to the issue of rebuilding nature's social union in a way that best reconciles our aspirations with those of the animals over whom we have dominion. I do not expect to achieve paradise but I will do my best to be fair.

Assessment of animal welfare: the five freedoms

Any proper discussion of animal welfare requires a comprehensive and unsentimental definition and analysis of welfare as perceived by the animals themselves. Single sentence definitions such as 'Welfare defines the state of an animal as it attempts to cope with its environment' (Fraser & Broom, 1990) tend to have the self-referential flavour of 'A rose is a rose' and do not really advance our understanding. Clearly, the welfare of an animal is defined by how it feels at the time but this is not enough. I may feel good while drunk but any short term benefits to my welfare are unlikely to be sustained. A horse that breaks into a barn and gorges itself on corn may pay a greater price for its pleasure. The welfare of an animal must be defined therefore not only by how it feels within a spectrum that ranges from suffering to pleasure but also by its ability to sustain physical and mental fitness and so preserve not only its future quality of life but also the survival of its genes. My best attempt at a single-sentence definition is that 'the welfare of an animal is determined by its capacity to avoid suffering and sustain fitness'.

When the Brambell Committee (1965) first reviewed the welfare of farm animals in intensive husbandry systems they proposed that all farm animals should, at least, have the freedom to 'stand up, lie down, turn around, groom themselves and stretch their limbs'. These minimal standards (which have yet to be achieved) came to be known as the 'Five Freedoms' and for many years dominated discussion of animal welfare in Europe. In my early years on the UK Farm Animal Welfare Council (FAWC), I suggested that this obsession with space requirements was very narrow-minded, since it concentrated almost exclusively on one aspect of behaviour (comfort seeking) to the exclusion of everything else that might contribute to good welfare, like good food, good health, security, etc. Preserving the concept of 'Five Freedoms', I attempted to produce a logical, comprehensive method for first analysis of *all* the factors likely to influence the welfare of farm animals, whether on the farm itself, in transit or at the point of slaughter. These definitions have evolved somewhat with time and have recently been revised by FAWC (1993) so that they now read:

(1) *Freedom from thirst, hunger and malnutrition* – by ready access to fresh water and a diet to maintain full health and vigour.
(2) *Freedom from discomfort* – by providing a suitable environment including shelter and a comfortable resting area.
(3) *Freedom from pain, injury and disease* – by prevention or rapid diagnosis and treatment.
(4) *Freedom to express normal behaviour* – by providing sufficient space, proper facilities and company of the animal's own kind.
(5) *Freedom from fear and distress* – by ensuring conditions which avoid mental suffering.

Table 1.1 illustrates how the concept of the five freedoms can be used to evaluate, in a systematic and comprehensive fashion, the welfare of animals in different environments; in this case to compare the welfare of egg-laying hens in battery cages and on free range. The approach is simply to create a matrix in which the rows define the freedoms (or subsets thereof) and the columns define the husbandry systems. As they stand, the single words or phrases in each box of the matrix in Table 1.1 are not intended as adequate descriptions of welfare, merely notes for discussion. Indeed, when comparing welfare in different husbandry systems in tutorial classes with students, I find it best to leave the boxes empty and let the students fill them up for themselves in a form and in as much detail as they think fit.

I discuss the issues raised by Table 1.1 at greater length in Chapter 8. I do

Table 1.1 An outline comparison of the welfare of laying hens in battery cages and on free range based on the concept of the five freedoms.

System	Battery cage	Free range
Hunger and thirst	Adequate	Adequate
Comfort: thermal	Good	Variable
physical	Poor	Usually good
Ill-health: disease	Low	Parasitism?
pain	Feet and legs	Injury
Behaviour	Very restricted	Cannibalism?
Fear and stress	Frustration	Agoraphobia

not wish to overcomplicate the argument at this stage, merely to illustrate how it operates. For example, we may assume that it is equally possible to provide adequate food and water in both systems. Out of doors on free range hens will sometimes be too hot, sometimes too cold. In a battery hen house, temperature is maintained at a comfortable 21°C. However, hens confined in a wire cage with a wire floor at a stocking density of 450 cm^2 per bird will suffer damage to their feet and osteoporosis, weakening of bones largely through inactivity, predisposing them to fractures. On the other hand, caged birds are remarkably free from infectious disease, partly because their droppings fall through the floors of the cages and are carried away. Out of doors, parasites such as *Coccidia* can build up in the ground and cause the birds not only to be unthrifty but to *feel* sick.

In cages, hens find it difficult to move at all and are denied even the primitive satisfaction of stretching their limbs. There is good evidence that this leads to frustration and that this frustration increases with time (see Chapter 4). Out of doors on a commercial free range farm with, say, 2000 birds, their behaviour may be unrestricted but their habitat is grossly abnormal. The domestic hen has evolved from jungle fowl that lived in social groups of perhaps six hens with one cockerel. Being small, almost flightless and very vulnerable the jungle fowl devised a strategy for survival which incorporated a healthy element of fear. During the day they sheltered under bushes to seek protection from predators in the air; at night they roosted in branches to escape predation from the ground. In groups of this size, a hen in the jungle or on a modern smallholding knows who her companions are, whether they present a threat, and where to run in the event of an emergency. When 2000 birds are run together on a so-called free range system they are not so much a social group as a dangerous mob. Hens are socially maladapted to crowding and problems may arise such as feather pecking which can proceed to cannibalism. Moreover, a sudden emergency, such as the arrival of a bird of prey, or a hot air balloon, can cause mayhem as 2000 birds scramble to get back indoors through 20 popholes. The problem here is not one of fear (a very useful trait for a hen) but loss of control. The individual hen is caught in the same predicament as the individual spectator at a football match when the crowd stampedes. I have observed commercial free range systems in which more than half the hens elect, sooner or later, not to go out of doors at all. If they were humans we would say they had developed agoraphobia.

This example of the application of the five freedoms illustrates three points of general significance:

(1)   When put to work, the five freedoms no longer appear as a counsel of perfection but become an attempt to make the best of a complex and difficult situation. Absolute attainment of all five freedoms is unrealistic, indeed they are to some extent incompatible. Complete behavioural freedom, for example, is unhygienic for all us animals! The criteria are comprehensive (if superficial) and so should prevent welfare issues being argued from incomplete premises, e.g. production traits only (1–3), a traditional fault of producers, or ethological issues only (4–5), a traditional fault of animal welfare advocates. They offer a set of first principles for an approach to the understanding of welfare as perceived by the animal itself and thus to the management of the environment so as to reconcile the proper, but not paramount needs of animal welfare with, in this case the proper business of producing cheap, healthy, nutritious eggs.

(2)   By revealing that all commercial husbandry systems have their strengths and weaknesses, the five freedoms make it, on the one hand, more difficult to sustain a sense of absolute outrage against any particular system such as the battery cage and easier to plan constructive, step by step, routes towards its improvement. I shall deal with the improvement of farming systems in Chapters 7–9. For now, let me reassure those who wish to see a ban on the battery cage that I, too, think it is unacceptable *in its present form*.

(3)   The discovery that hens suffer from agoraphobia illustrates the dangers of introducing anthropomorphism into the evaluation of animal welfare. Modern commercial free range systems for laying hens arose less from a desire to improve hen welfare than from the market opportunity created by those who wish to eat eggs with a clear conscience. If we are to create real improvements in animal welfare we have, first, to acknowledge that an animal's perception of its own welfare may be very different from that of the general (human) public, especially when public perception is based largely on media images, rather than the realities of regular day-to-day contact with animals. We have then to do our best to understand how animals view the world and finally try to educate public opinion towards a perception of welfare that is as close as possible to that of the animals themselves.

Although the five freedoms were devised as a check list for welfare in farming systems, they do, I believe, serve equally well for pets, laboratory animals and others for whom we make most of the decisions with regard to food and shelter. (Remember the rabbit.) Wild animals are responsible for most of their own decisions (within a habitat largely defined by us). However, they are motivated by the same needs – hunger, comfort, security, sex – and, for sound reasons, aim to achieve most of these things with the least effort though the hyperactivity of the rutting male is a rare exception to this general rule. The difference between wild and domestic animals is essentially one of degree. Because the environment carries more potential dangers, the wild rat in a larder will pay relatively less attention to food than Cordelia and more attention to its own security. It is romantic to think that wild animals sacrifice comfort to preserve their freedom but more realistic to conclude that most of their attention is directed towards actions essential for their immediate survival.

There is, however, one fundamental way in which the welfare of wild, or extensively ranched animals may be said to be superior to that of animals in the home, farm, laboratory or zoo. Life in the wild may involve a great deal of discomfort and fear but when problems arise the animals are at liberty to make their own decisions as to how to deal with them. If these decisions are successful they adapt to the problems of fear and stress because they learn that they can be controlled. (If they are unsuccessful then their problems are over.) The tethered sow, or the isolated chimpanzee, or the dog shut up all day in an urban flat, may have food, comfort, security and a total absence of fear but experience real suffering as a consequence of the inability to make any constructive contribution to the quality of their own existence. Experimental psychologists have an expression to describe 'adaptation' to such barren environments. They call it 'learned apathy'. I prefer to call it hopelessness. This may be one of the greatest of all insults to welfare.

Life, liberty and the pursuit of happiness

It was once pointed out to me that, by calling for five freedoms for farm animals, I was offering them one more than Roosevelt offered the American people. My reply was that since I was speaking for the entire population of sentient animals, the ratio did not seem overgenerous. I also thought (although not at the time) that the American people have already done rather well out of their Declaration of Independence, which promises 'life, liberty and the pursuit of happiness'. We can offer none of these things to the animals over whom we have dominion.

Of course, 'the preservation of life', to use the words of Thomas Jefferson's original draft, is a hollow promise. No living thing escapes death (although its genes can survive). Humans are a sufficiently sentient species to be aware of, and so fear death. Quite early in human development we began to devise solutions or, at least, palliatives to this problem that range from religious belief in the prospect of eternal life to the more rational (Buddhist, but not

quite) aim to conquer the problem of personal death by achieving trans-
cendence of the sense of self. It is necessary to ask whether other animals fear
the concept of death, and equally necessary to recognize that this is not the
same thing as experiencing fear in the context of acute mortal danger. The
answer to this question depends on the extent to which animals are *aware* of,
respond to and remember the implications of suffering and death in others
and must be addressed on a species-specific basis. A few species (primates
and perhaps elephants) may experience the concept of death in a way
somewhat similar to ourselves. There is however good evidence that most
species do not. For example, grazing animals like sheep or red deer are
unconcerned both at the time that one or more of their fellows is shot and
when they are subsequently left to lie about dead. Although it is a good
maxim, when in doubt, to give the animals the benefit of that doubt, I think it
fair to conclude that for most non-human animal species, the concept of
death is not a welfare problem. Being dead, is, of course, no problem at all.

If we object, on grounds of conscience, to the killing of animals (or
nominated species of animals) by man, we do not ensure the preservation of
individual lives, we merely change the method of death. Pursuing this logic
even more ruthlessly, if we elect not to eat animals, they will still get eaten. It
is the inescapable fate of all living animals to be consumed, sooner or later,
by something else and used largely for fuel. A rabbit may be killed and eaten
by us or by a fox. Most humans in history who escaped death at the hands of
their fellow humans or other obviously dangerous animals were eventually
killed and eaten by microorganisms. Today, the risk of death from infectious
disease (with conspicuous exceptions such as HIV) is not what it was and we
are more inclined to self-destruct from diseases like cancer, often after suffering the disintegration of a great deal of body and mind before the moment
of non-existence. We shall then be consumed by other life forms or by fire;
the chemistry is much the same.

During the course of this book, I hope to explore the concept of quality of
life as perceived by animals in sufficient depth to give some meaning to words
such as stress, fear, pain, awareness, suffering, pleasure and even happiness in
animals who cannot communicate these things to us through the medium of
speech (or art or music). Before closing this opening chapter I must, however,
return to the question of death and repeat my belief that whereas most
animals will do their best to keep themselves and their offspring alive (i.e.
preserve their genetic inheritance) they do not live in chronic metaphysical
fear of death as an end to existence. This means that longevity *per se*, is not
essential to their welfare. It follows from this that it is not cruel (i.e. does not
cause suffering) to kill an animal if it can be done without causing pain, fear
or any other form of distress. A particular slaughter method can and should
be condemned if it can be shown that animals are cruelly treated or terrified
before the moment of killing. Compassion in World Farming have been
particularly effective in drawing such abuses to the public attention. However, calls to vegetarianism based on images of blood and guts appearing in

the abattoir *post mortem* are mischievous since they deliberately confuse compassion with squeamishness. I am far more impressed by the moral courage of a lady farmer of my acquaintance who puts her beef cattle through 'pre-slaughter counselling'. This involves habituating her animals to handling and the short ride to the abattoir, then walking with them up the race to the stunning pen so that they remain calm and do not suffer right up to the point of non-existence. This may be an extreme position for a farmer but it illustrates quite beautifully the fundamental point that reverence for life is compatible with a realistic, dignified approach to death.

Part II
Analysis:
How Is It For Them?

An enquiry into the nature of animal welfare and animal suffering

'The question is not
Can they reason?
Can they talk? but
Can they suffer?'

Jeremy Bentham

2 Animal Mind and Animal Suffering

'How much of the mentality that we offer one another ought we to allow the monkey, the sparrow, the goldfish, the ant? Hadn't we better reserve something for ourselves alone, perhaps consciousness? Most people are determined to hold the line against animals. Grant them the claim to make linguistic references and they will be putting in a case for minds and souls. The whole phyletic scale will come trooping into heaven demanding immortality for the tadpole and the hippopotamus. Better be firm now.'

Brown, R. *Words and Things* (1958)

The five freedoms offer a useful set of rules for the definition and analysis of animal welfare. However, most of the needs defined within this simple list, for example, food, comfort, health and security, may be applied to all classes of animals from invertebrates to man and the higher primates. They do not address the question as to whether a particular animal suffers if one of these needs is not met and, if so, how much. The investigation of animal suffering requires a different approach from that used to define and analyse animal welfare. We may begin with three deceptively simple questions.

- 'What do animals want from life?'
- 'Are they aware of suffering?'
- 'How can we know?'

Feeling and doing

The first problem is that suffering is, by definition, a subjective sensation. It describes how we feel. I think I know how I feel, though I might be deluding myself. I can get some impression of how you feel. If you communicate your feelings by way of words and facial expression I can interpret your actions in the light of shared experience. This limited approach to understanding the feelings of others becomes more difficult when humans do not share a common language and practically impossible when faced by a creature as enigmatic as a goat. To illustrate these difficulties let us consider the link between something all animals do, namely eat, and a primitive sensation which we know we feel, namely hunger.

We may eat because we feel hungry, because our appetite is titillated by attractive food or because it is the socially acceptable thing to do (we have been invited for dinner). If we are genuinely hungry and have no prospect of food, perhaps because we have no money, we may suffer acutely from discomfort, and chronically from loss of body condition and physical fitness. We are also likely to suffer anxiety as to where our next meal is coming from. If we have children or dependent relatives in the same predicament we may worry about them and communicate that worry to the social services. If, when dining out, we are tempted by a delectable pudding after a large main course of meat and two veg., we will probably eat it because it is there (we have been motivated by an external stimulus rather than an internal drive) or we may eat it simply to please the cook. If we decide, for reasons of health or vanity to reject this pudding we may experience a mild pang of disappointment but if there had been no pudding we would not have missed it.

We can, of course, distinguish between the feelings and motivation of the starving man entering the soup kitchen and those of the diner faced by a pudding at the end of a social dinner and conclude that only the former constitute suffering. However, the *behaviour* of both individuals may appear to the observer to be exactly the same. Both are likely to eat with apparent relish, whether hungry or not, and both may communicate feelings of pleasure and gratitude to the hostess or cook which, finally, may or may not be sincere. A non-human observer, a visitor perhaps from another planet, or a dog, might surmise from our actions that we get pleasure from food but could only conclude with any certainty from observation of human health and human behaviour that we need food to survive and eat it when it is available. He has hardly begun to address the three questions listed above. Before I attempt to address them in a generic sense I shall examine the specific problem of interpreting the interaction between the sensation of hunger and the act of eating in a species other than our own.

Animals need food but do they want it?
Our observer has established that humans *need* food for their welfare. If food is present they eat it. The more percipient observer may also note that humans will work hard to produce food and conclude from this that humans *are aware that food matters*. Observing a tortoise wandering apparently at random, bumping into a lettuce and eating it because it is there, or a toad sitting motionless for days before striking at a fly that moved within reach of its tongue, the same observer might conclude from these observations alone that the tortoise and the toad react instinctively to the presence of food but have no profound awareness of its necessity nor even any conscious motivation to eat so long as they happen to exist within a habitat where food is in plentiful supply. Observing a cheetah selecting and stalking its potential prey within a herd of antelope then timing its final, furious assault, he might reasonably conclude that the cheetah, like the human, was making a series of complex strategic and tactical decisions as to how that food might best be obtained. The observer might

then divide animals into two categories: (1) those like toads and tortoises that simply react instinctively to the presence of food and (2) those like humans and cheetahs who are *aware* of the need for food and apply their minds to the problem. One might criticize our alien ethologist for generating a sweeping hypothesis from a very limited set of observations but he will not have been the first.

Do animals suffer hunger?

We know what we mean by suffering and we tell each other how we feel. The extraterrestial observer may not comprehend our capacity to suffer, perhaps because he does not understand our language or perhaps (like extraterrestials in the older science fiction stories) he appears to us to have no feelings. Our other observer, the dog, however, probably understands what it is to suffer hunger because he has experienced the sensation himself. He has also learnt how to communicate feelings of hunger (real or contrived) to us. He will observe that we, like him, eat, but may have difficulty in distinguishing the motivation of the starving man in the soup kitchen from that of the gourmand tackling his pudding. He does not have the information that will allow him to predict how long our food supply will last and whether we have any anxiety about the future. He may indeed have no concept of the future. To return to Burns and his timorous beastie,

> 'Still thou art blest, compared wi' me!
> The present only touches thee:
> But Och! I backward cast my e'e,
> on prospects drear!
> An' forward though I canna see,
> I guess and fear!'

I have chosen the dog as the second interpreter of human behaviour in terms of human feelings because most people feel that dogs have some empathy with humans. However, despite this empathy, the dog will have difficulty in understanding the full nature of human pleasure and human suffering partly through lack of communication and partly because he has a different palette of emotions. He may, for example, understand the concept of hunger but not pride.

Now the dog may be less, and the extraterrestrial more intelligent than us. The point at issue is that the welfare of an animal is defined not by what it does but by how it feels and it is inherently difficult for one animal species to interpret the behaviour of another animal species in terms of how they feel. If we fail to recognize suffering in other species we must not interpret this to mean that they do not suffer. It is merely one possibility. On the other hand, we must avoid the anthropomorphic projection of our own conception of suffering onto other species. We may believe it to be cruel (i.e. cause unnecessary suffering) to keep a tiger in a cage or a pig on a tether. However, if we, without prejudice, observe the behaviour of the caged tiger or tethered pig, and record that they are in good health and spend most of the time eating or sleeping, we are faced, on this evidence alone, with three possibilites, namely:

(1)   they do not suffer;
(2)   they suffer in a different way from us;
(3)   they fail to communicate to us how they suffer.

The objective scientific distinction between these three possibilities is difficult but the moral distinction is profound.

How can we know?

The most important point to be drawn from the argument so far is that while observation of the 'natural' behaviour of animals can tell us a great deal about their physiological and environmental needs it may not give us much, if any, indication as to how they feel. This requires a completely different approach, one which has been pioneered by Marian Dawkins and described in her books *Animal Suffering* (1980) and *Through Our Eyes Only* (1993). She examines different facets of the life of an animal such as a chicken and asks the questions '*Does it matter and how much?*' She applies economic theory to measure the cost that an animal will pay to achieve or avoid a particular commodity or experience. In essence, she examines their sense of values. In *Through Our Eyes Only* (pages 142–9) she writes:

> 'For us, one of the most crucial aspects of feeling an emotion is that it *matters* to us. We are not passive bystanders to our own emotions ... If we want to know whether other animals have emotions we have to look first for signs that they too care about what happens to them.'
>
> 'Money is not the only way in which people pay costs. The young pianist who gives up four hours per day all through her teenage years is demonstrating how much music matters to her ... What counts is not just what is done or obtained but what is given up to get it. Mattering is the cost of the action in terms of time, money, a marriage, reputation, etc.'
>
> 'If an animal will go to considerable lengths to make something appear or disappear then it is telling us by its actions that it values that commodity or its absence.'

The elegance of this approach is that it enables us to examine the concept of value in species other than our own without the need for a common (spoken) language. However, we cannot yet make a direct link between value and suffering in animals. The spider works hard to construct a web, but the action may be entirely instinctive and we should not necessarily assume that it suffers when it discovers that the web is broken or even if is subsequently runs short of food. The rank (human) capitalist may have an excellent sense of economic value but an atrophied awareness of suffering. A sense of value and the capacity to suffer are not the same but they are both indices of intelligent awareness, which is a property of mind.

Do animals have minds?

I do not wish to divert too far from my primary objective, which is consider what we should *do* (other than agonize) about the problem of man's dominion over the animals but I cannot, at this stage, avoid a little philosophy. We, the human race, are faced by the philosophical proposition that at least some of the other animal species whose lives we control may know the meaning of value and the meaning of suffering. Now one might reasonably argue that this proposition is too vague for analysis and ask that it be defined more specifically in terms such as 'Is a particular animal within a particular species (say a pig, dog or stick insect) *aware* of physical problems such as hunger, thirst, pain and exhaustion, and psychological problems such as fear and grief?' We might also conclude 'So what? The rat does not care for me so why should I care for the rat?' That would be harsh but logical. What I cannot accept is the basic premise that the property of mind is unique to *Homo sapiens*, especially when little attempt has been made to seek evidence to the contrary. Most philosophers and scientists have shied away from this question for fear of what they might find, a point acknowledged somewhat ruefully by the quotation from Brown which prefaces this chapter.

Descartes, after much thought in a stove-heated room (but very little experience in the field) gave credibility to the argument that the essential difference between man and the other animals was the existence of mind or consciousness. *Cogito ergo sum* – I think therefore I am – also implied *non cogitant ergo non sunt* – they don't think therefore they aren't. He saw non-human animals as automata, equivalent to clockwork toys, and therefore established a philosophical basis for treating them as commodities whose value was determined entirely by their usefulness to us.

This simplistic expression of the Cartesian argument cannot, of course, withstand the overwhelming body of evidence in favour of Darwin's theory of evolution by Natural Selection. A rational person may quibble with details of Darwinism but cannot deny the basic premise that all modern life forms have developed through selection for traits that favoured survival, traits determined by genes many of which are now known to be widely conserved and thus widely distributed among the animal kingdom. Most of these traits have been mechanical or chemical and unconscious, e.g. the neck of the giraffe that allows it to browse on vegetation out of the reach of other herbivores, or the rumen of the cow that allows it to live on a diet of grass. Man, though feebler than the lion and constitutionally unadapted to a diet of grass, has become extraordinarily successful (so far) mainly through evolution of his mind. Conscious decisions for actions based upon a proper awareness of the situation and an intelligent weighing of the options became progressively favourable for survival and so were progressively reinforced by natural selection.

While it is fair to say that the mind of man is outstandingly more complex than the mind of other animals this is only an expression of degree, akin to saying that the neck of the giraffe is outstandingly longer than that of other herbivores. We can no more assume that the properties of mind and consciousness arose spontaneously in a single species, *Homo sapiens*, than we can assume that the human eye appeared spontaneously in all its perfect complexity. We must assume that the human properties of awareness, consciousness and mind have evolved because they have been essential for our development, which has itself been essential for our survival. Since the need to develop mind is linked to such a primitive objective, i.e. survival, we cannot then deny the probability that it will have been part of the evolutionary strategy for species other than our own.

The evolution of mind

It is important to steer a cautious course between the rock of belief in the uniqueness of the human mind and the shallows of anthropomorphism. The human mind is very special, and one of its most special properties, namely the ability to benefit from an extended education, only became a dominant feature in natural selection within the primates. For most animal species two of the most important essentials for success have been (1) to grow to maturity and self-sufficiency as quickly as possible to minimize the risks of infancy and (2) to achieve that growth at least cost in terms of food energy to both offspring and parent. At a very late stage in evolution, the primates reversed this process, slowing down growth rate in the young and increasing the period of dependence on their parents. Clearly this was a success. The explanation of this needs a little arithmetic.

Figure 2.1 illustrates the relationship between mature size (M) and maturation rate in homeothermic animals, i.e. birds and mammals. Maturation rate is expressed as the time (in days) needed for the most rapid phase of sustained growth from 25% to 75% mature body weight, ($t(25–75)M$). As a general, and rather obvious rule, the heavier the animal at maturity, the longer it takes to mature. The three tonne elephant takes longer to mature than the 300 kilogram pig which takes longer than the 30 gram mouse. Figure 2.1 uses logarithmic scales partly to ensure that lightweight birds and mice, middleweight humans and pigs and heavyweight elephants can all be encompassed within the same graph and partly to illustrate a powerful general rule for comparing rates of growth between species differing greatly in mature size, namely,

time taken to mature (days) = $x \times$ mature weight $(kg)^{0.25}$

The different lines in Fig. 2.1 emerge from an exploration by James Kirkwood and me (amongst many others) of the biological relationships between body size, metabolic rate and maturation rate in different species of mammals and birds. The figure contains five lines relating maturation rate ($t(25–75)M$) to mature size (M). Reading from left to right, the first line,

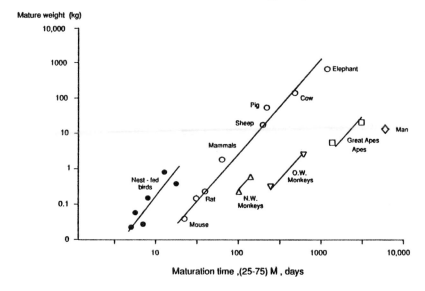

Fig. 2.1 Mature body size and time taken to mature in birds and mammals.

indicating most rapid maturation relates to altricial, or nest-fed, birds. The second includes all mammals excluding primates. The next three reveal a progressive slowing of maturation rates through three taxonomic groups of primates, New World monkeys such as tamarins and marmosets, Old World monkeys, such as macaques, the great apes and finally man, as a single point at the extreme right. The parallel lines in Fig. 2.1 indicate that the relationship (x) between mature size and maturation rate within each group is very similar. In other words, ($t(25-75)M$) when divided by mature weight to the power 0.25 is constant (full explanation of this concept is not necessary to the present argument but given by Kirkwood and Webster, 1984; and Kirkwood, 1985). Maturation rate, when scaled according to mature size is therefore the same for nearly all mammals. Nest-fed birds mature faster than mammals, but the relationship between maturation rate and mature size is the same.

Another, linked, universal law of biology is that, in homeotherms:

Food energy, E, requirement in megajoules (MJ) per day $=$
$y \times$ body weight $(kg)^{0.75}$

The relationship between the energy cost of growth, maturation rate and mature size becomes:

$$E = y \times (0.5M^{0.75}) \times t$$

Where E is the energy in megajoules required to grow from 25% to 75% of mature weight (M) and t is the time in days.

Alternatively,

$$E = (y \times 0.5M^{0.75}) \times (x \times M^{0.25})$$

which simplifies to

$$\frac{E}{M} = \frac{x}{y}$$

Put into words, this means that, within a particular group of animals (those defined by an approximately constant metabolic age or those which fall on the same straight line in Fig. 2.1), the food energy requirement for growth, expressed per kg of mature size is the same, or the energetic efficiency of growth is independent of mature size. One does not need a full understanding of the arithmetic to appreciate the evolutionary significance of this. Animals have evolved to achieve different optimal sizes and shapes to exploit different environmental niches. However, the great majority of mammals have coped with the biological problems of growth by adopting a similar strategy, which is to achieve maturity and self-sufficiency at least cost in terms of energy. This implies that natural selection in nearly all animals has been dominated by mechanistic attributes of biological efficiency that have nothing to do with mind. The very rapid maturation rate of the altricial bird relative to that of the mammals can also be explained on a functional basis. The growth rate of mammals is necessarily constrained by the fact that they have to be reasonably functional (seek food, run away from predators) throughout most of their growth period. The bird that is fed in the nest, like the eagle, cannot fly and dare not step out of the nest until it has reached almost its mature weight. In essence, it takes in nutrients very fast, reaches adult weight,though not adult form,very fast, then at the end of the period of rapid weight gain, metamorphoses even more rapidly into a fully finished and perfect flying machine.

It is obvious that humans mature much more slowly than other mammals of similar size. If humans conformed to the general rule for most mammals, we would mature rather more rapidly than a pig, with the consequence that children would become as big as their parents by two years of age. This prospect is enough to terrify most parents. It would certainly not allow enough time to educate children for self-sufficiency in the modern world. Figure 2.1 shows that humans are, indeed, far removed from the interspecies line for mammals. Remember the logarithmic scale which indicates that the maturation rate in man is 11 times slower than in a mammal of comparable size such as the sheep. We did not, however, arrive at this point from nowhere. Maturation rates show a progressive slowing with the 'advance' in evolution of primates, from primitive New World monkeys (tamarins and marmosets) to the great apes (chimpanzees) to man.

This is rather different from the usual psychological (e.g. Griffin, 1981) or philosophical (e.g. Singer, 1984) arguments for, or against, the uniqueness of the mind of man but it has the merit of avoiding any preconceptions as to what we mean by mind and how we can assess it in species other than our own. It simply suggests, on strict evolutionary ground, that mind as we conceive it (i.e. the ability to have abstract thoughts, benefit from education, and incorporate those thoughts and that education into strategic decisions, etc.), is not a unique property of *Homo sapiens*. However, it is only within the primates that selection for mind began to replace selection for simple biological efficiency as the primary evolutionary determinant of survival and development.

Generic and species-specific questions as to the nature and complexity of the animal mind are fascinating but not, in fact, critical to the problems of animal suffering and animal welfare. I have already suggested that conscious awareness of suffering (i.e. pain) would have been favoured by natural selection because it helps the animal to avoid further damage to the injured site and avoid the source of pain in the future. A more complex human mind that was aware of the basis of the pain and the likely prognosis might suffer more (or less) from this added understanding but could no more equate lack of understanding with lack of suffering in a piglet than in a baby. This is, in fact, the basis of Singer's accusation of 'speciesism'. I close this section therefore by repeating the quotation from Jeremy Bentham (1748–1832). The father of Utilitarianism, not usually considered a very moral philosophy, asked simply, 'The question is not, Can they reason, can they talk, but can they *suffer?*' This is a very good question, but not very specific. The difficult problem for welfare science is to break it down into a series of simple questions that animals can understand too.

Feelings, moods and cognition

I hope by now to have persuaded the sceptic that animals can have feelings, (even if many of them have simple minds) and dissuaded the romantic from the belief that they think and feel just as we do. Table 2.1 lists feelings and moods that a particular animal *may* experience, simply as a starting point for further investigation. Rather in the manner of Humpty Dumpty who said 'When *I* use a word, it means just what I choose it to mean, neither more nor less', I define feeling as conscious awareness of sensation related to a specific stimulus from the internal or external environment or both. For example, the sensation which we know as hunger, may be triggered by hypoglycaemia (internal stimulus) or the smell of bacon (external stimulus) or both. If we are intensely hungry the intensity of the feelings aroused by the smell of bacon or (I have been asked to add) some equally succulent vegetarian alternative, will be that much more intense. The word hunger only defines one end of the spectrum of our feelings about food which may range from extreme suffering due to severe hunger, through a neutral state which we may call satiety to extreme pleasure, during and after a delicious meal. Feelings, thus defined, constitute something which relate to specific stimuli which we and other animals can interpret and act upon, where possible, so as to make us feel better. Mood defines a state of mind, such as anxiety, that cannot necessarily be linked to a specific stimulus, nor interpreted as a reason for a specific action, but which is likely to modulate both the emotional and behavioural responses of an animal to a particular sensation. Cognition is involved when the response of an animal to a set of stimuli involves more than just simple or conditioned reflexes but mental processes by which it interprets incoming sensations from the internal and external environment within the context of its mood and its accumulated experience. Having 'thought about' the options, it can then take decisions as to the most constructive course of action.

Table 2.1 should not be considered to be a comprehensive list of all the feelings and moods that an animal may experience; nor should it be presumed that all animal species are aware of all these feelings and moods. However, I think it is appropriate to the birds and mammals whose lives we control the most – those my profession calls (with characteristic pomposity) 'animals of veterinary importance', i.e. pets and horses, animals on farms, in zoos and in laboratories.

Feelings about food, as indicated above, may range over the whole spectrum from extreme suffering through neutrality to extreme pleasure.

Table 2.1 (a) Possible feelings and (b) moods in animals.

(a)

	Feelings	
← Suffering	— Emotional range — Neutrality	→ Pleasure
Hunger	Satiety	Delight
Thirst	Satiety	
Heat, cold	Thermal comfort	Luxury
Exhaustion	Rest	Luxury
Pain	Comfort	Sensuality
Malaise	Health	Vigour
Fear	Security	

(b)

Moods	
Negative	Positive
Anxiety	Excitement
Apathy	Curiosity
Impotence	Libido
Hopelessness	Control

Within the central, neutral range, animals will experience the sensations of hunger, satiety or the appeal of a particularly attractive source of food and, if possible, adjust their food intake on the basis that (1) it makes them feel good at the time or (2) they know from past experience that it will make them feel better (or worse) in the near future. I shall discuss this in more detail in Chapter 3. In a satisfactory environment, most animals should be able to adjust their feelings to stay within the range between neutrality and satisfaction and so avoid distress. Suffering only occurs when an unpleasant sensation becomes particularly intense, particularly prolonged, or when the animal is denied the opportunity to take constructive action to relieve it.

Extreme thirst is an obvious source of suffering but the spectrum of feeling probably does not extend beyond satiety. When rats and men drink sweet or alcoholic drinks to excess it is not to quench their thirst! Extreme heat and cold stress are obvious sources of suffering. Most animals will work only to achieve thermal neutrality (Chapter 4) but heat (especially) can give hedonistic pleasure. Observe the human race on the beach or a cat lying on a radiator or perilously close to an open fire. An animal will feel the need to rest and sleep on a regular basis and take appropriate action. Suffering occurs only when this need is denied for an extended time, e.g. when lambs are transported illegally in lorries for over 15 hours. Some animals will lie down longer, and with more pleasure, if they can find a particularly luxurious bed. Once again, consider that supreme hedonist, the cat.

Animals will not, of course, normally consider any one of these feelings in isolation. The motivation to go out and seek food to reduce the sensation of hunger will be weighed against the motivation to stay in the lair or nest to achieve rest, comfort, security or even the pleasure of sloth. To avoid suffering the animal needs to establish a set of motivational priorities then act upon them. Once again, this suggests that one of the most effective ways to cause suffering is to deny an animal the opportunity to make a constructive contribution to the quality of its own existence.

Pain is obviously one of the most severe sources of suffering, Absence of pain is obviously a sufficient objective for any animal. It is, however, physiologically acceptable to put sensual satisfaction such as that experienced by a dog having its tummy tickled at the opposite end of the pain spectrum, not least because it largely involves the same nerve endings.

Being unhealthy is a powerful indication of poor welfare but it is not necessarily a source of suffering. The family breadwinner (of either sex) tucked up in bed with a cold and cosseted by his or her partner may well be rather more comfortable than if still at work. Suffering occurs when one *feels* the symptoms of illness. This sense of malaise is not only a source of suffering in itself, but may also exacerbate other feelings like cold, pain or exhaustion, and moods such as anxiety. This concept has profound implications for the veterinary approach to the symptomatic treatment of sickness in animals (see Chapter 5). Good health, like absence of hunger, may be considered a neutral but acceptable endpoint to the spectrum of malaise and health. However, in youth at least, the spectrum can extend to pleasure in a positive sense of vigour. Fox cubs at play are probably relishing their vigour, as are the calf or piglet that runs and skips in a field or straw yard. Close confinement of such animals in boxes or cages denies them the pleasure of expressing this sense of vigour, although, to anticipate the next stage of the argument, they may not be in the mood to skip in such barren environments.

A sense of fear has such obvious survival value that it must have featured strongly in natural selection throughout a wide range of the animal kingdom. Some aspects of fear have become 'hard wired' into the genes. Thus, some monkeys are innately frightened of snakes but penguins have no innate fear of man. Others are acquired (Chapter 6). In both cases, I define fear (as distinct from anxiety) as a conscious feeling provoked by an external stimulus after interpretation by the brain in a way defined by the animal's genotype and experience. Once again, it only constitutes suffering when carried to extremes or when the animal cannot do anything to reduce the state of fear. The healthy gazelle observes the cheetah on the African plains and moves to a safe distance. Similarly, both sheep and sheepdog know the rules that define flight distance and direction of flight. If the rules are obeyed, the sheep may experience but not suffer from a sensation of fear and respond in a constructive and orderly fashion. They only suffer a sense of panic when the rules break down. It is often alleged that sheep are stupid, usually by those who have observed them only in the presence of untrained humans or dogs, both of whom are instinctively viewed as predators and both of whom may be breaking the rules. My response to this is that none of us is at our intellectual best when in a state of panic.

All the feelings described above are relatively primitive. They are concerned with personal comfort, security and satisfaction and it is reasonable to assume that they have been involved, to a greater or lesser extent, in the natural selection of a wide range of animal species. I have deliberately excluded, at this stage, more refined feelings and emotions such as friendship and altruism which can contribute to the biological success of families and social groups, partly because these feelings are probably restricted to a very small number of species, and partly because they are not central to the main argument. One does not have to be nice to suffer.

The difficulties in interpreting how another animal feels when presented by a specific internal or external stimulus are as nothing compared to the difficulties of interpreting something so subjective as mood. However, there is good physiological evidence that non-specific moods such as anxiety, excitement, libido, curiosity, etc. arise from primitive, subconscious areas of the brain stem, which implies that they evolved well before the ascent of man. Moreover the enormous interest shown by the drug industry in developing mood-altering drugs for man (especially tranquillizers or anxiolytics) has, of course, generated an enormous body of evidence describing the biochemical and behavioural effects of such drugs on animals. I shall return to this subject in Chapter 6. For the present it is sufficient to state that mood is not unique to the human species and must be built into any evaluation of animal suffering.

I have attempted in Table 2.1 to pair opposing positive and negative moods such as curiosity and apathy, excitement and anxiety. It would, however, be a mistake to link these opposites and suggest that an animal attempted to steer a middle path between apathy and curiosity in the same way as it would balance its need for food against its need for rest. It is necessary only to accept that the conscious emotional state of an animal may be affected not only by a specific stimulus, its instinctive and cognitive interpretation of that stimulus, but also by the mood it happens to be in when it receives that stimulus.

Measurement of 'behavioural needs'

If we can accept that most animals are motivated most of the time to act in a strictly utilitarian fashion, i.e. to avoid suffering and achieve pleasure within the categories defined by Table 2.1, then it is possible to study their motivation by putting them into situations that will test their motivational priorities and strength of motivation. Table 2.2 outlines the sorts of questions that may be asked.

Table 2.2 Measurement of motivation.

Motivational priorities
Preference tests: short term, e.g. food selection
                   long term, e.g. food *v*. rest
Comfort *v*. companionship

Strength of motivation
What will I pay: to achieve, e.g. space, a nest
                 to avoid, e.g. cold, isolation
What will I sacrifice: to achieve, e.g. comfort, security
                       to avoid, e.g. pain, fear

Consequences of denial
Short term, e.g. displacement activity
Long term, e.g. 'rebound' behaviour
Stereotypic behaviour
Mood shifts, e.g. 'learned apathy'

Preference tests
The simplest of experiments is the short term preference test. A rat, for example, may be invited to select one food in preference to another, either directly or by activating a trigger (e.g. pressing a panel or interrupting a light

beam) that it has learnt to associate with a particular reward. A chicken may be introduced to a simple maze that offers it the choice of proceeding to cages with different types of floor, e.g. wire, solid wood, or deep litter. When properly designed, such experiments can be of great value so long as they are not over-interpreted or considered in isolation. Short term preference tests are obviously essential to a company wishing to develop and market a new cat food. Such tests have also been used to improve floor design in battery cages for laying hens. However they cannot, by their nature, give any indication of (1) strength of motivation, (2) changes in motivational priorities or (3) the wisdom of choice.

An animal such as a rat or chicken is likely to respond to a preference test rather like a young child motivated by the need to avoid pain and seek pleasure without the added complication of an acquired sense of right and wrong. A child (or a rat) may repeatedly select chocolates in preference to wholemeal biscuits, thereby indicating a clear preference but not necessarily one that is consistent with its long-term welfare. Children presented with different-coloured chocolate buttons may eat more red ones than blue ones, or more chocolate buttons altogether if they are given a range of six colours rather than a single colour. In each case the child displays a clear preference but not one that could be said to matter in a biological or psychological sense, though it matters, of course, to the manufacturer!

Motivational priorities

A longer-term version of the preference test can be a useful tool for studying the changing pattern of motivational priorities that make up a typical day in the life of an animal. A cow at pasture may be motivated by internal desires and external opportunities to eat, drink, sleep, mate, explore, feed her calf, seek companionship or seek solitude. In practice, most of her time will be devoted to grazing and resting (lying down) each of which may occupy eight hours in every twenty-four. The cow will select a first priority (e.g. grazing) from the available opportunities then stop grazing to lie down or feed her calf when her motivation to do these things exceeds that of continuing grazing. These decisions are usually clear-cut, which implies an intelligent, conscious control of conflicting priorities. If her behaviour were controlled simply by the relative strength of motivating forces she would 'dither' at the point when (say) the motivation to lie down exactly equalled the motivation to graze. MacFarland (1989) has analysed the basis of motivational priorities in much more detail than is possible here. Suffice it to say that most animals have the good sense not to dither.

Analysis of longer-term motivational priorities is a good and largely natural way to study strength of motivation. One can, for example, examine the extent to which a cow will sacrifice rest for feeding by first observing how she allocates her time between eating, lying and standing when none of these actions is restricted, then progressively restrict the time available for eating and lying to the point where she must decide how to allocate her limited resources of time between these and other essential activities. This application of economic theory to the study of animal behaviour asks the animal how it wishes to ration resources when these resources are limited.

Economic theory, necessities and luxuries
I have already outlined Marian Dawkins' application of economic theory to the study of animal motivation, which is to measure the value of a commodity by what the animal is prepared to pay for it in terms of time and effort. In its simplest form this can involve a rat or pig being asked to press a button repeatedly to achieve food or warmth. Alternatively, the animal may be compelled to work harder by pushing against heavier and heavier doors, or walking further and further to the desired goal. Ian Duncan, for example, measured the motivation of hens to seek a nest box in which to lay their daily egg by compelling them to walk in a circular corridor towards a nest box that never got any closer. Some birds would walk more than 1.5 kilometres which suggests that the motivation of the hen to seek a nesting site is very strong indeed. Dawkins suggested, cautiously, that a nest box is rated by hens as 'price-inelastic' or a necessity, but that a commodity such as a dust bath is 'price-elastic', or a luxury, since birds will use litter to dust bathe if it is there, but do not appear to be prepared to work for it.

Examples of this approach to defining the quality of the environment for animals in terms of necessities and luxuries will appear frequently throughout this book. At this stage I wish only to introduce the methods used by ethologists to measure the value that animals place on different activities, as an essential prerequisite to any discussion of 'behavioural needs'. I must also add a note of caution. For such experiments to have meaning, the animals need to understand the question. They must, first, be aware both of the goal and the way to achieve it. Second, they must not be unnerved by the experimental conditions to the point where they lose their powers of thought. Consider an animal that has been trained to work for a goal that is out of sight, e.g. push open a door to obtain food. The same animal may fail to push open the door when the 'reward' is the company of another animal, for security or even for sex. This may be because:

(1) it values company less than food so is prepared to work less hard;
(2) it appears to forget that the door leads to a companion (although it can remember that it leads to food);
(3) it simply does not think about other animals in their absence (even for sex).

This distinction is extremely important. The fourth freedom assumes that animals have a behavioural need for 'the company of their own kind'. If it can be shown that chickens, for example, simply have no conscious awareness of other chickens unless they are actually present (out of sight is truly out of mind) then it becomes difficult to justify including the fourth freedom within a Code of Welfare for chickens. However, the chicken's reluctance to work for companionship may be because it finds the door to be not only hard work but positively frightening, in which case we have underestimated the cost. Alternatively, although it cannot see either reward beyond the door, it may smell food but not another chicken, in which case our hypothesis about memory is incorrect. Finally, if the experience induces severe alarm or panic, it would be a heartless examiner who failed the bird for lack of intellect.

Early investigators of animal behaviour such as Pavlov and Skinner tended to pose questions of stark simplicity to animals in barren environments who were presented with a single choice and an immediate reward or punishment. Given such simple questions, it is hardly surprising that they got simple answers. However, as soon as we attempt subtler questions which are more appropriate to the trials of real life, i.e. those that allow the animal to apply some element of cognition and make decisions based on complex stimuli interpreted in the light of its experience, then we can no longer presume that the animal will respond to experimental stimuli according to our preconceptions. This is because the animal may be responding to a different set of signals from those we thought we had imposed – signals which we may have failed to notice. Communicating with animals is rather like communicating with foreigners. We must not assume that because we fail to understand them it is they who are thick.

In a satisfactory environment, an animal will normally perform constructive acts to control how it feels, i.e. achieve pleasure or avoid suffering. In many cases, therefore, the source of suffering arises not so much from the primary stress but from the fact that the animal is denied the opportunity to control it. Behaviour patterns classically associated with frustration include displacement behaviour, rebound behaviour, stereotypic behaviour and learned helplessness.

Displacement behaviour

When an animal is aroused by an intense stimulus such as food, or a confrontation between two males, and is then frustrated by being denied access to the food or forced to withdraw from the confrontation, it will frequently embark on an alternative activity which may be purposeful, such as grooming, but unrelated to the main stimulus. Animals appear to use such *displacement behaviour* to reduce the intensity of acute unpleasant feelings such as frustration, anger and pain and perhaps more chronic, non-specific moods such as anxiety. It is what we do ourselves. Consider the loser in a family argument who storms off to wash the car (or the pots).

Rebound behaviour

If an animal is prevented from performing a particular action designed to satisfy a behavioural need, we would expect it to devote an unusually long period of time to that action when, once again, it became possible. This is called rebound behaviour. To give an obvious example, an animal that is deprived of food for an unusually long period will eat more when it regains access to food, unless, of course, it has become weak and exhausted from starvation. Konrad Lorenz (1966) suggested that the motivation of animals to a wide range of behaviour patterns (such as exploration or hunting) builds up during periods of denial and expresses itself during deprivation as displacement activity and thereafter as rebound behaviour. This has largely been discounted as a general hypothesis but the search for rebound behaviour can be used to investigate welfare problems in farm animals (such as battery hens) confined so closely that they are practically unable to carry out comfort behaviours such as grooming and stretching (see Chapter 4).

Stereotypic behaviour
Animals in barren environments with 'nothing to do', i.e. little opportunity to make a constructive contribution to the quality of their own existence, may over a period of weeks, months or years develop stereotypic behaviour or stereotypies – the prolonged, obsessive performance of apparently purposeless activity. Horses are particularly prone to stereotypies, which include 'weaving', prolonged rocking from side to side of the head and (usually) front legs, and 'windsucking', repeated swallowing of air. Another classic stereotypy is the pacing of wild cats back and forth in their cages. Stereotypic behaviour has been over-simplistically described as a mechanism for coping with the frustration incurred by life in a barren environment. As we shall see, it is much more complicated than that. At this stage we may assume that it is a form of behaviour induced by chronic frustration although what has induced the frustration and whether stereotypies help the animal to cope cannot yet be resolved so simply.

Learned helplessness
Experimental psychologists have coined the term 'learned helplessness' to describe a loss of responsiveness to stimuli in animals, acquired after prolonged periods in which they have been denied the opportunity to perform constructive actions designed to achieve pleasure (e.g. food) or avoid pain (e.g. electric shocks). This is sometimes described as an adaptive response, an interpretation which I find chilling. Learned helplessness defines the state of mind in an animal that has given up. I prefer to call it hopelessness.

The nature of stress and suffering

My aim is to ensure a fair deal for those animals over whom we have dominion. This does not require the creation of a stress-free paradise. Indeed, there is no reason to assume that animals would appreciate a problem-free environment any more than we would. My favourite 'heaven' cartoon has two immortal gentlemen sitting, somewhat blank-faced, upon a cloud. The caption reads, 'I wish I had a magazine'. Any animal, in the course of a normal life is presented with a series of problems which it must tackle, in order of priority, by taking appropriate action – sometimes instinctively, sometimes after conscious thought. It is only when the problems become too severe or too complex for constructive action, or when the opportunity for constructive action is frustrated that these problems may stress the animal to the point of suffering. MacFarland (1989) has attempted to embrace motivational priorities and the concept of suffering within a multidimensional model of state-space. Figure 2.2 presents a simplistic illustration of this concept.

Try to imagine the state of mind of the animal as a multidimensional egg that exists as an island of serenity within a sea of suffering (any problems so far?). Stimuli and stresses from the internal and external environments will tend to move the state of mind of the animal towards the circumference or shell of the egg. These stresses include hunger, thirst, thermal stress (heat and cold), fear, pain and exhaustion. All these stimuli increase in magnitude from the zero point, at the centre of the egg towards the shell at which point the intensity of the stimulus becomes sufficient to induce suffering. It is theoretically possible for all these stimuli to operate simultaneously and to pull the state of mind of the animal away from the mid-point in six or more dimensions at once. This can be analysed mathematically, although it is impossible to draw.

The upper, right-hand quadrant of Fig. 2.2 illustrates responses to stresses capable of causing two sorts of suffering, hunger and exhaustion. An animal such as a cow which has to work hard for its food will commence grazing

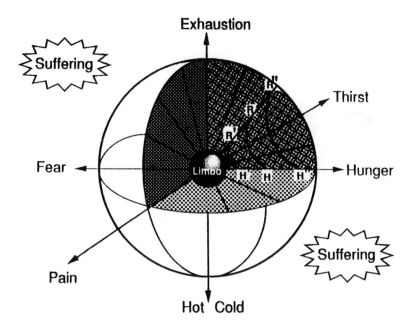

Fig. 2.2 McFarland's egg. Motivational priorities, suffering and limbo.

when it is hungry (point H in Fig. 2.2). As it grazes it moves its state of mind towards zero in the hunger dimension but away from zero in the dimension that carries tiredness to its limit of exhaustion. At point R, it concludes that the motivation to rest has overcome the motivation to eat so it stops grazing and lies down. The limits of the curve HR describe the state of mind of a cow on good summer pasture. They are well within the state-space that it recognizes as comfortable so, in these circumstances, neither hunger or tiredness can be said to constitute suffering.

The longer curve, H''R'' towards the shell, describes the condition of a cow during the northern winter or during the dry season in the tropics. The quantity and quality of the food are now inferior and the cow has to work much harder to avoid intolerable hunger. She may also have to reconcile these objectives with the need to reduce the stresses of cold or heat. In these circumstance, the cow may not yet actually experience suffering but she is finding it increasingly difficult to cope. As she nears the limits, her actions become (to quote MacFarland) 'increasingly desperate'. He refers to this state as purgatory which is an attractive use of the word, although not one that would satisfy a Jesuit. In Fig. 2.2 it is defined as 'suffering', the area outside the circumference of the sphere.

This model assumes only that the animal acts to move its feelings away from the state of suffering. It does not incorporate any positive mood towards a state of pleasure. It is, however, based on the premise that the animal is consciously motivated to act to improve its state of mind and therefore includes the possibility that it might suffer if denied the opportunity to make a constructive contribution to the quality of its own existence even if it is presented with no obvious environmental stress. Consider, finally, curve H'R' in Fig. 2.2. This could illustrate the state of mind of a adult sow confined in an individual pen. She is regularly provided with all the food she needs, (if not all the food she desires) in a form than can be eaten quickly and digested easily. She can satisfy hunger with minimal effort, is protected from heat, cold and fear, and is unlikely to experience exhaustion since she can do little but stand up and lie down. In these circumstances she may enter what MacFarland calls a state of limbo. He writes:

'Does the animal suffer in limbo? If the animal is in a state which it persistently attempts to reduce or avoid ... I would want to suggest that it is suffering.'

This raises the question: 'Do animals attempt to escape from limbo?' If the normal routes of escape (like exploring for food or a mate, or simply for curiosity) are unavailable, the animal may have to devise alternative, apparently non-constructive activities simply to improve its state of mind. This is, of course, an attractive interpretation of the motivation that underlies stereotypic behaviour. It is also reasonable to ask whether an animal in limbo, with nothing constructive to do or occupy its mind, might not experience other sources of suffering, like chronic pain, to an exaggerated degree. The answers to these questions are not easy but they are of crucial importance to our assessment of the quality of life experienced by animals closely confined and with very little to do, whether on farms, in zoos, in the laboratory, or in a hutch at the bottom of the garden.

Conclusions

Many animals, including those species whose lives we control the most, demonstrate properties of mind which may be far less complex than ours but are sufficiently advanced to feel suffering and pleasure. However, feeling is a subjective experience which can only be communicated indirectly. Methods exist for measuring the value that animals attribute to different commodities (necessities and luxuries) that may determine the quality of their life and the consequences of frustration. Non-human animals are motivated by strict utilitarian principles designed to avoid personal suffering and/or achieve pleasure. Suffering should not be equated with stress. Suffering occurs when the intensity or complexity of stresses exceeds or exhausts the capacity of the animal to cope, or when the animal is prevented from taking constructive action. Suffering may also occur when an animal is in a state of limbo, free from any obvious source of environmental stress but denied the opportunity to make any sort of constructive contribution to the quality of its own existence. Prolonged exposure to sources of suffering may induce abnormal behaviour patterns such as stereotypies or profound changes of mood, including the development of a sense of hopelessness.

Once we accept that the animals over whom we hold dominion have the capacity to suffer, then we too have problems. These are moral problems but they require pragmatic solutions. These involve, first, an analysis of the nature of stresses to the bodies and minds of animals and the extent of their ability to cope with these stresses, then advocacy and adoption of practical ways to prevent these stresses from intensifying to the point of suffering. We are under no obligation to give animals everything they want, but we cannot begin to be fair until we know what they want.

3 Hunger and Thirst

'L'on a le temps d'avoir les dents longues, lorsqu'on attend pour vivre le trépas de quelqu'un.'
[You have time for hunger when your life waits on the death of someone else]

Molière, *Le Médecin Malgre Lui* (1666).

Hunger and thirst are the two most basic, primitive and unremitting of all motivating forces. Sex can be equally powerful but for most species there are periods of remission. On the basis of the argument advanced in the previous chapter, I shall assume that sentient animals, by which I include, at least, all the birds and mammals, experience pleasure both when they eat food and when they confidently anticipate that food will arrive. This implies that they can suffer both directly from the absence of food and indirectly when they are prevented from doing things that they anticipate will lead them to food. When we care for animals we seek to provide them with freedom from hunger and thirst by giving them access to clean water and sufficient food, often scientifically formulated to provide a correct balance of nutrients. We should not forget, however, that these animals evolved satisfactorily without benefit of nutritional science. The science of animal nutrition only became necessary when we took animals away from their natural habitat (or took the habitat away from the animals), so denying them the opportunity to choose for themselves what to eat and how much. This chapter is not, therefore, concerned with how we should meet the nutrient requirements of sentient animals (hereafter when I write 'animals' I mean 'sentient animals') but with their perception of appetite, hunger and thirst, the factors that motivate them to seek food and drink, their ability to recognize and select a 'sensible' diet and their potential for suffering if these needs are not met.

I need to create some more Humpty Dumpty-type definitions. Many scientists will find these definitions incomplete, particularly those who have expanded any of them into a whole book. It is, however, necessary to my argument to draw clear distinctions between words that often appear as synonyms in common use:

● *Hunger*. Hunger is a primitive sensation induced by integration of signals from a range of sensory nerves recording information concerning the balance between supply and demand of nutrients to the tissues of the body. This definition implies that it is a simple indicator of physiological state or homeostasis, triggered only by signals arising from the internal environment. As such, it may be called, more correctly, *metabolic hunger*, and can refer to the desire for food *per se* primarily to meet energy needs or to the desire for a single nutrient as specific as sodium. Even the most primitive animals experience the *sensation* of metabolic hunger and act accordingly. We can have no idea at what stage in evolution animals began to suffer from conscious *awareness* of this sensation but we can, I think, assume that all vertebrates, at least, can *suffer* from hunger, not least because of the complexity of their approaches to seeking and storing food, and the risks they are prepared to run to get it.

● *Appetite.* Appetite is a complex conscious sensation induced by a variety of stimuli arising from the internal and external environment. These include the internal stimulus of metabolic hunger (as defined above) which exists whether food is present or not, direct external stimuli such as the sight, smell and novelty of food, and social stimuli such as competition or social meal-taking. Appetite, accompanied by the expectation that it will be satisfied, can be highly hedonic and an obvious source of pleasure. Frustration of appetite, in the absence of metabolic hunger, can hardly be called suffering.

● *Satiety.* Chambers defines satiety, unhelpfully, as the state of being satiated, itself defined as 'fully gratified'. I shall define it as the motivational opposite of hunger, i.e. the (largely internal) drive that motivates an animal to make the conscious decision to stop eating and do something else (which can include simply standing around not eating).

● *Oral satisfaction.* In the natural state, animals such as horses, cattle and pigs need to spend many hours eating relatively low quality, fibrous food in order to meet their nutrient requirements. However, the horse in a stable, the sow installed on concrete, or the veal calf fed entirely on a liquid diet may be fed in such a way that they can consume all the nutrients they need to avoid metabolic hunger in less than ten minutes per day. Such animals are particularly prone to develop *oral stereotypies*, the compulsive, prolonged performance of apparently purposeless oral activity, e.g. crib biting and windsucking in the horse, bar chewing in sows, solo tongue rolling and mutual tongue-sucking in calves. These activities, which I shall later describe in detail, are commonly quoted as indices of frustration in animals given diets that may meet their nutrient requirements but which fail to overcome their motivation to go through all the behaviour patterns associated with nutrient intake in the natural state. These may include not only eating and ruminating but hunting or searching for food. This argument is contentious, as we shall see. It does, however, require a distinction to be made between satiety, which is the motivational opposite of the physiological sensation of hunger, and oral satisfaction, which becomes the opposite of the more complex psychological sensation of appetite.

● *Thirst.* Thirst may be defined quite simply as a physiological need for water triggered by nerves sensing an increase in the osmotic pressure of the blood, which is usually but not always a sign that the body is becoming dehydrated. The rat that drinks large amounts of water to obtain sugar in solution, and the human that drinks large amounts of beer to obtain alcohol in solution are not motivated by thirst. Satisfaction of thirst is an obvious source of pleasure but I would not call it hedonic.

Metabolic hunger and conscious appetite

I have defined metabolic hunger as a sensation which recognizes the balance between supply and demand of nutrients to the tissues of the body. Hunger and satiety are the *on* and *off* switches whereby animals regulate food intake approximately according to their needs. The scientific literature is awash with theories of appetite control and the origins and interpretation of the sensation of hunger in animals. Short-term sensations of hunger and satiety, leading to tactical decisions to start and stop eating, have been attributed both to events within the gut, e.g. impulses from nerves sensing gastric and duodenal filling and emptying, and to nerves sensing concentrations of nutrients such as glucose and amino acids at various sites in the blood, such as entering and leaving the liver. Impulses signalling a short-term nutrient deficiency are integrated, subconsciously, within the hypothalamus, which may initiate autonomic or hormonal signals to mobilize nutrient reserves from (especially) fat, and/or initiate the conscious desire to eat. The mobilization of energy reserves will proceed automatically but the conscious response to this signal will depend on other aspects of the animal's motivational state. The fox running away from hounds may well be receiving signals that its blood sugar is low but has more pressing needs than the satisfaction of hunger.

There is also a longer-term *strategic* element of appetite control in animals based upon the perception that body condition (e.g. muscle and fat development) is not what it should be. In humans this may involve higher elements of self-awareness such as vanity or long-term health fears. This is superimposed upon a more primitive (but more subtle) ability to regulate nutrient supply not only according to the needs of the moment but to meet genetically programmed targets during pregnancy and growth, or during recovery from illness or undernutrition. One good example of this is the phenomenon known as 'catch-up' growth in farm animals. If young cattle, for example, are brought off grass in the autumn and given free access to a relatively low quality diet such as grass silage, they will eat to appetite and continue to grow but at slower rate than their genetic potential. At the end of the winter the animals will be larger,but leaner than they were in the autumn. Specifically they will contain less fat and muscle tissue relative to their skeletal size. When they are turned out to good quality grass in the spring they will eat much more and grow much faster than an animal which does not sense that it is thin or underweight for its age. Two further examples of the same phenomenon are the elevated appetites of adult animals during pregnancy or during recovery from a debilitating illness. In all three cases, the appetite regulator is reset, not to maintain homeostasis or the *status quo*, but to bring about a change in body state.

It is not particularly helpful to the present argument to elaborate on the relative importance of the various short- and long-term regulators of appetite control in animals. Suffice it to say that the intensity of metabolic hunger depends both on acute signals from the internal environment and on the longer-term perception of body state, however these things may be transduced. Figure 3.1 attempts to illustrate, in a strictly mechanistic sense, the factors that may contribute to metabolic hunger and conscious appetite in an animal. It makes no attempt to incorporate the specific physiological stimuli to hunger (e.g. low blood glucose concentrations), the anatomical location of the hunger and satiety regulators (e.g within the hypothalamus) nor the specific effector mechanisms (e.g gene switches and hormones). These are quite fascinating but another story. (For further reading on the physiology of appetite control see Forbes (1988) and Winick (1988).)

I repeat: metabolic hunger is the sensation which recognizes the balance between supply and demand of nutrients to the tissues of the body. An animal may eat a variety of foods (A, B, C and D in Fig. 3.1) which are digested to yield available nutrients to meet the requirements of the body. Indigestible material is excreted in the faeces. By far the greatest proportion of the available nutrients (75–95%) is used as a source of metabolizable energy which serves as fuel for work essential to life and is dissipated as heat. The nutrient requirements of an animal may be partitioned, somewhat abitrarily, as follows:

(1) *Maintenance:* metabolic processes essential to the maintenance of homeostasis and body mass in the adult animal. An animal is said to be at maintenance when the supply of available nutrients exactly balances their loss in metabolism. In the case of energy metabolism this occurs when metabolizable energy intake equals metabolic heat production.

(2) *Work:* this defines the requirement for nutrients to meet the extra (energy) costs of the work of foraging, escaping predators, shivering in cold environments, etc.

(3) *Anabolic processes:* growth, pregnancy, lactation. The nutrient requirements for these processes are regulated by a biological programmer which sets targets which are defined by the genetic constitution and physiological state of the animal (e.g. growing, pregnant, lactating).

Available nutrients taken in excess of these requirements contribute to body reserves. Energy is primarily stored as fat but the body will also store reserves of protein, minerals and some (fat-soluble) vitamins for use in times of need. The body also sets its own priorities for nutrients. Obviously, the requirement for maintenance largely, but not entirely, overrides the priority for growth. However, the demands of pregnancy and, to a lesser extent, lactation will override those of maintenance, up to a point.

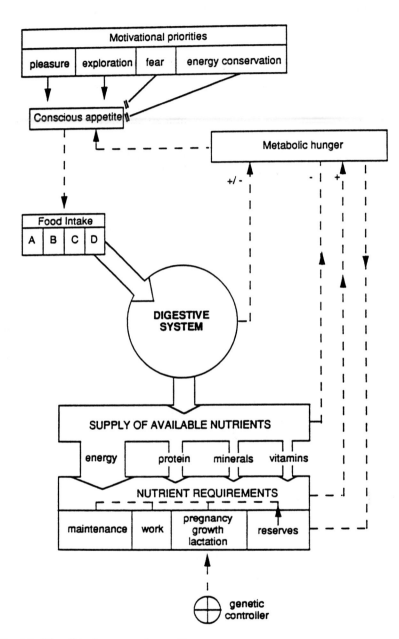

Fig. 3.1 Stimuli to hunger and appetite.

Thus an animal will contribute its own body reserves to the development of its offspring but only until the point where its own survival becomes seriously compromised.

Metabolic hunger, sensed subconsciously at the level of the hypothalamus, depends on integration of short-term sensations from:

(1) the digestive tract – indicating, for example, the fullness of the stomach and the supply of digesta to the duodenum.

(2) the supply of available nutrients from the gut to the liver via the hepatic portal system.

(3) the uptake of specific nutrients from the circulation into the cells and tissues of the body at rates which are determined both by the inevitable demands of maintenance and by the genetic programme for anabolic processes such as growth, lactation, wound healing etc.

Having integrated these sensations, the hypothalamus sends out signals which seek to balance supply and demand in the short term, either by triggering appetite, the conscious desire to eat, or by mobilizing nutrient reserves. This mobilization of reserves cannot, of course, continue indefinitely. As the nutrient reserves progressively diminish, so the intensity of the signal to the conscious controller of appetite must increase. Simply put, the thinner the (healthy) animal is at the time of an acute nutrient demand, the greater will be its appetite and the more likely it will be to suffer if this appetite is not satisfied.

In the sentient animals, conscious appetite involves complex and, usually, rational decisions which recognize the powerful stimulus of metabolic hunger but do not respond to it instinctively. Such animals make decisions when to start and stop eating, what to eat, and where to eat by interpreting their metabolic hunger for energy and other specific nutrients in the light of other conscious motivational priorities. In Fig. 3.1 I listed pleasure, exploration, fear and exhaustion. Eating is a source of pleasure. Palatability is a measure of the pleasure derived from food, which may either be achieved immediately if the food tastes good, or after some delay when the animal discovers that the food makes if *feel* good. The corollary to this is that food may prove to be unpalatable either because it tastes foul or because the animal eats it, later feels unwell, and so associates this taste with discomfort (or malaise) rather than pleasure.

Most animals are motivated by the urge to explore the environment in search of reward. Since food is one of the most pleasant rewards, animals are motivated, according to their digestive systems, to forage or hunt. The simple visceral sensation of hunger is therefore modulated by the sense of pleasure that an animal derives from the pursuit of food, provided, of course, that it has a reasonable expectation of reward. A pig, for example, inveigled into an experiment, may press a panel fifty times to obtain a pellet of food. More realistically, it will root for hours in the ground if it has the reasonable expectation of finding a worm or something similarly succulent every fifteen minutes or so. They are not achieving much by way of nutrient supply but they are deriving great oral satisfaction.

For most wild animals there are powerful deterrents to the pursuit of satiety and oral satisfaction. These animals have to reconcile the demands of hunger and thirst against the fear of predation. The conflict faced by a thirsty bushbuck at a waterhole occupied by lions is an obvious source of stress, although one that can usually be resolved by constructive action before it intensifies to the point of suffering. Most wild animals, whether hunters or foragers, also have to resolve the tricky paradox that they need food to provide energy to do work to find food. This requires strategic decisions to ensure that the food energy gain from hunting or foraging exceeds or at least matches the energy cost of the exercise. For wild animals that fend for themselves, the resolution of hunger and thirst is not only one of the most demanding of activities but one of the most complex. Carnivorous hunters, for example, have to learn, and learn fast, what foods are good and bad for them, where their prey live and hide, how to kill them without getting killed or maimed themselves, and whether the probability of hunting success in a particular territory will justify the energy cost of the hunt.

I close this section with four truisms regarding wild animals faced by the problems of hunting and foraging to satisfy their own hunger and thirst.

(1)   Wild animals seldom get fat.
(2)   Wild animals are regularly faced by the problem of hunger, which cannot be addressed in isolation but in the context of other stressors such as fear and exhaustion.
(3)   In a sustainable natural habitat, wild animals may be under near-constant stress but, so long as they remain fit and well, they possess both the skills to resolve these stresses and the opportunity to use these skills. Most of the time they can take effective action to avoid suffering.
(4)   In a sustainable natural habitat any wild animal that becomes sick or lame is unlikely to suffer for long.

The allure of domestication

Since animals are motivated most of the time to achieve pleasure and avoid suffering with minimum expenditure of effort (the amorality of true innocence) and since hunger and thirst are the most unrelenting of drives, it is hardly surprising that they can be attracted to places where the food is good and cheap. Man domesticated animals primarily by offering them easy access to good food, first at a distance and then within the compound. This powerful and reliable reward was sufficient to overcome their instinctive (and learned) fears of novelty, confinement and the presence of man. Some animals are easier to domesticate than others and these species-specific differences in 'domesticatability' will have increased with time. Individual animals within potentially domesticatable species like the dog, cow or goat, that responded with least fear to man's offer of food would have been best fitted for survival in this changed environmental niche and this fitness for domestication will have been favoured by selection in successive generations. At the other extreme we have the supremely non-domesticatable tiger, which stays well away from man and has learnt to treat 'easy' food (often bait for a trap) with the utmost suspicion. Much of this behaviour is instinctive but it, too, has been reinforced by generations of experience. The tiger behaves the way we expect a tiger to behave not just because it is a tiger but also because man, over the centuries, has been motivated by the desire not to domesticate it but to kill it. Some large, potentially aggressive species of bears that have evolved on remote arctic islands away from direct contact with man the hunter or competitor, appear to regard modern, non-aggressive biologists as unthreatening and therefore of little consequence.

This preamble prompts an important, if contentious, argument. There are obviously large, genetically based differences in behaviour between (say) the tiger and the spaniel. The former is the quintessence of wildness, the latter the quintessence of domestication. The romantics among us view the tiger as the noble savage who has rejected man's dominion. We may love the spaniel, perhaps for the love it gives us, but we seldom respect its independence. We have categorized these two animals, respectively, as wild and domestic. If we are animal lovers, we are then inclined to conclude that the wild animal should be set free and the domestic animal treated with tender loving care.

Now compare the mountain chamois with the domestic nanny goat. The former is secretive, wisely afraid of man and, by all criteria, truly wild. The latter can be as amiable as the spaniel and far more insouciant. In this case, however, the physiological difference between the two species is quite small but they have been conditioned by environmental pressures into entirely different patterns of behaviour.

Finally, consider the English fox. For generations, the fox was viewed by the Englishman as a competing carnivore, pursuing the same prey, (chickens, pheasant, etc.). Other competing carnivores, like wolves, were hunted to extinction but the Englishman (or, at least the Englishmen with power) decided that hunting the fox was 'fun' and foxes should therefore be preserved. At this point, the fox species became more valuable to the Englishman alive than extinct, using value as defined in Chapter 2. The country gentlemen ensured both the preservation of a habitat which *they* thought fit for a wild animal and continued to hunt and harry the said animal, thereby ensuring that it stayed wild.

In more recent years our life styles and sensibilities have changed and the fox has been quick to spot the difference. We have both succumbed to the allure of suburbia. Big suburban gardens and big-hearted suburban sensibilities, brimming dustbins and all-night fried chicken outlets have created a splendid environmental niche for the fox. We might say that they are becoming tamer. I suggest however that the word 'tamer' describes our perception of their changed behaviour, rather than any fundamental change in their own motivation. Food is of the highest importance, not only for survival but as a source of pleasure. It is simply that the suburban fox has discovered that discarded portions of fried chicken are tastier than insects and yield more nutrients relative both to the work done and the risks involved in foraging through the streets at night.

Thus while the behaviour of wild and domestic animals may appear to us to be entirely different, their motivational priorities are essentially similar. In the context of hunger and thirst, they are powerfully motivated both to seek and obtain the rewards of food and water. This involves complex decision making, the expenditure of effort and the assessment of relative risk. Animals, however, subscribe to no puritan work ethic (except when feeding their young). If the reward can be achieved with minimal effort, so much the better. This premise has, I suggest, profound implications for our approach to animal management and I shall return to it more than once. For the moment, let me illustrate only the extremes of the argument. We should not assume that because we define an animal as wild, our sole responsibility is to set it free (animal liberators please note). It may prefer an easier life style. Equally, we should not assume that because we define an animal as domestic, our sole responsibility (in the context of this chapter) is to keep it fed and watered. It may prefer to contribute to its own welfare. McFarland's approach to motivational analysis (Fig. 2.2) implies that animals are best satisfied in an environment where they can work moderately hard for a just reward, thereby avoiding both suffering and limbo.

Hunger for specific nutrients

Since animals eat food primarily for energy to fuel the work of the body, and since all the digestible organic matter in the food they eat can be used as a source of energy, it follows that the sensation of hunger usually reflects a simple need for energy and a non-specific desire for food to meet that need. However, on grounds of commonsense, one would also expect animals to recognize a need for certain specific nutrients like amino acids to meet their targets for growth, or minerals such as sodium, vital to the maintenance of the volume of blood and extracellular fluid. In the first example the animal, lacking amino acids for optimal growth, is hungry because it senses that it is underweight for age. In the second example it experiences both malaise and thirst. The question arises: 'Are they able to select the type of food most appropriate to their needs?' We know that sentient animals have evolved complex foraging strategies to acquire food energy at optimal efficiency and least risk and we know that this information involves learning, by trial and error or observation of parents or peers. It is reasonable, therefore, to assume that animals can learn and communicate the fact that some foods meet their needs for some nutrients better than others. This does not require any profound degree of nutritional wisdom, merely the ability to associate a particular choice of food with feeling better or worse. The sodium-depleted animal that licks salt and then drinks water will feel better almost at once. It is not, therefore, surprising to discover that animals will regulate their salt intake with precision when given the chance. What is impressive is their ability to detect the presence of sodium by smell. Young cattle, in the laboratory, can detect sodium in air at concentrations so low as to be almost beyond the limits of resolution by the most sensitive scientific instruments. In the Rocky Mountains of western Canada, the vegetation tends to be sodium-deficient and natural salt licks are few and far between but when game wardens have moved Rocky Mountain goats into new areas, these animals have been known to scent and move unerringly to natural salt licks from distances of up to 10 kilometres.

Some of the most interesting aspects of current research into appetite and feeding behaviour of animals concern food selection and the ways animals resolve their demands for specific nutrients. Scientists who chose to use the laboratory rat for much of this work did so largely for convenience but they could hardly have selected a more fascinating species. The wild brown rat (*Rattus norvegicus*) has adapted with remarkable success to high-density living in unhygienic environments which give access to a wide range of potential food sources but at a high risk that they might be carrying diseases or poisons laid down by man. In order to survive, the rat has to discover quickly which are nutritious and which are harmful. Wild rats are neophobic, i.e. they approach all new things with extreme caution. If a rat feels any sensation of malaise after consuming food or water from a new source, it will avoid that source in the future, *if it can*. A striking demonstration of this skill comes from an experiment in which laboratory rats were provided with drinkers containing either ordinary (H_2O) or 'heavy' water (D_2O). Within 24 hours, all but one rat had recognized the difference and learnt to avoid the heavy water. One rat who failed to discriminate died 18 days later. The lesson to be drawn from this experiment is not that D_2O is toxic but that the rats spotted it so quickly.

Another admirable feature of wild rats is their ability to communicate the information that a new food source may be dangerous. When a new, slow-acting rat poison was added to an attractive food source such as grain and introduced at a single site within a population of wild rats, a small proportion of the population discovered the bait and sampled it. Within 24 hours, not only were those rats less inclined to eat the poisoned grain but so too were a significant proportion of other rats within a radius of approximately 1.5 km who were experiencing the food source for the first time. The signal had gone out that the food source was dangerous. We do not, of course, need to postulate that the rats went round 'telling each other' that the food was poisonous. Possibly rats that ate the poisoned bait carried the smell of the poison, or some other chemical specific to the food source on their fur or whiskers. They then became ill and transmitted the smell of sickness. Other rats in the vicinity associated the smell of the new food with the smell of sickness and concluded that they should give it a miss (Galef, Mainardi and Valsechhi, 1994).

Two aspects of this study are particularly relevant to the nature of animal mind and animal suffering. First, an animal such as the rat can, without recourse to language, transmit and interpret information which we would consider complex, The received message is, in effect, 'I haven't tried this food but I think it's poisonous'. Second, the rat has demonstrated that it is aware that another member of his species is suffering, or at least, not feeling well. I am not suggesting for a moment that a rat would be moved to compassion by this awareness of suffering in another. It is, however, powerful evidence in favour of the argument that concepts such as mind, awareness and suffering are necessary to the evaluation of consciousness in an animal that behaves as intelligently as a rat.

Much of the science of animal nutrition has been directed towards the development of balanced, compound rations, designed to meet all nutrient requirements, e.g. for growth in the pig or chicken. These rations are then fed to animals in pelleted form with the express intention of preventing selection. In the early years of intensive agriculture, when pigs and chickens were first brought off the land, confined indoors in cages and denied any opportunity to forage for themselves, we saw the emergence of a new series of diseases, associated with deficiencies of specific nutrients, especially trace elements and vitamins. Induced deficiency of Vitamin E, for example, gave rise to previously unrecognized conditions such as 'crazy chick disease' in poultry and 'round heart disease' in pigs. Such 'production diseases' can usually be solved quite quickly by the application of science, *retrospectively*. However, we cannot deny that they arose because the animals were denied the opportunity to select foods for themselves. This suggests that we might learn a lot about the needs of animals for specific nutrients simply by 'asking' them what they want.

The motivational basis of food selection in animals is too complex a topic to discuss here in depth and I should stress at the outset that there are few easy answers. I shall, however, describe two series of experiments which I find particularly fascinating. In the 1970s I was studying the nutrient requirements for growth in animals and wished to distinguish between the energy costs of fat and protein deposition. To this end, I set up a colony of Zucker or 'fatty' rats. This inbred strain carries a single recessive gene which causes obesity. When carriers of the gene are allowed to breed, three out of four rats are normal but one, the homozygous recessive 'fatty' becomes progressively obese from the moment of birth. It was thought initially that these 'fatties' had uncontrolled appetites but it soon became clear that they controlled their appetites very well. John Radcliffe and I formulated a series of diets, offered them *ad libitum* to lean and fatty Zucker rats and measured what happened. The diets included protein at inclusion rates of 300 and 700 g/kg, high and low concentrations of fat (200 and 20 g/kg), and, in two cases, 150 or 300 g/

kg indigestible fibre. Some of these diets are unusual to say the least. They contain all the nutrients neccessary for lean tissue growth but rarely in the correct proportions. Table 3.1 (from Webster, 1993) indicates the rates at which female lean and fatty rats laid down protein and fat during growth from 34 to 66 days of age.

Table 3.1 Gains in protein and fat during growth from 34 to 66 days of age in female lean and 'fatty' Zucker rats offered different diets *ad libitum*.

Diets (g/kg)	Lean rats		Fatty rats	
	Protein	Fat	Protein	Fat
300 protein + 20 fat	25	29	24	135
700 protein + 20 fat	24	20	24	78
300 protein + 200 fat	27	34	25	178
700 protein + 200 fat	25	27	25	135
300 protein + 150 fibre + 20 fat	26	23	26	153
300 protein + 300 fibre + 20 fat	26	22	25	128
Coefficient of variation, %	3	21	4	27

Note at the outset how much more fat was deposited by the fatty rats than by the lean individuals (78 to 178 g as against 20 to 34 g). This simply reflects the fact that the fatties ate far greater quantities of all diets than the lean rats. Note next the far more interesting observation that, despite these large differences in food intake, both lean and fatty rats deposited protein (i.e. grew lean tissue) at exactly the same rates on all diets. The fatties were compelled to eat far more than the lean rats to achieve their targets for lean tissue growth because they were genetically programmed to partition an abnormally large proportion of food energy, including energy from protein, into adipose tissue. Both lean and fatty rats

(1) ate least energy and deposited least fat on the 700 g/kg protein + 20 g/ kg fat diet;
(2) ate most energy and deposited most fat on the 300 g/kg protein + 200 g/ kg fat diet;
(3) increased intake of food (but not intake of metabolizable energy) to sustain lean tissue growth when diets were diluted with indigestible fibre.

What has this to do with hunger and suffering? I argue that it offers powerful evidence that, during the period of rapid growth, the prime force driving metabolic hunger was the demand to grow the vital, lean body mass at a rate programmed by the animal's genes and its physiological state. When rats were offered single, unbalanced diets but allowed to consume them *ad libitum* the amounts of food, and food energy they needed to eat to satisfy their metabolic hunger varied enormously according to the composition of the diet. Furthermore, the rats appeared to be completely unconcerned how fat they got so long as they achieved their programme for lean tissue growth. Although the absolute rate of fat retention in the fatties was over six times greater than that of the lean rats, the coefficient of variation between diets in fat deposition was similar for both groups (21% *v.* 27%).

This presents a pretty paradox. The fatty rats did not get too fat because they overate, they overate because they were too fat. They were born with a genetic fault that partitioned nutrients abnormally between protein and fat. Given this problem, they regulated food intake with the same precision as the lean rats to satisfy their metabolic hunger for nutrients to meet their target for lean tissue growth, which was the same as that for the lean animals. When their food intake was restricted to that of lean rats, their lean tissue growth was stunted although they were still relatively obese. One must assume that on a 'normal' food intake they were abnormally hungry.

Extrapolating this argument to more general circumstances, I argue that we can impair the welfare of an animal or cause it to suffer metabolic hunger in at least three ways:

(1) by offering an insufficient quantity of food (obviously);
(2) by offering an unbalanced diet;
(3) by imposing an abnormal metabolic demand.

In the first example the animal suffers hunger and a progressive deterioration in welfare as its body condition deteriorates. In the second example, the animal may overcome metabolic hunger for a specific nutrient but only by eating abnormally large amounts of food energy and so impairing its long-term welfare. The Zucker 'fatty' provides a good, if obscure, example of an animal that is compelled by the abnormal metabolic demands of its tissues to eat an abnormal ration, grow obese and die young. There are however, more common, and more serious examples of animals compelled by abnormal metabolic demands to overeat to the extent that they compromise their own physical welfare. Heavy strains of broiler chickens have been selected by man, not for balanced growth and development of muscle and skeleton to produce a healthy adult, but simply for rapid growth of lean tissue to the point of slaughter at approximately six weeks of age. This not only creates bone and joint problems associated with birds 'outgrowing their strength' (see Chapters 5 and 8) but the abnormally large nutrient demand of growing muscle generates an intensity of metabolic hunger that the birds cannot satisfy without compromising their welfare.

The second series of experiments that I shall describe in detail deals with the ability of young pigs to recognize the need for specific nutrients to meet their target for lean tissue growth. Kyriazakis and Emmans (1991) initially took early-weaned pigs at 9 kg and fed them low (130g/kg) or high

(280g/kg) protein diets until they reached 16 kg (Table 3.2). At this stage they had no choice of diet but could eat as much as they wanted. On the low-protein diet the pigs ate more food but took longer to reach 16 kg (17 days *v.* 11 days) and were much fatter. Like our Zucker rats in similar circumstances, they were overeating for energy in an attempt to meet their protein requirement.

Table 3.2 Food selection and growth in pigs, first given low or high protein diets to 16 kg bodyweight and allowed free choice of diets thereafter (from Kyriazakis and Emmans, 1991).

	Low protein		High protein	
	Male	Female	Male	Female
Time (days) to grow from:				
16 to 33 kg	12	13	17	18
9 to 33 kg	29	30	28	29
Food selection from 16 to 33 kg				
Food intake (kg/day)	1.26	1.57	1.24	1.39
Protein intake (g/day)	332	319	238	220
Selected protein concentration (g/kg)	263	203	192	158

After reaching 16 kg all pigs were then offered free access to both rations (130 and 280 g/kg protein). The pigs previously restricted to the low protein diet showed extreme compensatory growth and had caught up with those previously fed the high-protein ration at a body weight of 33 kg. The males (in particular) achieved this not by consuming more food but by selecting food of a higher protein concentration. At first they ate almost entirely from the feeder containing the 280 g/kg ration but as their weights and weights-for-age converged with the previously unrestricted pigs so too did their choice of diet. The average protein concentrations selected by the normal and previously stunted males during this period were 192 and 263 g/kg. Females showed similar, but less marked, trends in choice of protein concentration and an increase in food energy intake following the period of growth restriction. Females are physiologically programmed for a higher fat:protein ratio than males so must consume more energy to meet their primary target for lean tissue growth.

Taken together, these two studies suggest that the main source of metabolic hunger in rats and pigs, during growth, is the impetus for protein deposition. Given the opportunity, they may select foods 'wisely' to meet this metabolic need. All this really implies is that they select foods that induce the maximum reward with the least expenditure of effort. If they are unable to control food quality they may be compelled by hunger for a specific nutrient to expend more effort to eat and metabolize non-essential nutrients and this may compromise both their short-term sense of satisfaction and their long-term welfare.

It is tempting but dangerous to get carried away by dramatic experiments such as these. The general picture is far more fuzzy. All we can say for sure is that some animals select some nutrients with extreme precision in some circumstances. Rats and pigs can select foods to meet their needs for protein during growth. Within inbred strains of rat the accuracy of selection may be high and the variation between individuals very small. In other words, all members of the (inbred) population may select a diet almost exactly according to their nutritional needs. However, in experiments with the more genetically diverse pig, the variation between individuals tends to be much greater. Thus, while a population of pigs may select foods according to their average needs, the variation in food intake and therefore in growth rate and body composition may be too great to make a feeding system based on free choice commercially viable.

There are probably many nutrients, for which animals can neither recognize a need (even when in a deficient state) nor identify a source. Although cattle have an exquisite ability to sense and act upon their need for sodium, they have, apparently, no comparable wisdom with regard to magnesium, even though acute magnesium deficiency can be fatal in a matter of hours. This may be because sodium deficiency has always been a problem for grazing animals, whereas magnesium deficiency is a relatively recent condition arising from the intensification of grassland production. If so, there will not have been time for magnesium wisdom to have been favoured by selection.

The laboratory rat, given a standard, balanced diet or a limited choice will eat wisely for growth, maintenance and lactation. However, it too can be seduced into 'bad' eating habits if it is presented with a 'cafeteria' offering a wide choice of attractive foods (chocolates, sweet biscuits etc.). Such rats overeat and get fat. It may be that in rats and most animals there is no metabolic regulator – or a very weak regulator – for fat deposition simply because it was unnecessary in the wild state. However, if rats are to be persuaded to overeat, it is usually necessary to ensure that the cafeteria diet is not only attractive but constantly varied. Rats may overeat cafeteria diets partly because the individual foods are changed so often that they are unable to associate their taste with any subsequent sensations of satisfaction or malaise.

While I think it most unlikely that research on food selection will ever lead us to the stage where we can turn farm or laboratory animals loose in a modest cafeteria and expect them to eat wisely and economically, I do believe that this research can teach us a lot about the nutritional and behavioural needs of animals. At the very least, we owe it to the animals within our dominion to ask them what they want, even if we then decide, paternalistically, what is best.

Thirst

The basic, primitive sensation of thirst must be common to all sentient animals. It is an instinctive response to dehydration, triggered primarily by a rise in the osmotic pressure of the blood. I think it fair to assume that for any animal with sufficient sentience to suffer at all then water deprivation must constitute the most severe source of suffering. The nature of this suffering will include, in all cases, the intense desire to drink water and the malaise consequent upon dehydration. This sense of malaise will involve a progressive sense of weakness and disorientation and, almost certainly, a progressively severe headache (of the 'hangover' type). In higher mammals this desire for water and sense of malaise will be compounded by a sense of anxiety if the animal sees no clear prospect that its thirst will be assuaged.

It is self-evidently cruel, indeed criminal, to deny an animal access to water. It is, however, normal to restrict access to water for many animals, often for good reasons, e.g. to prevent a horse from drinking too much cold water and upsetting its digestion. But there are occasions when the normal ration of water may no longer be sufficient. This can be due to

(1) excessive water loss, through sweating, panting or diarrhoea;
(2) excessive intake of minerals, especially sodium;
(3) unpalatability or fouling of the water supply.

In hot environments, animals attempt to keep cool by the evaporation of moisture from the skin or respiratory tract (sweating and thermal panting, Chapter 4). This inevitably leads to an increase in water requirement. Some of the worst cases of dehydration caused by heat stress are seen when animals are left in vehicles parked in the sun on a hot day, be they chickens in commercial lorries or dogs in family cars. Chronic diarrhoea causes not only severe water loss but also the loss of electrolytes such as sodium. Since sodium is the prime osmotic regulator of the volume of the blood and extracellular fluid, this compounds the problem of dehydration. The sodium-depleted animal may suffer less from thirst than an animal with simple water loss but is at far greater risk of collapse and death from circulatory failure.

Some food and water sources are naturally rich in sodium or have salt added to make them more palatable. The more sodium an animal eats or drinks, the more water it needs to excrete this sodium via the kidneys. Piglets taken from their sow at three weeks of age can be killed by a condition known as salt toxicity. This occurs when they are presented with a dry, slightly salty weaner ration and have not yet learnt properly how to get access to water, usually from a nipple drinker.

While most problems of thirst in wild animals arise from a simple absence of water, many problems in domestic animals arise from the fact that the water source is fouled or otherwise unpalatable. If cattle in yards foul their water bowl with their own faeces, they may not drink for over 24 hours. One might argue ruthlessly that if this is the case then their suffering is not too intense. They will also during this time, restrict their food intake, since thirst overrides hunger, and this is in nobody's interest. Moreover, when the water supply is cleaned up, they are likely both to drink a large quantity of water and eat a large quantity of food. This 'rebound' behaviour not only indicates how much they were missing but can lead to digestive disorders like ruminal bloat.

Among the many enigmatic features of cats is their fastidious approach to drinking water. There are many cats who simply will not drink tap water out of typical water bowls. The same cats will probably drink rain water from puddles or tap water from pottery bowls (often the toilet bowl). Unless overhot, or overworked, the wild cat can obtain much of its water require-ment from the prey it eats (since animals contain over 70% water). The urban, or entirely confined cat, fed canned meat (also containing 70–75% water) is in much the same position. Some such cats when given dry food have been known to restrict their water intake to the point where they compromise their own welfare by inducing kidney damage.

Because the problem of thirst is so obvious, the business of providing water for animals is often taken for granted. I have briefly illustrated just a few of the problems that may be overlooked. The general message must be that anyone with responsibility for the care of animals as individuals or *en masse*, should make sure not only that all their animals have access to sufficient clean, potable water but also that they are all drinking as much as they need.

Oral satisfaction and oral stereotypies

Animals are motivated to eat and to forage for food both by metabolic hunger and by the pleasure they derive from eating. It is quite reasonable to argue that if our responsibility to animals extends only to the avoidance of suffering then we need do no more than provide them with access to all the nutrients essential for maintenance of life, work, growth, pregnancy and lactation. If they can experience the pleasures of successful foraging and the taste of good food, so much the better but this may be considered a luxury rather than a necessity. Ethologists will argue, however, that there is a fundamental difference between satiety and oral satisfaction, as defined at the beginning of this chapter. Many animals confined on farms, in zoos or laboratories, with no opportunity to hunt or forage, are given their daily ration in a form which can be eaten in a matter of minutes. This may satisfy their nutrient requirements but it clearly does not conform with the normal eating behaviour of the animal that fends for itself in the wild. This may well be frustrating, and particularly frustrating if the rest of their experience is so barren that eating becomes almost the sole source of satisfaction. The critical, and as yet unresolved question is 'Can an animal whose nutrient requirements have been met, experience a intensity of frustration, induced by failure to satisfy achieve oral satisfaction, so severe as to cause genuine suffering?'

We are compelled to ask this question by the fact that some animals denied oral satisfaction in barren environments develop forms of stereotypic behaviour, namely unvarying, repetitive behaviour patterns that have no obvious goal or pattern (Lawrence and Rushen, 1993). Stereotypic patterns of behaviour in animals can take many forms (Table 3.3) and arise for a number of reasons. While it is always dangerous to overgeneralize, it is probably fair to say that most 'naturally occurring' stereotypies can be linked to some form of environmental deprivation. This does not, of course, say *why* animals perform them. Individual patterns of stereotypic behaviour may be

(1)   a mechanism for coping with environmental deprivation, (thereby avoiding suffering);
(2)   an outward and visible sign of distress;
(3)   neither of these things, merely a relatively harmless way of passing the time.

Table 3.3 Examples of stereotypic behaviour in animals.

Type	Species
Movement stereotypies	
Weaving	Horses, polar bears
Pacing	Carnivores
Looping	Mink, voles, chipmunks
Rocking	Primates, including man
Oral stereotypies	
Bar chewing	Pigs, cattle
Crib-biting/windsucking	Horses
Tongue rolling, sucking	Cattle, especially veal calves
Thumb-sucking	Primates, including man

The list of stereotypies in Table 3.3 is by no means comprehensive. For fuller details see Lawrence and Rushen (1993). I have distinguished two categories, movement and oral stereotypies. Perhaps the classic movement stereotypy is the compulsive pacing of the caged tiger (often just before feeding time). Similar patterns of behaviour are also seen in smaller wild animals confined well away from the public gaze. Mink, voles and chipmunks in barren cages develop compulsive repetitive patterns of behaviour which include standing somersaults or looping runs up the sides and across the roof of their cages. It is generally assumed that these stereotypies represent a displacement activity induced by frustrated attempts to escape from the barren, confined environment and I shall discuss them in more detail in Chapter 4.

I have included within the movement stereotypies the compulsive rocking behaviour (sometimes accompanied by head-banging) seen in some children who are autistic, emotionally disturbed, or who have been subjected to severe environmental deprivation. A similar pattern of behaviour can develop in young chimpanzees and for much the same reasons. It is the similarity between the repetitive, pointless behaviour patterns seen in confined animals and in clearly disturbed children that gives obvious cause for concern.

The induction and performance of stereotypies may be related to the presence, or absence of stimuli from the external environment but they are also regulated by (and regulate) the internal state, i.e. mood, as outlined in Table 2.1. States of mood such as boredom or arousal, anxiety or excitement can be linked to the chemistry of the brain and modulated by drugs. Some of the movement stereotypies in children and animals can be triggered or exacerbated by psychomotor stimulant drugs like amphetamines. Bar chewing in pigs, a classic oral stereotypy, can be reduced or abolished by naloxone which is a specific antagonist of opiate receptors in the brain. This observation gave rise to the attractive hypothesis that stereotypic behaviour might act as a form of self-narcosis. Since animals are known to release endogenous opiates in response to the stress of pain, it is argued that stereotypies stimulate animals to release opiates in the brain, these opiates reduce the effects of stress, thus stereotypies are a mechanism for reducing the effects of stress.

There are several flaws in this argument. Pain is only one sort of stress and since opiates are painkillers they may be a specific response to pain. Bar chewing in sows (which was inhibited by naloxone) is only one form of stereotypy. The evidence linking stereotypies to the stimulation or inhibition of endogenous opiate systems is scant and inconsistent, the latter presumably because the nature and origins of stereotypies are so diverse. It is however reasonable to argue, less specifically, that animals use stereotypies to affect mood. Moreover, all the activities listed under movement stereotypies in Table 3.3 can be linked to moods influenced by environmental deprivation and so should be a cause for concern.

Oral stereotypies may be another matter. Confinement may or may not cause distress but eating is unequivocally a source of pleasure. I realise that I am setting a trap for myself by lumping all oral stereotypies within a single category but if stereotypies are a mechanism for manipulating mood, then it is equally valid to assume that

(1) animals receiving short, sharp meals are denied oral satisfaction and perform oral stereotypies to reduce stress;
(2) animals receiving short, sharp meals perform oral stereotypies to enhance the pleasure or to aid digestion (or both).

The most studied stereotypies in farm animals are bar-chewing in pregnant sows and tongue rolling or mutual tongue sucking in veal calves. Both animal types are typically confined in individual stalls and both are given food in a concentrated form that can be consumed very rapidly, leaving the animals with nothing much else to do until the next meal. Compulsive bar-chewing develops in some pregnant sows fed a restricted diet to support maintenance and the modest nutrient requirements of pregnancy. If they are given more to eat, a bulkier diet or access to straw they will spend less time bar-chewing, which suggests they are motivated, at least in part, by a combination of hunger and boredom. However, the greatest intensity of bar-chewing usually occurs after, rather than before, the daily meal. One can interpret this by saying that both hunger and desire for oral satisfaction have been aroused but not satisfied by the short, relatively small meal, i.e. the short meal has produced an increased sense of frustration. It is equally possible to argue that the meal was a source of pleasure which the sow has learnt to enhance by a form of postprandial activity in much the same way as we, in a more innocent age, may have smoked a cigar. A more topical and more exact comparison would be chewing gum.

Veal calves typically get two liquid feeds per day. These feeds are consumed very quickly but provide a very large quantity of nutrients. Veal calves given no access to solid food necessary for rumen development undoubtedly lack oral satisfaction and are prone to a number of digestive disturbances. However, they are not hungry for nutrients. Once again, the greatest intensity of oral stereotypies is seen immediately after the meal. These include tongue-rolling, compulsive licking of fixtures and fittings and perhaps, compulsive grooming. The mutual tongue-sucking behaviour of kissing calves after a liquid feed may be too brief to be a true stereotypy. It certainly looks more like a source of pleasure rather than an expression of suffering (Fig. 3.2).

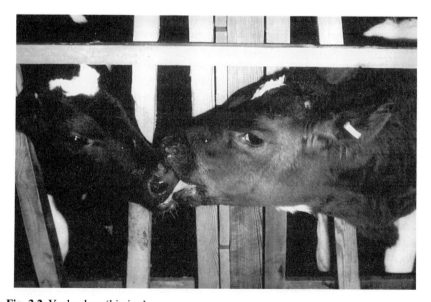

Fig. 3.2 Veal calves 'kissing'.

Whether animals perform oral stereotypies for pleasure or to reduce frustration, we may assume that, initially at least, they derive satisfaction from the activity and would be dissatisfied (in extreme cases to the point of suffering) if the activity was prevented. This is an argument for allowing sows to chew bars to their hearts' content and for grown men to go around sucking their thumbs. The argument fails if a particular stereotypy can be shown to be harmful, or in other words, if a particular form of self-indulgence can be shown to impair welfare in the longer term. This may involve either a direct physical consequence of the behaviour itself or an indirect, longer term deterioration in the mental state of the animal as the stereotypic behaviour becomes progressively dissociated (or 'emancipated') from the original stimulus. I shall consider these possible changes in mental state when I return to the discussion of movement stereotypies in Chapter 4.

Oral stereotypies can be physically harmful. The most compulsive bar-chewers among sows may increase their energy expenditure by 30–40% and will lose condition unless food intake is increased accordingly. Veal calves can spread infection by licking one another or develop hair balls in the rumen by licking themselves. However, these problems arise mainly because the fundamental approach to feeding and housing veal calves is so abnormal. The rearing of calves for white veal in stalls, on diets deficient in iron and totally lacking in fibre abuses each of the five freedoms (see Chapter 9). Within the long catalogue of abuses to veal calves we may include permanent muzzling and even, at one time, tongue amputation to prevent calves from tongue-rolling, tongue-sucking, licking the furniture, or even grooming themselves, This is a particularly extreme example of how man has created problems of health and welfare by imposing unnatural conditions on animals and then 'treated' the problems he has generated by recourse to procedures that cause even greater distress. If the principles enshrined by the five freedoms had been built into animal welfare legislation, the conventional form of white veal production (now banned in the UK but not elsewhere in Europe) would never have got off the ground.

The most common form of oral stereotypy in horses involves crib-biting and windsucking. The crib-biter grasps and gnaws the crib, stable door or other suitable fixtures. This action alone causes severe wear to the incisor teeth. However, it is typically accompanied by windsucking, a practice whereby the horse repeatedly swallows air into the gut. It is generally believed that windsuckers have poor appetites, are prone to digestive disorders like colic and lose condition (see Chapter 10). A number of methods have been devised to prevent windsucking. These include the windsucking collar which is designed to constrict the neck as tightly as possible, except for a loop to allow free passage of air through the trachea (Fig. 3.3). An even more radical approach involves surgery to sever the neck muscles used by the horse to swallow air.

It is easy to condemn the muzzling of veal calves, because there are obviously more humane ways of preventing potentially harmful effects of oral

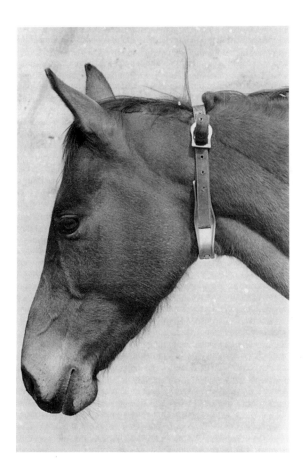

Fig. 3.3 A windsucking collar for horses.

stereotypies. The windsucking horse presents a more difficult problem, mainly because, as yet, it is a problem we do not understand. Crib-biting and windsucking are classically described as 'stable vices' and attributed to lack of oral satisfaction in a species adapted to grazing on the short grasses of the prairies or steppe. However, they are seen (albeit much less frequently) in horses at pasture, even in foals while still feeding from their mothers. We know that windsucking, like other oral stereotypies, tends to be induced by short-sharp meals or even a single peppermint but this does not explain *why* horses do it. We do not know why some windsuckers lose condition. It could be due to reduced food intake, increased energy expenditure, impaired digestion or any combination of these three. Pending some good new research, I really do not know how best to manage the windsucking horse.

This uncertainty carries its own message. The incidence of oral stereotypies such as bar-chewing has been a major element of the welfare case against the confinement of sows in stalls. I am very critical of the sow stall for a variety of reasons which include chronic discomfort, pain and ill-health (see Chapter 8). However, I cannot condemn any system as cruel simply on the grounds that it predisposes to oral stereotypies. I am unconvinced that they are necessarily a sign of stress (or even frustration). If they are, then animal lovers must accept the fact that the problem is at least as great in the idolized horse as in the factory-farmed sow.

4 Housing and Habitat

' 'Tis very warm weather when one's in bed.'

Jonathan Swift

Environmental requirements

The second of the five freedoms, 'freedom from discomfort' can be achieved according to FAWC by 'providing a suitable environment including shelter and a comfortable resting area'. The expression 'a suitable environment' is a somewhat all-embracing term. A geneticist would define it as everything that is not written into the animal's genome, or genetic identity. This chapter will deal, rather more specifically with housing and habitat, namely the immediate physical environment of animals whether in or out of doors and restrict the argument to those features of housing and habitat that are likely to *matter* to the animal. Table 4.1 lists the environmental factors most likely to affect the sense of wellbeing of a sentient animal and thus motivate it to behave in such a way as to achieve 'pleasure' (in the form of comfort, security, etc.) or to avoid suffering.

Table 4.1 Major environmental requirements of animals.

Comfort:	thermal – neither too hot nor too cold
	physical – a suitable resting place
	– space for grooming, limb stretching, exercise
Security:	of food and water supply
	from death or injury due to predation, aggression, floods etc.
	from fear of predation, aggression, etc.
Hygiene:	to avoid the discomfort of squalor and the danger of disease
Education:	to acquire the knowledge necessary to achieve comfort and security during independent, adult life

The environmental requirements listed above range from the primitive physiological need of all homeothermic (and some poikilothermic) animals to control body temperature, to the more subtle needs of higher animals to acquire the education necessary to achieve reasonable comfort and security during independent adult life. Universal physical stresses like heat and cold provoke primitive reflex responses, like sweating or panting in the heat and shivering in the cold, but they also produce conscious decisions to seek the warmth of the sun, for example, or the shade of a tree. Indeed, some animals which we consider to be primitive, like the lizards, have evolved particularly subtle patterns of behaviour to optimize body temperature. In the morning, they move out into the sun to warm up and so improve mobility prior to hunting. At night they cool down to conserve energy. I am neither suggesting nor rejecting the idea that lizards have sufficient sentience to experience suffering and pleasure (I simply don't know). The general point I wish to make is that when a free-living sentient animal experiences a primitive sensation like heat, cold or hunger, it usually puts its mind to the problem. Reflex physiological responses like shivering in the cold, or mobilization of fat reserves during cold and hunger, occur when the animal is unable to, or elects not to resolve the problem by conscious action.

Consider cattle standing in the tropical sun. If shade is close at hand they will seek it. If there is no shade, they cannot regulate body temperature by taking conscious action, so reflex physiological mechanisms are triggered to increase heat loss through evaporation of water by sweating and thermal panting. If there is shade but at a distance, the cattle will make a conscious decision as to the relative discomfort involved in walking to that shade or staying out in the sun until it cools down at night.

To ensure physical comfort an animal needs a suitable site to rest and sleep in any position it fancies, and sufficient space to groom itself and indulge in modest, relaxing exercise, like limb stretching and wing flapping. When the Brambell Committee first reported on the welfare of farm animals in intensive systems, they recommended that minimum housing standards should include sufficient space for the animals to 'stand up, lie down, turn round, groom themselves and stretch their limbs'. As I explained in Chapter 1, I believe that the Brambell Committee's criticism of intensive husbandry systems was based on an inadequate definition of welfare. It would, however, be unreasonable to deny their basic premise that any animal confined by man for his own use should be given, at the very least, sufficient space to achieve these basics for physical comfort. Thirty years after the Brambell report, there has been some, small progress towards meeting these minimum standards for pigs, calves and hens in some countries of Europe but the march of reason is painfully slow.

The motivation to seek personal security is obviously primitive, innate and universal amongst sentient animals. In nearly all species of mammal and bird, the breeding female extends this instinct for survival to protect her offspring until they have grown up and learnt self-sufficiency. This instinct is also primitive and has evolved as the best female strategy for genetic success, particularly in those species which produce small numbers of offspring per year. For males, paternal devotion is only one route to genetic success. In most mammals, male promiscuity has proved to be a better strategy.

All animals, from the lowliest amoeba, take immediate action to avoid harm, and most act in such a way as to reduce risk by seeking or building shelters from predators and foraging for food at times or places of relative safety. Most of these behaviour patterns in most species are automatic, 'hard-wired' within the central nervous system, and can go very wrong if the signals are confused, like the moth that flaps mindlessly into the lamp. In my attempt to restrict discussion of animal welfare to those species which have the capacity to suffer I set myself two almost impossible questions:

(1) At what stage in the evolution of animals did behaviour directed towards security become more than automatic and begin to involve a sense of awareness of relative risk leading to tactical decisions designed to avoid harm and strategic decisions designed to reduce risk?

(2) At what stage in evolution did this sense of awareness begin to involve suffering in the form of (i) fear of imminent danger and (ii) longer-term anxiety?

Let us try to enter the mind of a kitten, newborn to a wise old farmyard cat. She, the mother, has already lost two litters to the farm dog and has elected to give birth, this time, two bales deep into a straw rick. (I knew this cat. The dog, incidentally, was a lurcher.) The kitten is helpless but safe, totally inexperienced but already in possession of the necessary genetic apparatus for an animal that will learn to live by its wits. If it is to succeed it has to become as wise as its mother without getting itself killed in the process. This requires two conflicting motivating forces, curiosity, the motivation to explore the environment and so acquire an education, and anxiety, the motivation to stay out of trouble.

As the young kitten begins to explore, play with its brothers and sisters and practise hunting skills it is powerfully motivated by curiosity and minimally constrained by anxiety. This balance of motivating forces is built into the genetic pattern for development of advanced species whose early life is spent under parental protection. Curiosity, exploration and play not only build survival skills like hunting and foraging, but also provide an education as to what is, or is not, important and/or dangerous. With increasing age comes an increasing sense of fear. This cannot be attributed simply to unpleasant experiences. There is evidence to show that as an animal matures and ages its behaviour in response to a novel stimulus is modulated progressively more by anxiety and less by curiosity. If an animal, as it grows up under the protection of its mother (or owner) can gain experience of most of the things likely to happen to it in adult life, it can educate itself to distinguish between dangers that are real or imaginary (see Chapter 6). Such animals will feel reasonably secure in a familiar environment that they recognize as safe and will not be motivated strongly either by anxiety or curiosity, having mostly 'been there and done that'.

As an animal grows up in a barren environment having learnt nothing of what is and what is not dangerous, it loses its sense of curiosity and becomes progressively more likely to be motivated by anxiety, because it does not know what it should, and what it need not, fear. Pigs, or veal calves in crates in darkened rooms, or rats isolated in cages in a silent laboratory can rest at peace whilst the silence is preserved but may panic at the slightest noise. The UK Codes of Welfare for Farm Animals recommend that all animals should be exposed to 'the sights and sounds of normal farm activity'. This clause has sometimes been mocked as a sentimental luxury, merely the expression of a wish to make life more entertaining for our farm animals. It is far more serious than that; it is essential to prevent the terror that can arise from total ignorance.

Thermal comfort

Birds and mammals are homeotherms who regulate internal body temperature at a level (37°C to 40°C) which is close to the upper limit for survival of body cells and tissues (about 46°C). The warmer the tissue the faster it can work but the greater its need for energy. The evolutionary advantages of increased mobility for both predator and prey outweigh any disadvantage implicit in a high energy demand but commit most homeotherms to work constantly for their living, seeking food. There are some exceptions to this general rule, for example the special strategy of hibernation, which requires not only the ability to reset the body thermostat but also the ability to overwinter in a spot secure from predation since hibernating mammals are usually defenceless.

[A diversion. One of the biggest problems in writing a book which attempts to develop general, relatively simple practical rules to help us to understand animals better and so care for them better, is that there is an exception to almost every rule. I originally finished the above paragraph with the phrase 'hibernating animals are defenceless' then I remembered the hedgehog, then I remembered a Labrador bitch who would pick up hedgehogs, carry them carefully to the Grand Union Canal, drop them in then kill them when they unrolled and began to swim for the bank. It is this need to qualify everything that can make the good scientist worthy but dull. Note that I write 'can make'. I am qualifying this too.]

To achieve homeothermy a bird or mammal must balance the heat it produces in metabolism (H_p) against the heat it loses to the environment, (H_l). The temperature balance equation may be written as follows,

$$H_p \pm H_s = H_l = H_n + H_e$$

H_s = heat storage within the body.
H_n = heat loss by convection, conduction and radiation, often described as sensible or 'Newtonian' heat loss (hence H_n)
H_e = heat loss by evaporation of water from the skin and respiratory tract.

Figure 4.1 illustrates the heat exchanges of a sheep standing in the sun.

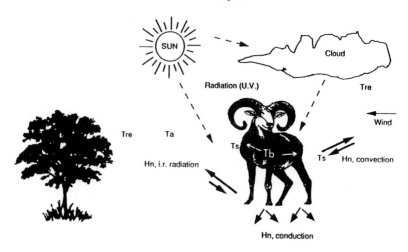

Fig. 4.1 Heat exchanges of a sheep standing in the sun.

Heat is exchanged first by convection between the heat sources in the body at deep body temperature (T_b) and the surface of the skin (whose temperature is T_s), then by convection between skin and air or by conduction between the surface of the body and other surfaces, usually the ground. In most circumstances the skin is warmer than the air or ground and heat is lost, e.g. by convection, at a rate proportional to the temperature gradient between the skin and the air ($T_s - T_a$). (T_a is the temperature of the air.) Increasing air movement (draughts) increases the rate of convective heat loss relative to ($T_s - T_a$). Radiant heat exchanges are more complex. There is exchange of radiant heat within the infra red spectrum between the surface of the animal and other surfaces in the environment (T_{re}), which may be walls, trees or even the sky. Once again this is proportional to temperature gradient, in this case defined by ($T_s^4 - T_{re}^4$). There is also, during the hours of daylight incoming solar radiation whether direct or diffused through cloud, which always constitutes a heat gain.

The sensible heat exchanges of an animal at a given ($T_b - T_a$) are determined by its physical form, in particular the thickness and thermal insulation of its coat of hair or feathers. The shaggy musk ox of the Arctic islands is far more tolerant of the cold than the sleek Brahma cattle of India, and the Arctic fox is more cold tolerant than the whippet. Size is not very important. For a fuller picture of responses and adaptation to heat and cold in animals see Curtis (1983), Wathes and Charles (1994). Sensible heat exchange at a given ($T_s - T_a$) is also affected by features of the environment such as wind and rain both of which reduce the insulation of the coat. Free-living animals can usually act to modify sensible heat exchanges by seeking shelter from wind, rain and sun, by huddling together for warmth or by spreading their limbs to cool down. Housed, closely confined animals may be spared the worst excesses of wind, rain and snow but if they do experience thermal discomfort (e.g. when isolated in a draughty pen or crushed in an overheated lorry) there is little they can do in a physiological sense to regulate sensible heat loss; it is dominated by Newtonian Law, in this case relating H_n to $(T_s - T_a)$.

A particular species of animal may be adapted, largely by virtue of its anatomy, to life in hot or cold climates (i.e to lose more or less heat at a given air temperature) but, in the short term, it has limited physiological ability to prevent H_n from varying with air temperature. If it cannot manage to maintain homeothermy by behavioural means, it must adjust those elements of the heat balance equation which can be regulated physiologically, namely metabolic heat production (H_p) and evaporative heat loss (H_e).

Homeothermic animals may be divided, somewhat arbitrarily, into two categories, those that, in their natural environment, normally regulate heat production to keep body temperature *up* to the set-point on their thermostat and those that normally regulate evaporative heat loss to keep body temperature *down* to the set point. The heat exchanges of these two categories of homeotherms are illustrated in Fig. 4.2 (from Webster 1984). Type I (regulators of H_p), is by far the bigger category since it probably includes all the birds, small mammals (under 5 kg) such as rodents, rabbits etc., and many larger mammals including, certainly, the well-studied pig and, probably, most of the carnivores.

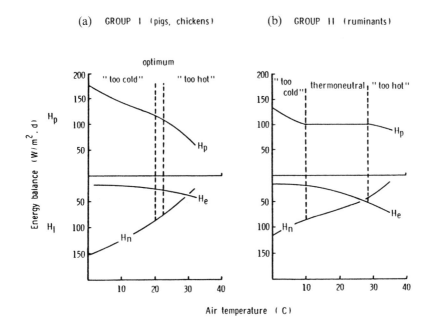

Fig. 4.2 Heat exchanges in Type I and Type II homeotherms.

An animal loses heat by evaporation when water on the surface of the body vaporizes on exposure to air. All animals lose some heat by continuous evaporation of water from the skin surface and from the respiratory tract as they exhale warmed, moistened air. However, they differ greatly in their ability to regulate H_e either by active secretion of sweat or by thermal panting. Type I homeotherms are those with a limited ability to regulate H_e. This means that environmentally induced changes in H_n must be accommodated by physiologically induced changes in H_p, (Fig. 4.2(a)).

Type II homeotherms include man, the higher primates and most of the large grazing animals of the tropical and subtropical savannah and steppe. Man and the horse (to give but two examples) are excellent sweaters. The woolly sheep cannot sweat effectively but has an exquisite mechanism for regulating heat loss by rapid shallow respiration over the turbinate or scroll bones within the nose which act as highly efficient heat exchangers. Cattle and wild deer rely on a combination of sweating and thermal panting. As a result of their ability to regulate H_e over a wide range at negligible metabolic cost, Type II homeotherms (with the notable exception of civilized man) have a wide *thermoneutral zone* wherein their metabolic heat production is independent of air temperature (Fig. 4.2(b)).

The expressions *thermoneutral zone* and *zone of thermal comfort* are often used synonymously and this can create confusion. One of the primary specifications for controlled environment buildings for pigs and poultry (Type I animals) is to regulate air temperature so as to be within their thermoneutral zone. It can be argued that this has been done for welfare reasons although the real reason is to minimize feed costs. The optimal temperature for caged laying hens has been demonstrated, with great precision, to be 21°C. Undeniably, the thermal comfort of the laying hen at 21°C is good but it would be ridiculous to claim that it was any better than that of a well-fed, well-feathered hen strutting in a dry, sheltered barnyard at 10°C. The barnyard hen will produce about 20% more heat than the hen in the battery cage but achieve this by the perfectly comfortable mechanism of eating 30% more food and using it to generate 20% more heat through the normal processes of metabolism. She is not suffering from cold stress, she is simply costing the farmer more money for food. In this example, the expressions *thermoneutral zone* and *zone of thermal comfort* do not have the same meaning. However, if the hen outdoors were exposed to more severe conditions (e.g. freezing temperatures or strong winds) then it would be forced to shiver in order to achieve the increase in H_p necessary to maintain body temperature. The hen would now begin to *suffer* from the stress of cold. If the food intake of the barnyard hen at 10°C were restricted to that of the hen in the battery cage it would be presented with three stresses:

(1)   it would have to shiver to keep warm because it could not produce more heat by eating more food;

(2) it would lose condition because H_p has increased but the metabolizable energy (ME) intake remained the same;

(3) it would become increasingly susceptible to cold as it lost both the energy reserves and insulating properties of body fat.

Expanding the argument from this specific example to general principles of suffering as illustrated by McFarland's multidimensional egg model (Fig. 2.2), we may infer that an animal can accommodate without distress small changes in the intensity of heat or cold, where possible by taking the decision to adjust its microenvironment or its food energy intake. As the intensity of heat or cold are increased the cost of thermoregulation by sweating and shivering increases to the point where the animal approaches, and finally exceeds the threshold of suffering from:

(1) directly unpleasant sensations of heat or cold;

(2) acute hypo- or hyperthermia;

(3) exhaustion of energy reserves following prolonged shivering or inadequate ME intake, exhaustion of water and electrolyte reserves following prolonged sweating or thermal panting.

Several important welfare issues emerge from an inspection of Fig. 4.2. For Type I animals there is no true thermoneutral zone (i.e. in Fig. 4.2(a) the slope of the line relating H_p to T_a is never horizontal). This is a direct consequence of their limited ability to regulate H_e. In moderately cold environments Type I animals can maintain comfort and welfare by eating more (given the chance). In hot environments they must eat less in order to reduce H_p. This may be incompatible with welfare and there is a basal level below which H_p cannot fall if life is to be sustained. Because of their limited ability to regulate H_e, Type I animals tend to be more susceptible than Type II to both heat and cold stress.

This creates an important welfare paradox. Much of the criticism of 'factory farming' has been directed at systems of intensive housing for pigs and chickens. One of the great incentives for this development was the fact that savings on food costs achieved by confining pigs and chickens in temperature-controlled buildings outweighed the capital costs of the buildings, especially when capital grants for buildings were more generous than subsidies on animal feeds (see Chapter 8). The optimal air temperature for intensive pig and chickens is not necessarily the air temperature that the animal would choose for itself, particularly if it had a generous supply of food, but a temperature close to the upper limit of the zone of thermal comfort, i.e. one that it senses as warm. Most of these buildings are well insulated and rely on the large amount of heat produced by densely-stocked animals to maintain a warm temperature within the house over the 'normal' range of environmental conditions experienced out of doors. If it gets exceptionally cold outside, it is easy to turn on supplementary heaters. However, most intensive pig and poultry houses in the UK are not designed to cope with exceptionally hot days in mid summer. Thus the animals whom we house at great expense to keep them out of the cold are those we are most likely to kill from heat stress, by stocking them too densely in circumstances where they cannot dissipate the heat they produce in metabolism.

The problem of heat stress is particularly acute when Type I animals like pigs and poultry are packed densely into vehicles for transportation. Five thousand broiler chicken in a poultry vehicle produce heat at a rate of about 75 kilowatts (the equivalent of 25 3 kW convector heaters). Most poultry vehicles are not fan-ventilated and rely largely on air movement as the vehicle is in motion to dissipate this enormous amount of heat. When the vehicle is stationary, air temperature in the immediate vicinity of the birds is usually more than 10°C higher than that outside the vehicle. Transportation can (although need not) stress animals in a variety of ways that I shall consider in Chapters 8 and 9. At this stage, I would simply suggest that more animals found dead on arrival at their destination are killed by heat stress than die from any other cause.

Adaptation and acclimatization to heat and cold

The welfare of any animal is determined by its ability to adapt to its environment and to environmental change without suffering. The adaptation of animals to heat and cold has been studied more comprehensively than any other aspect of environmental physiology, partly because of its innate importance but also because it offers an attractive approach to the study of stress in general. Stresses of heat and cold are definable, measurable and can be administered repeatedly without causing lasting harm. The clear message that emerges from this work is that animals are amazingly adaptable creatures. Most textbooks and Codes of Welfare for farm and laboratory animals tend, however, to ignore this capacity to adapt and define optimal thermal environments in very precise terms based on measurements made in the laboratory. For example, the UK Home Office requires that rats kept for scientific procedures be housed at an air temperature between 20–25°C. Wild nocturnal rats in the UK will seldom, if ever, experience air temperatures as high as 25°C. Anyone who wished to expose a laboratory rat to the thermal conditions naturally experienced by wild rats would need to justify his action to the Home Office on grounds of scientific necessity or run the risk of prosecution for causing unnecessary suffering.

Now the anatomy and physics of heat exchange in wild and laboratory rats are very similar. Does the wild rat suffer constantly from cold stress or is the laboratory rat unnecessarily pampered? I suggest that the answer to both questions is no. Both classes of animals have adapted successfully to the environments to which they are habitually exposed. To explain this further, I need to clarify my definition of adaptation according to the conventions of

environmental physiologists who make precise distinctions between the
words *adaptation, acclimatization* and *habituation.*

- *Adaptation* describes anatomical, physiological and behavioural changes
  that have evolved over several generations within a species, or population within a species that make it better fitted for life in a particular
  habitat.
- *Acclimatization* describes anatomical, physiological or behavioural
  changes that occur within an individual that make it better fitted for life
  in a particular habitat.
- *Habituation* describes a gradual loss of conscious perception of, or
  behavioural response to a repeated stimulus that permits the animal to
  disregard stimuli that it discovers to be irrelevant.

Adaptation or acclimatization to heat is inherently more difficult than
adaptation or acclimatization to cold since it is easier to elevate heat production, especially when there is no shortage of food, than it is to reduce
heat production below the level associated with metabolic processes essential for the maintenance of life. Most homeotherms (Type I animals) have
evolved in circumstances where heat stress either was not a threat to the
survival of the species, or was a problem they could resolve by taking constructive action. There are relatively few places in the world where animals
are compelled to expose themselves to air temperatures in excess of 40°C.
When these conditions do occur during the day, most small, free-living
birds and animals can reduce heat load by seeking the shelter of a nest or
underground burrow, by wallowing in mud or, at least, getting out of the
sun. In these circumstances there has been little selection pressure to
increase evaporative heat loss by sweating or thermal panting. These
animals can also seek shelter in nests, burrows, etc. from the chilling
effects of cold air, wind, rain and snow.

In those Type I species that have adapted to survival in environments
where winter air temperatures may be 40°C or more below body temperature, there has also been strong selection pressure for physiological adaptation to cold. This involves not only an enhanced ability to increase heat
production on demand but also an enhanced ability to regulate blood flow
through the superficial tissues of the body, to conserve heat where possible, but also, in conditions of extreme cold, to increase the convection of
heat to extremities, to preserve comfort and prevent tissue damage. Arctic
birds standing on the ice are doing something that would not only cause
us great pain but actually destroy our feet with frostbite. Such birds may
be uncomfortable, although they do not give that impression. They are
certainly not freezing their feet.

Type II animals (Fig. 4.2(b)) are those that have evolved a substantial
capacity to regulate heat loss by evaporation of sweat or from the respiratory
tract. Most species within this category are the ruminants and equidae, the
large grazing mammals of sunny, exposed grasslands such as the tropical

savannah. Cattle and deer, horses and zebras have a limited ability to shelter from heat, especially the heat of the sun. (They don't build nests!) Their survival depended therefore on enhancing their ability to regulate evaporative heat loss and so dissipate heat produced as an inevitable consequence of metabolism even in circumstances when the net flow of sensible heat (H_n) is into, rather than out of the body. An increased ability to dissipate heat by evaporation makes it possible to increase insulation against H_n without incurring heat stress and so increase tolerance to cold. Ruminants and horses are therefore better adapted, in a physiological sense, to both heat and cold stress than Type I animals like the pig and chicken. One can argue that this physiological adaptation is a less comfortable (or more stressful) solution to the problems of heat and cold than behavioural adaptation and has arisen only because the size of Type II animals and their habitat made a behavioural solution impossible. It is, however, to their advantage in circumstances where man has removed the possibility of behavioural thermoregulation. Sheep and cattle can tolerate conditions of heat and cold during transportation that would kill a pig or chicken. In this example, their greater capacity to survive is, of course, a dubious advantage, since it means that the unscrupulous haulier can submit them to appalling conditions during transportation and still get paid for delivery of a live animal.

The ability to regulate evaporative heat loss by thermal panting, which is seen to greatest effect in the ruminants, carries a further advantage. Cooled venous blood leaving the heat exchangers in the turbinate bones of the nose passes through another vascular heat exchanger, the carotid rete, where it directly and specifically cools the arterial blood supply to the brain. When a wildebeest is chased by a lion on a hot day, the energy expended by both animals causes their average body temperature to rise sharply. However, the wildebeest, unlike the lion, is able to maintain a cool head, since only it possesses the carotid rete mechanism that specifically cools the blood supply to the brain. Watchers of wildlife spectaculars are aware that big cats that fail to catch their prey quickly give up, for a number of very sensible reasons which include the problem of brain hyperthermia. The ability of ruminants to run for longer distances than the carnivore on the hot open plains has not only contributed to their survival, it must also have contributed to their sense of security.

It is tempting to spend more time on the fascinating physiological mechanisms that animals have evolved in response to different environmental pressures. I must, however, use them only as illustrations to the main theme of this section of the book 'How is it for them?' – exploring the things which matter to an animal because they are interpreted as a source of pleasure or suffering. As scientists we try to interpret subjective experiences in animals in an objective way (e.g. by measuring the value they put on a particular pattern of behaviour). It is impossible, however, to ignore our own subjective human experience, particularly when the sensations are something we think we all understand, like heat and cold. In fact, our perception of heat and cold is very far removed from that of the other animals for reasons that can be attributed to adaptation, acclimatization and habituation.

Man is a Type II animal, a good sweater and, like the ruminants, very well adapted to work in the heat. This will have carried some evolutionary advantage, although it should not be overemphasized, since it does not begin to compare with the benefits of increasing wisdom. However, civilized man, unlike other Type II animals, has become uniquely intolerant of cold. At first sight, we might attribute this to absence of body hair. However, pigs, and whales and (especially) white men resolve this deficiency by laying down insulation inside the skin in the form of body fat. This, of course, takes time and energy. Marine mammals and birds like seals and penguins give birth on land to offspring which are protected from cold at birth by external insulation in the form of fur or down-feathers. As they feed and grow, they lose their coats and lay down fat which is, of course, a much more effective form of insulation in the water.

Man's loss of cold tolerance has largely been a matter of culture. He discovered early on that sitting before a fire with a fur coat round his shoulders amounted to much more than a simple absence of suffering, it was a positive delight. Today we design our houses and adjust our clothing to ensure that we are comfortably warm (unless presented by a conflict of motivation, such as the wish to appear sexually attractive). Moreover we derive sensual pleasure from exposure to radiant heat. The European lies in the sun not just to tan but also because it feels good. I believe we can extrapolate these sensations of thermal pleasure to animals. The cat that lies over a radiator or dog that creeps ever closer to the fire are exposing themselves, for a while, to much more heat than they actually need for the sheer pleasure of the experience. Eventually they decide they are too hot and slope off to cool down. Being warm, but not too warm, feels good. We should therefore assume that while the barnyard hen may be perfectly comfortable at 10°C, she would experience pleasure if she could expose herself to 21°C (the optimal temperature for caged hens) at least some of the time. Pigs that have been trained to provide themselves with supplementary warmth by pressing buttons to switch on infra red heaters, will work during the daytime to achieve a degree of warmth that gives them sensual pleasure. At night, they are less inclined to work for heat. This change in behaviour can be attributed in part, and obviously, to the fact that they are more inclined to sleep than press buttons. There does, however, appear to be a real shift in their thermal preference such that they actively prefer a cooler environment at night time (see Curtis, 1983). This is an elegant example of one of my central themes, namely that we who are responsible for animal husbandry could often make life more comfortable for our animals *and* save ourselves money by first asking animals what they want and then providing them with a habitat that allows them to express their preferences in a constructive way.

We must accept, however, that civilized man and the laboratory rat, have become soft; we have acclimatized to the sensual pleasures of warmth and failed to habituate ourselves to cold. Less than 100 years ago, aboriginal man, North America Indians, Australian aborigines and, most spectacularly, the Alalacuf Indians of Tierra del Fuego routinely exposed themselves near naked to environmental conditions that would kill the average, heat-acclimatized European within hours. The survival of these individuals involved a large degree of habituation, in the form of a decreased awareness of the sensation of cold in the skin. This enabled them to reduce blood flow to the skin and thus conserve energy in what may be called a *stoic* form of acclimatization. They were, however, very fond of fires, hence Tierra del Fuego. The Eskimo adapted to cold in a much more cultural fashion, partly by eating huge amounts of food energy in the form of fat, but also by designing highly effective forms of clothing. Thus the Eskimo kept his body comfortably warm. He did, however, retain a form of acclimatization to cold which urban man has lost (but could regain since I am referring to accli-matization rather than adaptation). The Eskimo can stand for hours over a hole in the ice holding a fishing line in his bare hands. This requires an enormous increase in blood supply to the fingers, which urban man could not achieve – his hands would be frostbitten in minutes. This form of adaptation to cold may be called *hedonic*. The well-fed, well-clothed Eskimo is not faced by a problem of energy conservation so can afford to turn on his internal convector heaters in order to preserve the comfortable sensation of warmth even in the most severe cold. This is an example of acclimatization rather than habituation. Both the stoic (habituation) and hedonic (acclimatization) responses to cold can be said to improve welfare and avoid suffering. Only the hedonic response could be thought of as comfortable.

This diversion into adaptation to cold in primitive man is intended to discourage two opposing fallacies in our discussion of the environmental needs of animals. On the one hand, we should not assume that the so-called optimal temperatures for farmed or laboratory animals (21°C for the hen, 20–25°C for the laboratory rat) are essential for their welfare. On the other hand we should not assume that animals will necessarily be 'happier' in natural conditions out of doors. Much of the impetus to our own domes-tication has been the desire to improve our thermal comfort and seek thermal pleasure. We have plenty of evidence to suggest that other animals feel much the same.

Comfort, hygiene and security at rest

All sentient animals need, from time to time, to rest and sleep in peace. To achieve this, they need an area which is comfortable, hygienic and secure. The relative importance of these criteria differ according to the design and age of the animal. Table 4.2 selects a range of animals over whom we exercise particularly strong dominion and assesses their needs according to the fol-

Table 4.2 The relative importance of the different criteria that define a suitable resting area for different animals.

	Dryness	Hygiene	'Give'	Warmth	Security from assault	
					deliberate	accidental
Poultry, broilers	***	*	0/*	*	0	0
Poultry, layers	**	*	0	0	**	0
Birds of prey	**	*	0	0	?	0
Pigs, weaners	**	**	*	**	*	*
Pigs, dry sows	**	*	**	**	***	0
Cattle, young calves	***	**	*	**	0	*
Cattle, dairy cows	**	**	**	0	0	**
Small rodents	***	**	0	*	*	0
Rabbits	**	**	*	*	*	0
Dogs	***	**	*	*	*	0
Horses	**	**	*	0	*	*
Neonates, general	***	***	*/0	***	***	**

lowing properties of the resting area: dryness, hygiene, warmth, 'give' (or cushioning ability) and security.

Most free-living birds perch and sleep in branches, which are dry, good for the feet and offer some security against nocturnal predators on the ground. They do not require features which we would consider essential in a good bed, such as warmth and the 'give' of a cushion or mattress because they are well insulated and very light-weight. When rearing young, they build nests, first to insulate their eggs during incubation, and then to provide security for their offspring until they are fully mobile. Broiler chickens, grown rapidly for slaughter at about six weeks of age, are usually kept on a deep litter of wood shavings which absorbs and is slowly digested by their droppings. When managed properly, this creates a warm, dry bed with some 'give'. Since heavy strains of broilers, in the last days of their short lives, do suffer from pain in their legs and spend a lot of time lying down, they probably appreciate this slight cushioning effect. If the litter is properly dry, the birds will breathe very dusty air; if the litter is damp the heavy birds are more prone to 'hock burn', chronic inflammation or ulceration of the skin of the legs.

Note that, in the above paragraph, I avoid making any definitive statement as to whether I consider deep litter to be good or bad. This may appear as an example of the sort of liberal indecision that infuriates the most ardent (i.e. least cool) advocates of animal welfare. Table 4.3 illustrates, however, that it is an inevitable consequence of applying the logic of the 'five freedoms' to the analysis of the welfare of any animal in any environment.

Table 4.3 Welfare aspects of deep-litter housing for broiler chickens.

Five Freedoms (Nos. 2–5)	Subdivisions	Quality
2. Comfort	Thermal	Good warmth from bedding
	Physical	Some cushion for painful limbs
3. Pain and disease	Surface hygiene	Normally good, risk of hock burn
	Air hygiene	Very dusty
4. Normal behaviour	Space	Very confined in final weeks
	Enrichment	Some dust-bathing, foraging
5. Security	Deliberate assault	Very low risk
	Accidental assault	Very low risk

In this table, I have assumed that the birds enjoy the first freedom, from hunger and thirst. I have subdivided freedoms 2 to 5 (and these are not necessarily the only important subdivisions) and then assessed the quality of deep-litter systems according to these subdivisions. Assuming the litter itself is of good, dry quality, it is comfortably warm and provides some cushioning for painful limbs. The litter is, of course, teeming with microorganisms but these will be harmless unless a pathogenic organism is introduced into the building. The air above the litter is very dusty, and much of this dust consists of bacteria and fungal spores. This may contribute to cardiorespiratory problems in broiler birds (such as ascites). During the first four weeks of life the birds have reasonable space but latterly they do not have the space to spread their limbs or flap their wings in reasonable comfort. The litter does provide a degree of environmental enrichment. The birds can 'dust bathe' after a fashion, although they are known to prefer dust to wood shavings and they can forage, rather unfruitfully, in the litter. The broiler house itself confers, of course, excellent security from foxes and other predators. Within the house, the deep litter does not contribute in any direct way to the security of the birds. However, broiler birds at this size and age do not present an significant threat to each other's welfare, whether by accident or deliberate assault.

Adult hens are another matter. Traditionally they were allowed to roost at night on perches, which allowed the birds to sleep in comfort and security, and their droppings to fall 'hygienically' to the ground or into a pit. The battery cage is as hygienic as a perch, or better, since the droppings fall through the wire floor. The cage floor is, at best, less comfortable to the feet than a perch and can, at worst, cause severe injury (some floors are worse than others). The adult hen is not, however, secure from its neighbours. Adult hens, for complex reasons we do not fully understand, develop the habit of feather pecking which can, in its most extreme form, lead to cannibalism. The problem is greater when birds are kept in large colonies, whether in barns or on free range, than when they are confined in groups of four or five in a battery cage. It is therefore usually necessary to trim the beaks of free-range but not battery hens to prevent cannibalism. However, beak-trimming can cause chronic pain (see Chapter 5). Once again, the proper analysis of the components of alternative husbandry systems reveals that there are few easy answers.

To return to Table 4.2. The most important properties of a resting area for young, early-weaned pigs are dryness, warmth and good hygiene. If the adult sow is to be comfortable she needs a warm bed with 'give.' Sows compelled to lie on concrete under most British conditions can suffer from excess heat loss (by conduction through the concrete) and chronic physical discomfort leading in some cases to chronic injury especially around the bony joints of the knees and hocks. These injuries can become infected. A chronically uncomfortable sow may adopt an unnatural 'dog-sitting' position, with her vulva on the soiled concrete, thereby exposing herself to the risk of an ascending infection of the urinary tract. I can think of absolutely nothing good to say about housing sows on concrete. The individual stall does, however, secure the sow from attack. Sows can be aggressive creatures and when they fight they can hurt, vulva-biting being a particularly unpleasant example of the damage they cause to each other.

Young calves need warmth, a well cushioned bed, and especially, good hygiene, since they are very vulnerable to, and cannot be isolated from, pathogenic bacteria. For adult dairy cows the two most important properties of a good bed are good hygiene and an excellent mattress. They seldom get both. Good hygiene is necessary to reduce the risk of microrganisms entering the teat canal and causing environmental mastitis. There has, until recently, been little incentive to provide dairy cows with a mattress because it confers no obvious economic advantage. However, when asked, cows show an overwhelming preference for beds which have the 'give' of a mattress, which is hardly surprising, given their weight and the design of their limbs. In the UK most dairy cows are housed over winter in individual cubicles. A few enjoy the luxury of a well-bedded, dry straw yard. Some endure the squalor of a poorly strawed, wet bed of muck. All cow cubicles offer good security against deliberate assaults from other cows. When cows are dehorned, bullying causes little direct harm but can unnerve a submissive cow to the extent that she is reluctant to lie down, becomes overtired, loses condition, lowers her milk yield and possibly damages her feet. A well-designed cubicle also protects cows from accidental damage – usually and most painfully caused by having another cow trample on one of her teats.

The other examples in Table 4.2 should, by now, be self-explanatory and you should be able to apply the principles to any animal of your choice. I would point out finally that all properties that may define a satisfactory resting area are essential to the newborn animal (with the possible exception of 'give'). Security is of paramount importance. In many animals this security is provided by the presence of the parents. Alternatively, parents may hide their offspring and stay at a discrete distance except at feeding time. The most extreme example (to my knowledge) of this 'hiding' strategy is the rabbit, who normally returns to her new-born offspring only once daily to suckle them for less than five minutes. Those that fail to find a teat during any feeding period in the first two weeks of life are probably doomed, but the majority of the litter will probably survive, and rabbits can afford to lose a few anyway.

The need for space

The need of animals (particularly farm animals) for space has attracted more debate than any other single issue in animal welfare. This is because it presents perhaps the most clear-cut example of the conflict of interest between economic forces and our moral obligation to provide a reasonable standard of living for the animals in our charge. Once an egg producer discovered that he could legally make more money by cramming five hens into a battery cage originally designed for four, other producers had to follow suit or go out of business. Politicians, on the other hand, wishing to be seen to be doing something in response to public pressure to improve welfare standards for farm animals, have clutched at minimal space requirements as a form of legislation that they could both define and enforce. The producer with a quarter of a million birds stocked at five per cage when four is the legal limit can hardly hide 50 000 birds when the inspector appears unannounced. However, the process of transferring the modest proposal of the Brambell Committee (1965) that farm animals in intensive systems should be given sufficient space to 'stand up, lie down, turn round, groom themselves and stretch their limbs', into effective legislation has been painfully slow. European legislation for the 'protection' of laying hens has been particularly cynical. When (typically English) brown hens are caged in groups of four or more, there is now a legal requirement that each bird be given 450 cm^2 of shared floor space. This law is a sham; a law that serves only to protect producers currently operating at the physical limits of stocking density. The area of the two pages of this book open in front of you is 690 cm^2. Current European law states that the welfare of caged hens will be 'protected' if they are provided with an amount of shared space equivalent to two-thirds of the area of this open book for the whole of their adult lives.

   In Part III, 'What we can do for them' I shall consider the scope and limitations of legislation as a route to improving animal welfare. However, in Part II, 'How is it for them?' I am still asking questions, rather than attempting to provide answers. More precisely, I am attempting to resolve complex, emotional issues of animal welfare into a series of discrete questions that can have an answer. Restricting the argument therefore to the need for space *per se* without reference to the quality of that space the questions become:

(1) How much space does an animal require to adopt the postures and perform the exercises necessary for physical comfort?
(2) How much space does an animal require for security from deliberate or accidental assault, or the threat of such assault?
(3) How much space does an animal actually want?
(4) What are the physical and psychological consequences of denying animals access to the space they need?

These questions have been mostly addressed to the laying hen and the laboratory rat. The hen performs a number of activities that can be called 'comfort behaviours'. These include grooming, stretching the limbs and neck, tail wagging and wing flapping. Given 450 cm^2 per head of shared space in a cage, hens cannot possibly flap their wings and have difficulty performing any of these actions. If all birds were motivated to flap their wings simultaneously, they would each need approximately 2000 cm^2 free space. All other activities can be performed within an area of approximately 1400 cm^2. The UK Farm Animal Welfare Council (FAWC) has recommended this as the minimal space allowance for laying hens in colony systems, on the basis that birds wishing to flap their wings can operate on the time-share principle. This is, of course, three times the legal minimum for birds in cages, which exposes FAWC to the double criticism of double standards and sloppy logic, since there is inherently more space available to a bird in a colony of 400 than in a cage of four when average stocking density is the same.

The space needed by an animal to achieve reasonable freedom from attack, or fear of assault depends, of course, on the perception and reality of the threat. A wildebeest cow needs, perhaps, a clear run of a mile to escape the lion. If she found herself within a confined area of the bush without an escape route she would be justifiably anxious. Adapted to life in a zoo, or game park, out of sight and smell of the lion, she would, no doubt, feel secure in a paddock that allowed her to escape the unwelcome attentions of other members of her own species, or at least ritualize these aggressive encounters in such a way that neither party got seriously hurt. The same principles apply to animals such as hens, pigs and rats, densely confined in cages for commercial use by man. In this case, the threat to security is entirely from conspecifics. Hens, pigs and rats, like most other animals, use aggression to establish a dominance hierarchy within social groups and, of course, to protect their own offspring. They have also evolved behavioural mechanisms for escaping or avoiding aggression, by getting out of the way or by a suitable display of submission. Although antagonistic behaviour such as fighting, or apparently mindless behaviour such as feather-pecking are largely instinctive in origin, the consequences of such behaviour, i.e. fear and pain, can be a real source of conscious suffering. Even when we confine a single species in isolation we can only define their need for space, in terms of freedom from pain or fear, by reference to their behaviour and mood; i.e the innate behaviour, aggression and fears of that species in a 'natural' environment and the way these things appear to have been modulated by the physical and social conditions they experience in environments created by man.

Once again, the analysis expands in geometric fashion. In addressing a single element of housing design for a rat, hen or pig, namely 'The need for space, subsection 2, the need for security' I introduce a whole raft of new questions. For example, what are the effects of stocking density and population size on:

(1) the incidence of antagonistic encounters between individuals?
(2) the nature of antagonistic encounters; do they lead to withdrawal, ritual submissive behaviour or fights?
(3) the establishment of a stable or unstable dominance hierarchy?
(4) deaths and injury directly attributable to fighting?
(5) physiological indices of fear and anxiety, e.g. increased adrenal activity, chronic differences in body condition, fertility, and/or life expectancy?

The third question in the first-stage analysis of the need for space – 'How much space does an animal want?' – can be addressed by measuring strength of motivation as described in Chapter 2. Hens have been shown to work for space up to an area of approximately 900 cm^2. This is less than the space they require for unimpeded performance of all comfort behaviours, which suggests that they are prepared to compromise. The final question, 'What are the physical and psychological consequences of denying animals access to the space they need?' is extremely complex and dangerously open to misinterpretation. It is, for example, relatively easy to relate poor growth or increased mortality in animals to overcrowding. Two good examples are laboratory rats and farmed salmon. Rats have been shown to develop classic stress-induced hyperactivity of the adrenal cortex leading in some cases to adrenal exhaustion and death, which can be attributed to the psychological effects of overcrowding *per se*. Overcrowding causes problems of erratic growth and increased mortality for farmed salmon, and some of these problems may be psychological. However, it is necessary for the welfare of the fish and their owners to establish a more precise diagnosis that also considers secondary effects of overcrowding such as abnormal competition for food, bacterial infections or infestation with external parasites.

One possible consequence of denying animals the space to do the things they need to do is that they may be even more highly motivated to do it when they get the chance. Christine Nicol has studied this 'rebound' behaviour in hens (see her chapter in Charles and Wathes, 1994). She maintained a group of hens in the same room but confined in individual cages with 800 cm^2 floor space. At four-week intervals these hens were given extra space (1600 cm^2) and spent more time than previously unconfined hens in activities such as tail-wagging and wing-flapping which had previously been difficult or impossible. This rebound behaviour suggests, unsurprisingly, that hens have an innate motivation to perform these activities. However, she also observed that most hens showed a progressive increase in the amount of rebound behaviour after successive periods of confinement up to about 16 weeks. Thereafter two subgroups tended to emerge, one that continued to show more activity when space was available and the other which abandoned this practice. Single experiments should be interpreted with caution but this one does suggest that the hens did not, in the first 16 weeks habituate to an environment that denied them the opportunity to perform comfort behaviour. If rebound behaviour is an expression of frustration, their frustration appeared to increase with time. After 16 weeks, some birds still gave vent to their frustration while others gave up, or developed 'learned helplessness'.

Everything about this elegant experiment suggests that hens have an absolute behavioural need for space *per se*. The legislator is then entitled to ask 'How much?' This creates a major dilemma for the scientist who studies animal welfare for a living. On the one hand, it is simply not possible to say that hens 'need' 450, or 900, or 1440 or 2000 cm^2 of floor space (the above discussion could be used to justify any of these figures), since each recommendation is based on a different definition of need. On the other hand, scientists studying animal welfare for a living must not allow their perennial cry for 'further research in this area' to be used by governments as an excuse for doing nothing. I shall not attempt to answer this question here. However, I shall not dodge the issue. I believe that attempts to address our moral obligation to ensure animal welfare in terms of minimal space requirements have been grossly oversimplistic. These are important questions but they do not, on their own, form an adequate basis for legislation. I shall develop this argument in Part II.

The problem of barren environments

Consider the lot of two very different mammals placed in rather similar circumstances – the mouse in a cage in a laboratory and the tiger in a cage in a zoo. An honourable attempt has been made to manage each animal according to the principles of the five freedoms. Both have been given sufficient food and water. Both have a suitable, warm, dry bed and sufficient space to groom and stretch their limbs. Both are free from injury or disease and neither is faced by any tangible source of fear or stress. The mouse is alone in its cage but within the reassuring sight and smell of other mice. The tiger is also alone in its cage although it can see carnivores in other cages. It is also known to be a solitary animal.

These are clearly barren environments that permit the tiger and mouse to do little more than go through the motions essential to continued existence, such as eating and sleeping. Now many will claim that it is simply not 'right' to keep a tiger in a barren cage. Fewer, perhaps, will champion the rights of brother mouse. The devil's advocate will say 'What harm is done by caging mouse or tiger?' Both are far from the region of purgatory or suffering at or beyond the limits of MacFarland's welfare egg. (Fig. 2.2). Both may be in limbo, but is this a source of suffering? This question is , once again, too big to be swallowed whole:

(1)   What (if anything) does the caged animal consciously need but cannot get (e.g. a sense of security, social contact, the pleasure of food or sex, the need to explore, or simply the need to escape boredom)?
(2)   How hard are the mouse or tiger prepared to work to satisfy these needs, i.e. how much do they matter?
(3)   Will the denial of any of these specific needs or simply the constant boredom become a source of suffering or will the animals learn to cope?
(4)   What evidence can we obtain to address these questions?

Locomotor stereotypies
Most of the evidence used in support of the case that animals do suffer in barren environments is based on observations of stereotypic behaviour (Table 3.3). Everyone who has visited an old-fashioned zoo will have seen the big cats compulsively pacing back and forth behind the bars of their cages. This is a classic locomotor stereotypy. Laboratory mice do not typically develop locomotor stereotypies. However, wild rodents such as the bank vole (*Clethrionomys glareolus*) tend to develop compulsive patterns of jumping or looping behaviour if isolated and confined in the standard type of cage for the laboratory mouse. In the case of big cat and small vole, this stereotypy has been interpreted as a redirection of behaviour originally designed to escape the confines of the cage into 'purposeless' activity. This is a logical guess, although difficult to prove. Weaving in stabled horses has been attributed to boredom and lack of social contact in a naturally gregarious herd animal. Primates, such as chimpanzees and children, develop rocking stereotypies when reared in barren environments without maternal care. Rocking and other stereotypies are also seen in humans with severe psychological disorders such as autism and schizophrenia. If stereotypic behaviour is a sign of mental distress or mental disorder in man we are right to feel concern when we observe similar behaviour in animals.

Interpretation of the causes and functions of stereotypic behaviour in man and animals is a lively area of research, abounding in hypotheses and counterhypotheses (Lawrence and Rushen, 1993). I shall attempt to simplify the arguments, secure in the knowledge that you cannot satisfy all of the scientists all of the time. The first, non-contentious point is that one cannot ascribe all stereotypies to the same cause, even when the cause is defined extremely loosely by a term such as 'distress'. In Table 3.3, I distinguished between locomotor and oral stereotypies and suggested cautiously that since oral stereotypies are directly linked to eating (a positive source of pleasure) they could be either a way of reducing suffering associated with lack of oral satisfaction or a way of increasing or sustaining the pleasure to be gained from a quick meal. Locomotor stereotypies may peak when a caged animal is anticipating its daily meal, this being a time of high arousal, but they are primarily associated with confinement and barren environments. While confinement in a barren cage may offer some comfort and security it cannot, by any stretch of the imagination, be ranked with food as a positive source of pleasure. Thus the locomotor stereotypies listed in Table 3.3 can reasonably be considered in a group and defined as responses to the aversive effects of isolation and confinement in a barren environment.

The next question becomes 'Are locomotor stereotypies a visible expression of:

(1) conscious distress in an animal rationally aware of its frustration or anxiety?
(2) a successful strategy for coping with the effects of, for example, boredom?
(3) mental disturbance provoked by prolonged distress associated with frustration or anxiety?'

The first alternative could be likened to the parent who paces back and forth while awaiting the outcome of an operation on his or her child. The parent is anxious, knowing the source of distress but unable to do anything about it. An example of the successful strategy 2 might be the sedentary clerk who copes with chronic boredom by becoming a compulsive jogger. However, when a pattern of behaviour like rocking behaviour in the autistic child becomes compulsive, it is usually interpreted as a sign of mental disturbance whatever may have been the original cause. It is therefore fair to assume that an animal which develops a compulsive pattern of purposeless, repetitive behaviour which has become emancipated from its original stimulus may also have become disturbed in its mind.

We cannot, as yet, be sure which of these three explanations best fits the classic locomotor stereotypies of confined animals. Majority opinion (see Lawrence and Rushen, 1993) favours the idea that they are coping mechanisms designed to reduce unpleasant forms of arousal, e.g. frustration felt by the tiger with an intrinsic motivation to go out and hunt, anxiety felt by the vole unable to satisfy its intrinsic motivation to create a burrow, or the sheer grinding boredom felt by a horse shut up alone in a stable. In other words, they are an adaptive mechanism designed to improve the animal's perception of its own welfare in an unsatisfactory environment. Within MacFarland's welfare egg (Fig. 2.2), they constitute a strategy for moving out of limbo.

But at what cost? We cannot ignore the evidence that locomotor stereotypies in humans can signify a mind that is disordered, if not necessarily distressed. My colleagues Jonathan Cooper and Christine Nicol (1991) observed the development of locomotor stereotypies in bank voles kept in barren cages. The individual voles were also given preference tests in which they could select between a barren cage and an enriched environment in the form of a hay box. At the start of the experiments all voles chose to spend most time in the hay box. However, those individuals that developed stereotypies progressively lost their preference for the enriched (probably more secure) environment of the hay box. Either they were no longer aware of the difference in environmental quality between the two boxes, or they were still aware but no longer cared. No longer caring may be an effective mechanism for coping with the stresses of life. True loss of awareness of enviromental quality implies an acquired disorder of mind. Neither explanation leaves us with a clear conscience. Locomotor stereotypies are a sign that something is wrong.

Environmental enrichment

The general reader may well feel that it should be obvious that sentient animals would prefer not to live in a barren cage and the study of stereotypic behaviour is no more than a ruse for employing scientists to complicate the issue. Some such criticism may be valid but it is not constructive. It is reassuringly easy to state the obvious, i.e. sentient animals should not be kept in barren cages. It is less easy to decide what to *do* for the best. Ethological studies of the motivation of animals to seek enriched environments and physiological studies of changes in brain chemistry associated with stereotypic behaviour can help us towards a more specific understanding of what they are missing (security, companionship, the pleasure of food) and how they are feeling (anxious, lonely, peckish). We can then use this information to enrich environments in a way that is best suited to provide the things they miss most. Designers of modern zoos have to compromise between what looks right to the visitor and what feels right to the animal. The latter are unlikely to be impressed by scenery in an aesthetic sense but may, for example, welcome the security of a shelter that kept them out of the public view.

Since most practical decisions to enrich the environment for animals in zoos, laboratories, pet cages etc., will have to be taken without recourse to directly relevant research, we need some general, simple guidelines. I offer two suggestions that are indeed simple, but may be satisfactory for most animals (other than higher apes) with minds content simply to seek reward and avoid suffering and untroubled by such concepts as conscience and duty, except, of course, to their offspring, whom they see as an extension of themselves.

(1) Reduce anxiety. The main source of anxiety is a sense of insecurity. Depending on the species and its experience the animal may feel insecure if:

(a)   it cannot retreat to a 'safe' shelter;
(b)   it lacks the sense of safety in numbers, i.e. the reassuring presence of other animals, ideally of its own species;
(c)   it has not learnt to distinguish between danger that is real or merely apparent because it was denied the opportunity to explore and gain experience while young.

The primate that grows up alone in a laboratory cage and the puppy that grows up alone in a shed are faced by all three problems and both are likely to develop neurotic behaviour. Both may suffer anxiety as a direct consequence of exposure to barren environments. All three sources of anxiety are avoidable.

The insecurity felt by a female animal in a barren environment is likely to be most acute at the time she is about to give birth. The hen will work hard to seek a nest for her eggs and the sow work hard to build a nest for her piglets, each powerfully motivated by the need to *do something* to improve the

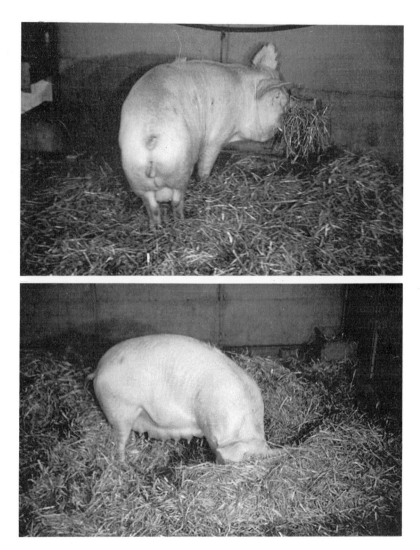

Fig. 4.3 A sow gathering straw to build a nest at farrowing time.

security of her offspring and undoubtedly anxious if this need is frustrated. Solutions to these problems are simple enough. However, most hens and sows will not be offered them.

(2) Reward endeavour. Science, commonsense and sensibility tell us that animals are innately curious. They are motivated to explore and to make a constructive contribution to the quality of their own existence, i.e. they will work to stay out of limbo. Their motivation to explore a novel object will fade once they have discovered what effect it may have on their lives. In most cases this investigation involves little more than 'Is it dangerous? Can I eat it? Can I use it to scratch, obtain food, or otherwise pleasure myself?' If the answer to all questions is no then the animal will lose interest since there is no obvious reward. Most 'toys' offered to animals in barren environments are ignored after a brief period of investigation because the animals perceive them to be useless. However, facilities or gadgets that allow animals to work to obtain food or bedding material can entertain them for hours because they provide a continually satisfying reward for endeavour.

The sow that is given a straw bed at the time of giving birth will feel more secure (and more comfortable) than the sow that is compelled to farrow on concrete. The sow that is not given a bed, but given a bale of straw and left to make her own nest (Fig. 4.3) will have not only the material needed for comfort and security but also the reassurance of having something constructive to do at a very worrying time. If you doubt this, ask mothers. They will understand.

5 Pain, Sickness and Death

> 'Pain remains a biological enigma;
> so much of it useless; a mere curse.'

Sir Charles Sherrington; letter to Lord Adrian, 1940

The question 'How is it for them?' now addresses issues which are, to us, the most intense sources of suffering: the feeling of pain, usually associated with injury; the feeling of sickness, usually associated with disease; and the problem of death. Man has a moral and legal responsibility to protect sentient animals from 'unnecessary suffering' associated with the first two of these three tribulations but the last is inescapable, for them and for us. We can elect, personally, not to kill animals, or eat animals that man has killed, but we cannot protect them from death. UK law protects (some) animals from acts or omissions likely to cause pain or unnecessary suffering but gives (some) people the right to kill them. The Protection of Animals Act (1911) first defines cruelty as 'cruelly to beat, kick, ill-treat, over-ride, over-drive, over-load, torture, infuriate or terrify any animal'. This clause reads as if it were drafted to strike a spark of sentience into ageing peers by suggesting that people were being nasty to horses in the street. It does, however, recognize that a sentient animal such as the horse can suffer not only from pain but also from fear and exhaustion. The 1911 Act refers to 'any animal' but is usually interpreted to mean only those species we wish to protect because they are 'the friends of man'. It may be used to prosecute youths torturing a cat, or even a wild rat that they had captured but it may not, of course, be used to prosecute adults who elect to over-ride, terrify and torture the fox. This is, to put it mildly, morally inconsistent.

Unnecessary suffering

The second definition of cruelty in the 1911 Act is 'to cause unnecessary suffering by doing or omitting to do any act'. The two attractions of this 'catch-all' clause are that it covers both sins of commission (e.g. torture) and omission (e.g. neglect) and that it can accommodate an evolving interpretation of what constitutes animal suffering. Its major problem lies in the interpretation of the word 'unnecessary' since it poses the questions 'when can suffering can be said to be necessary, and necessary for whom, man or the animal?' These questions form a major theme in Part II 'What we can do for them'. At this stage I shall illustrate it by way of a single example. Man elects to dock (cut short) the tails of lambs and some breeds of dogs. We assume that this will cause some pain, but not for long. Any suffering experienced by the lamb is deemed to be necessary *for the lamb* because it reduces the risk of blowfly strike which leads to a painful infestation with maggots. Any suffering experienced by the puppy is deemed to be necessary primarily *for the owner* who wishes to enter that puppy within the show ring.

Both these practices are permissible within English law, although the Royal College of Veterinary Surgeons has formally expressed their disapproval of the latter. A.P. Herbert wrote 'The common law of England has been laboriously built about a mythical figure – the figure of the Reasonable Man'. Most law is not designed to lay down absolute rules but to strike a fair balance between the differing aims of reasonable people. In this case, the law recognizes that suffering may sometimes be necessary. The acceptable limit to animal suffering cannot be defined only in terms of its effect on the animal but must be assessed by balancing the cost to the animal against the likely benefit to society, or to the animal itself.

The law relating to the mutilation of animals therefore applies a cost:benefit analysis to each individual procedure. Tail-docking of lambs is permitted in circumstances designed to minimize pain because the benefit to lambs is likely to far exceed the cost. Docked lambs have a far lower risk of suffering the far greater pain of 'blowfly strike', i.e. infestation by maggots. Mutilation of deer by removal of their antlers while 'in velvet' is prohibited partly because the pain and stress are presumed to be more severe and partly because the procedure is not carried out for the benefit of the deer but to make money.

English law still permits docking of the tails (but not the ears) of dogs. Breeds such as the springer spaniel may have been docked originally for their own benefit, to reduce the risk of injury while beating game birds out of the undergrowth, but this argument cannot possibly be applied to, say, the boxer breed, or indeed the great majority of modern spaniels. This form of mutilation of a non-consenting party in the interests of fashion is tolerated because it is assumed that the pain associated with docking in the first week of life is slight and does not last. The benefit (to anyone) of tail docking is minimal but so, too – the law assumes – is the cost. If it could be shown, however, that docked dogs 'miss' their tails, or suffer chronic pain or hypersensitivity in the amputated stump then the practice could be said to constitute unnecessary suffering. Since we already have good evidence that hens experience chronic hypersensitivity and discomfort following partial amputation of their beaks (Gentle *et al.*, 1990) this possibility should not be dismissed lightly.

All animals used for scientific purposes in the UK are now protected by the Animals (Scientific Procedures) Act (1986) which requires that all procedures involving laboratory animals be subjected to a cost:benefit analysis to determine whether the cost to the animal in terms of 'pain, suffering, distress or lasting harm', can be justified in terms of the potential benefit to mankind or, of course, other animals. The permissible cost to the animal will be greater if the potential benefit is a new cancer drug than a new cosmetic. I shall discuss the implications and interpretation of this Act in more detail in Chapter 12.

English law also licenses man to kill protected animals so long as the animal is 'slaughtered instantaneously or rendered instantaneously insensible to pain until death supervenes' (Slaughterhouse Act 1974 as amended by Section 5 of the Welfare of Animals at Slaughter Act 1991). The basic intent of this law is admirable, namely to minimize any pain associated with stunning and to prevent any recovery of consciousness before brain death is achieved. However, this law is, in my opinion, in many ways inferior to the Cruelty to Animals Act (1911) since it is designed only to avoid acute pain at the point of slaughter. This is not the only welfare problem that faces an animal in its last hours of life and a quick stun is not ideal if it is only achieved after the animal has had a frightening or distressing journey to the stunning point, urged on by goads or suspended upside down on shackles.

Since the laws relating to 'unnecessary suffering' are not absolutes but based on what appears reasonable to the reasonable man, it follows that they need to be kept under review in the light of advances in reason and I shall in Part III be making several specific suggestions for change. However, the central principle of all these laws is that pain does constitute a source of suffering to a sentient animal so that the infliction of pain, whether by design or neglect, is an act of cruelty.

The care of animals involves more than just the absence of cruelty. The third of the five freedoms exhorts us to prevent pain, injury and disease in animals and to ensure prompt diagnosis and appropriate treatment should they occur, *not just to restore fitness but also to make the animal feel better*. As always, this is easier said than done. If we are to convert this laudable aim into effective practice we need to consider how animals may feel pain when they are injured and how they may suffer when they are sick.

What is pain?

When we hurt ourselves, we know what pain is. We know what it feels like to have toothache, indigestion or lower back pain. We can describe the sort of pain we feel from these conditions and rank them on a scale of comparative intensity. Those of us who have experienced chronic lower back pain can recognize the symptoms in a fellow sufferer: spine twisted in protective spasm, extreme difficulty of movement, pallor and probably a deterioration of mood. We can also ask the sufferer to describe how bad it feels today. We then interpret the nature and intensity of pain in the other person in the light of our own experience. A radiologist may trace the source of the pain to damage and inflammation at the site of an intervertebral disc. Given this diagnosis, a physician may then prescribe anti-inflammatory drugs to reduce the pathology that is giving rise to the pain and analgesic drugs to reduce our conscious perception of how bad it feels.

The official definition of pain (in man) is 'an unpleasant sensory and emotional experience associated with actual or potential tissue damage and described in terms of such damage' (Iggo, 1984). All single-sentence definitions run the risk of stating the obvious. In this case, use of the word 'unpleasant' just manages to avoid saying 'pain is painful'. However, the adjectives 'sensory' and 'emotional' are important because they indicate that pain is more than just an acutely unpleasant sensation (e.g. the taste of something bitter on the tongue); it is also, for humans at least, likely to have a marked effect on mood. It may, for example, induce anxiety or depression. A rather wordier definition of pain might be 'an unpleasant sensory and emotional experience induced by sensations arising from noxious stimuli to nerve endings in tissues that are stressed or damaged mechanically, chemically or thermally. Signals are carried up sensory nerves to the central nervous system (CNS) wherein their nature and intensity is modulated by chemical messengers of other priorities (e.g. fear, excitement) before impacting upon the conscious mind'.

Acute, unexpected pain, e.g. picking up a very hot plate, may cause us to grimace and cry out. We shall almost certainly, reflexly, drop the plate. The patient suffering chronic severe pain that he knows to be associated with a terminal disease may weep with despair. For the mother in labour, intense pain may be accompanied by the exhilaration of birth. Individuals who have experienced damage to, or removal of prefrontal lobes of the cerebral cortex have reported that they continue to feel pain but they do not find it to be distressing. The conscious awareness of pain in man is not therefore a simple function of tissue stress or tissue damage or even of the strength of the signal from receptors in the damaged site, but depends on a complex series of modulating processes within the conscious and subconscious regions of the CNS. The suffering we experience from the sensation of pain is modulated by the effect of pain on mood, and *vice versa* and by our conscious (cognitive) awareness or expectation of its consequences. Hence the official definition of pain as 'an unpleasant sensory and emotional experience'.

All this means that pain in man is highly subjective. We know how we feel. We can gain some idea of pain in others from what they do and what they say but we cannot be sure how they feel. We must accept, therefore, that it is even more difficult to interpret how a particular non-human animal may feel pain without knowing something of its state of mind. This cannot be based on behaviour alone. The amoeba will change direction to avoid chemical damage but we assume it does not feel pain because it has no higher nervous system. The frog or cat will withdraw its foot if pinched after its brain has been destroyed. This is a reflex action operating at the level of the spinal cord. The conscious cat that burns its foot on a hot kettle may cry out, limp for some time and learn to avoid the kettle in future. We could reasonably interpret this behaviour as evidence that the cat was aware of the sensation of pain and had used that awareness for its own protection. We assume that the cat suffers pain by interpreting its behaviour in the light of our experience.

The Animals (Scientific Procedures) Act 1986 presumes that all vertebrates suffer pain, but invertebrates do not, a presumption that is becoming increasingly untenable as we learn more of the behaviour and neurobiology of species such as the octopus and squid (Wells, 1978). Patrick Bateson (1991) suggests that 'humans would think twice before attributing pain to an exquisitely made robot that flinched before it was hit, howled when the blow came [no Terminator, this robot!], clutched at the affected part and did lots of other life-like and appropriate things that minimized its chances of being further damaged'. If our presumption of pain in another was based simply on how similar its behaviour was to our own, we would empathize with the robot at least as much as with the cat, and much more than with the octopus. We cannot interpret pain in other species on the basis of behaviour alone.

Indices of pain in animals

Most features of the fundamental anatomy and physiology involved in the reception, transmission and central processing of information arising from noxious stimuli are common to all vertebrates (Fig. 5.1). Physiologists use the term 'nociception' to describe these phenomena and distinguish them from 'the (conscious) unpleasant sensory and emotional experience' that is pain. We can begin our enquiry into the nature of pain in vertebrate animals on the basis that their machinery is similar to ours. Thereafter, as with most complex questions of animal mind and animal suffering, we need to adopt the technique of triangulation (see Chapter 12), i.e. address the question from at least three different directions (Table 5.1).

Table 5.1 Approaches to the assessment of pain in animals.

Behaviour
Acute responses: withdrawal reflexes
                       distress; vocalization, facial expression
                       autonomic; sweating, panting
Protective responses: restricted movement, limping, contact aversion
Learned responses: aversion, fear

Mood
Anxiety, depression

Pain thresholds
Responses to mechanical or thermal stimuli

Pharmacology
Responses to anti-inflammatory drugs
Responses to analgesics – administered or self-selected
Responses to antidepressants

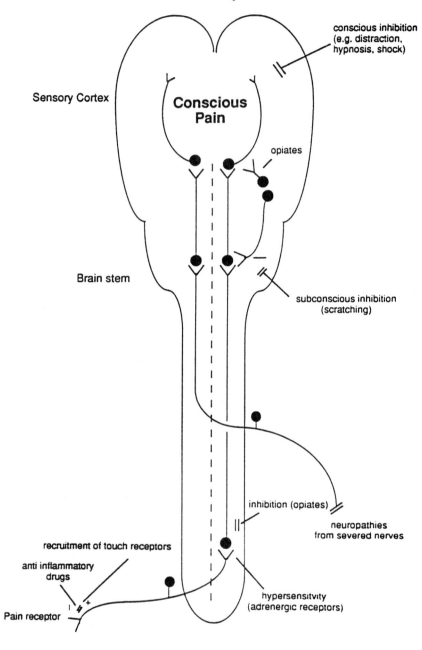

Fig. 5.1 Mechanisms involved in the conscious perception of pain.

When an animal touches something painful it withdraws its foot. We assume that this reflex withdrawal is associated with a conscious sensation of pain but know from experiments that it operates at a subconscious level. It does not *require* conscious sensation. Signs of distress, like crying out, limping, or running on three legs with the injured foot off the ground suggest to us that the animal is in pain but we should be cautious about using them as indices of the intensity of pain. Pigs, puppies and rabbits are more likely to cry out when in pain and fear than, say, cattle or wild ruminants. Screaming (or not screaming) usually serves a purpose. The puppy that yelps is trying to attract help, or at least sympathy from its mother or owner. The wild scream of the rabbit or pig may unnerve its predator or alert its siblings to the existence of danger. Many of the species that scream the most are those born in litters rather than as singletons. If a rabbit screams when it is captured its siblings may escape, and some of its genes may be preserved. The deer calf on the African plain is on its own. If it cries, limps or displays other obvious signs of distress it becomes the individual marked out by the lion as easy prey. It is likely that the domestic cow and sheep display similarly Spartan behaviour, i.e. they try not to reveal how much it hurts.

Both man and animals show similar autonomic responses to acute and chronic pain: sweating, increased respiration rate, increased secretion of adrenal hormones. These responses do not correlate particularly well with the conscious perception of pain in man, nor with responses to analgesics. This implies that they are unlikely to be a good 'objective' indicator of the intensity of conscious pain in animals.

Limping and other indices of lameness in animals are clearly designed to protect the damaged limbs. Our empathy with animals tells us that this is a sign of suffering but it is not conclusive evidence. It could just be a sensible precaution. More convincing evidence is provided by the behaviour of the 'debeaked' hen. Normal hens use their beaks not only for eating but as a most useful organ for actively investigating their environment. Hens with partial beak amputation show a marked aversion to using their beaks for anything but eating. This persistent contact aversion is associated with the development of neuropathies in the amputated stump similar to those seen following limb amputation in man (Gentle *et al.*, 1990). This strongly suggests that while debeaked hens may not be in pain all the time, their beaks have become hypersensitive so that what is sensed by a normal hen as touch becomes to them a source of pain.

Sentient animals also demonstrate learned aversion to painful stimuli, i.e. they remember what caused them pain and avoid the source and site of that unpleasant experience in future. They may also demonstrate fear when a repeat of the painful experience appears inevitable. One has only to observe dogs returning to the veterinary surgery.

In animals, as in man, pain is not just a sensory but also an emotional experience; it can affect and be affected by mood. In animals, as in man, drugs that are antidepressant but not analgesic (i.e. not pain killing) can affect the behavioural response to (especially) chronic pain. It appears to hurt as much but not to matter as much.

One excellent approach to the study of pain in man and animals is to apply a device to measure thresholds to pain from mechnical or thermal stimuli. Man can switch off the device as soon as it begins to hurt. If a similar device is placed on the leg of a trained animal, it will flinch as soon as it begins to hurt and this movement can be used to switch off the stimulus. Classically, this method has been used in man to measure the effectiveness of analgesics, differences between individuals and effects of modulators of conscious sensation such as mood, activity, acupuncture or hypnotism. Studies with animals by Avril Waterman and her colleagues (e.g. Ley, Livingstone and Waterman, 1989) reveal that horses, cattle and sheep have broadly similar pain thresholds to each other and to man. When in pain, the cow may display less distress than the horse or man, but this evidence suggests that she may well experience the same intensity of pain.

Pharmacology offers a powerful approach to the study of pain in animals. If the behaviour (e.g. locomotion) or mood of an animal improve when the source of pain is reduced, e.g. by the administration of anti-inflammatory agents, or the transmission of nociceptive stimuli is inhibited by drugs acting within the CNS, we may conclude that the animal has obtained relief from an unpleasant sensation and emotion, from which we must infer that it can suffer pain. However, different analgesic drugs have different effects in different species and this provokes the criticism that interpreting pain in terms of response to analgesics may be a circular, or subjective argument, i.e. the 'effective' analgesic is the one that produces the behavioural response we would expect to see in ourselves. Perhaps the most convincing pharmacological evidence for conscious awareness of pain in animals is the fact that injured rats will elect to drink water containing an analgesic in preference to their usual favourite, which is sucrose solution.

None of the individual indices of pain listed in Table 5.1 is, by itself sufficient evidence to conclude that animals feel pain in the same way as we do. Taken together, however, we have – I believe – overwhelming evidence to suggest that all vertebrate animals should be given the benefit of any remaining doubt. We have also the methodology required to study (in a humane fashion) where the main problems are likely to occur in practice and how to avoid them, not only where the problems are obvious, such as chronic lameness in farm animals, but also in cases where we do not know, or have so far chosen not to ask. Verheijen and his colleagues at Utrecht have obtained convincing evidence that fish display acute behavioural, autonomic and learned aversion responses similar to those seen in mammals not only when they are hooked (which may trigger both pain and mechanisms to avoid capture) but also when they receive electrical stimuli to the roof of the mouth transmitted while they are free-swimming (see also Chapter 11). The angler may decide that pain in fish is not his concern. However, the angler who claims that fish do not suffer pain is not only advertising the fact that he is prepared to pass judgement on the basis of total ignorance; he is, in the light of new evidence, almost certainly wrong.

Acute and chronic pain

The sensation of pain arises from noxious stimuli to pain receptors when tissues are injured but in man the intensity of acute pain often bears little relation to the amount of injury. We may experience intense pain if we hit our thumb with a hammer or have a tooth drilled without anaesthetic. However, people who have been shot, stabbed or even had a limb amputated by machinery often report little or no sensation of pain at the time. It is later that it really starts to hurt. Similarly animals may show few, if any signs of pain when acutely injured during fight or flight. Pain is, in the words of Sir Charles Sherrington, an enigma. The physiological and psychological mechanisms that govern nociception and the conscious perception of pain are complex, imperfectly understood and beyond the scope of this book. Figure 5.1 attempts only to analyse the nature of pain (and what we should do about it) in three stages:

(1) pain reception at the site of injury
(2) subconscious modulation of pain within the spinal cord and brain stem;
(3) conscious modulation of pain within the sensory cortex.

The acute sensation of pain is determined first, by the intensity of the peripheral stimulus and the number of nerve endings transmitting that stimulus. The fingertips of man or the nose of the pig have a much higher concentration of nerve endings than for example, the middle of the back. Physiologists usually distinguish between nerve endings sensing touch and pain, but the distinction is not absolute. Hitting one's thumb with a hammer is particularly painful partly because of the concentration of nerve endings at the site and partly because the thumb nail restricts swelling and removal of fluids lost from damaged cells. Laminitis (or 'founder') in horses and cattle is extremely painful for the same reasons and compounded by the fact that the animals are forced to stand on the inflamed digits. To appreciate the pain of laminitis in a horse or cow, it helps to contemplate crushing all one's fingertips in a door and then attempting to walk around on them.

Acute injury leads to inflammation at the site usually accompanied by further damage to cell walls and this is one reason why the intensity of pain tends to increase. In acute, severe pain it may help to reduce blood flow to the site (e.g. hosing the feet of laminitic cattle with cold water). Chronic pain associated with inflammation at the site of injury can be reduced by anti-inflammatory drugs or by *increasing* blood flow to aid removal of the noxious products of inflammation.

Modulation of incoming signals from pain receptors can occur at several levels within the central nervous system. Man and, presumably, animals have a powerful ability to suppress the sensation of acute pain arising from injuries experienced during fighting or other vigorous action. In essence, the mind elects to concentrate on other priorities. This mechanism for the suppression of pain which is at least partly conscious, can also be elicited by hypnosis or placebo drugs taken by humans under the impression that they are pain-killers. This is achieved, in part, by stimulating nerves to release endogenous opiates (morphine-like substances such as β-endorphin). The physiology of the endogenous opiates is fascinating and important. It is equally important, however, not to exaggerate their contribution to animal welfare.

To illustrate this point, let us consider the time-honoured procedure of 'twitching' the horse. For hundreds of years, vets and others wishing to restrain horses while they carried out potentially painful or distressing pro-cedures like rasping teeth or 'firing' limbs, have applied a twitch to the horse's nose, i.e. twisted a rope to squeeze the sensitive skin of the nose and upper lip (Fig. 5.2). The technique is undoubtedly effective, in the sense that the horse tends to stand still and it was traditionally assumed, on grounds of commonsense, that the pain from their nose made them reluctant to move and took their minds off what was going on elsewhere. The unsurprising discovery that twitching stimulated the release of endogenous opiates prompted some to suggest that twitching acted as a true painkiller like morphine and so was a humane alternative to the use of analgesic or anaesthetic drugs. This is clearly nonsense. Endogenous opiates do suppress the intensity of pain. They can be released in response to conscious stimuli other than pain, or to things consciously assumed to alleviate pain (like placebos). However, they are mainly designed to deal with pain itself. Twitching the horse stimulates endorphins because it hurts.

Pain, unlike other somatic sensations like touch and pressure, is not adaptive. We rapidly habituate to the sensation of touch from our clothing or pressure on the soles of our feet but we do not switch off the sensation of pain. Indeed there are mechanisms within the CNS, especially at the level of the spinal cord which can create hypersensitivity to pain, not only by amplifying signals arising from pain receptors in damaged tissues (Fig. 5.1) but also by reinterpreting signals arising from touch receptors so that touch itself becomes a source of pain. The problem of chronic pain cannot therefore be attributed simply to sustained damage and release of noxious substances at the original site of injury but also to chronic changes in the mechanisms for processing pain signals within the CNS. Ley *et al.* (1989) have demonstrated reduced thresholds to mechanical pain stimuli in sheep suffering with chronic footrot. This implies that even if the severity of the damage to the foot does not increase with time, the severity of the pain will increase.

The deliberate imposition of chronic pain must constitute one of the most severe and unacceptable forms of cruelty to animals. Current law protects animals from acute pain associated with beating or torture but does little to protect sheep from chronic pain associated with footrot and nothing at all to protect broiler chickens and turkeys that are misshapen or have outgrown

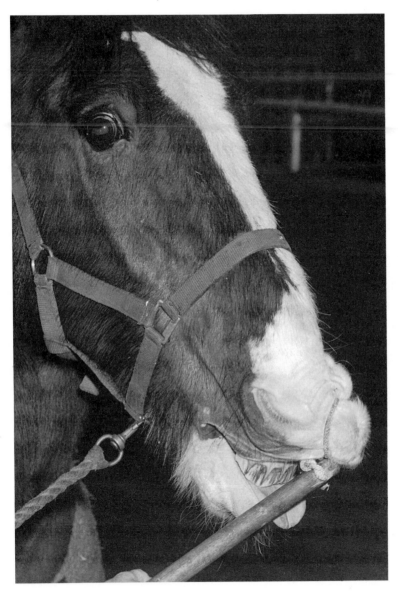

Fig. 5.2 'Twitching' the horse.

their strength from chronic pain associated with disorders of their bones and joints. As evidence accumulates that the severity of pain associated with conditions such as chronic lameness increases with time, then the need to reduce lameness and other forms of chronic pain in animals becomes ever more acute.

What is pain for?

At first sight, the reason for pain is obvious. It is a powerful signal designed to direct the behaviour of animals so as to avoid injury and promote recovery from injury. I list below a more comprehensive series of reasons drawn largely from Bateson (1991). Pain is necessary

(1)   to distinguish between harmful and non-harmful stimuli;
(2)   to provoke animals to give high priority to escape or remove harmful stimuli;
(3)   to teach animals to avoid harmful stimuli in future, or to decide what degree of pain (or harm) is acceptable in the pursuit of information or reward;
(4)   to inhibit activities likely to delay recovery from injury.

The first two reasons do not necessarily depend on the conscious aware-ness of pain. However, the latter two require memory and conscious deci-sion-making based not on pain itself but on the expectation of pain. Once again, as with other aspects of mind, we must accept that conscious aware-ness of pain evolved because it contributed to survival of the fittest. It cannot be considered as a unique property of man. We have no alternative therefore but to assume that sentient animals experience pain in much the same way as ourselves.

The difficult, unanswerable questions are 'why is all pain so distressing and some pain so pointless?' Presumably the intensity of distress associated with acute pain is necessary to ensure that the motivation to avoid injury overrides most other ambitions and so favours survival. The temporary inhibition of acute pain by endogenous opiates also acts to favour survival when the need to escape overrrides the need to avoid further injury. The need to protect tissues from further injury explains why pain stimuli are non-adaptive. However, it is difficult to see how the goal of Darwinian fitness is assisted by CNS mechanisms designed progressively to increase the intensity of chronic pain. It is also difficult to see what is the 'point' of intense pain associated with internal disorders such as cancer or kidney stones. Such pain may persuade us to seek effective medical assistance and so enhance our chances of survival but this (to quote Bateson) 'can hardly explain its evolution'. Presumably 'useless' pain sensation in deep tissues evolved as an inevitable accompaniment to that designed to enhance survival by reducing injury and enhancing healing in the skin and limbs.

There is another, bleaker interpretation of the unyielding nature of chronic pain (or emotional stress), namely that it favours survival of the fittest by accelerating the demise of the sick and injured (Gray, 1987). Nature is effi-cient but not compassionate. To quote John Collee, it is not 'natural' for an old woman to die in bed surrounded by loving relatives. It is 'natural' for her to collapse under a pile of sticks and be eaten by wolves. Any time we feel inclined to guilt at the extent of man's dominion over nature, it is of comfort to remember that one of our greatest achievements has been our ability to protect both our families and other animals from 'natural' suffering.

Sickness

Although the welfare of an animal cannot be defined by any of the five freedoms in isolation but requires an effective compromise between them all, I would personally rank good health, or freedom from pain, injury and disease as the first among equals. This is not, however, the place to discuss the prevention, diagnosis and treatment of specific diseases of animals – a huge subject that already overloads the five-year curriculum for veterinary students. The important question in the context of this book is how does an animal *feel* when it is sick and what can we do to make it feel better.

Our perception of sickness is highly subjective. A veterinary surgeon presented with a calf with a respiratory infection may prescribe an antibiotic in the knowledge that it will not affect the primary viral pathogen but will reduce the risk of secondary bacterial invasion of the damaged lung and so increase the probability of a full recovery. If her daughter has a respiratory infection she will probably send her to bed and give her an analgesic and anti-inflammatory drug like paracetamol. If she develops the symptoms herself she may carry on working during the day but self-prescribe at least one large whisky before bedtime. She has treated the calf with antibiotic because she was taught that infections are caused by germs and she wishes to control at least some of those germs. She perceives her daughter to be weak and fevered and sends her to bed with a tablet because she wants her to *feel* better while her natural defences effect a cure. Having rather less concern for her own welfare than for that of her daughter, she pours herself a whisky in the certain knowledge that it will have no effect upon the progress of her disease but because, once again, she knows that it will make her feel better. In the case of the calf, she has attempted to control the disease, in the case of her daughter and herself she has attempted to control the symptoms. Since the animal's subjective perception of its own sickness is likely to be no more profound than that of the veterinary surgeon, we may reasonably assume that it, too, would feel its welfare to be well served by action designed to relieve the symptoms of sickness *in addition to* any action designed to remove the specific source of infection.

An animal may feel sick when all or part of the body is physically damaged or chemically poisoned by:

(1) external injury or damage to internal organs;
(2) pathogenic microorganisms or their toxins;
(3) deficiencies or excesses of normal dietary constituents or products of their digestion or metabolism;
(4) poisonous plants or chemicals.

The main generalized or systemic signs of sickness associated with these sources of physical and chemical damage are fever, pain, dullness and depression, reduced appetite or anorexia, and loss of body fluids. In addition, an animal may have distressing local symptoms specifically related to the primary source of infection or disease, e.g. local pain or difficulty in breathing. Some of these symptoms may be life-threatening, e.g. loss of body fluids from chronic diarrhoea or vomiting. Others, such as pain and depression, may be distressing to the animal but have little impact on the prognosis of the disease. The owner of a pet or farm animal and his veterinary surgeon are therefore faced by two distinct questions:

- 'How much am I prepared to pay to restore this animal to health?'
- 'How much am I prepared to pay to relieve the distress caused to this animal by sickness and pain?'

As always, there are no absolute answers. We must, however, attempt to enter the mind of the sick animal. Although the feeling of sickness or malaise in man may be modulated by rational thought, anxiety or the fear of death, the basic sensation is as primitive as hunger, which implies that it is much the same for them as for us. When we are sick, we apply a cost:benefit analysis to the treatment of our own symptoms. We give ourselves as much nursing as we can afford (in terms of time and money). Our approach to the relief of distress caused by sickness in animals should be the same. We may ultimately decide that the cost to us is too high. We cannot, however, pretend that they would not benefit.

Relief of sickness

Table 5.2 lists the main sources of distress associated with sickness in animals and gives examples of how they might be alleviated by medicines or by nursing. Fever is a controlled elevation of body temperature induced by pyrogens, produced by invading bacteria or by the cells of the body's own immune system, which re-set the animal's thermostat within the hypothalamus. It is a natural manifestation of the defence mechanisms that animals have evolved to fight infection and must therefore be a good thing, in a Darwinian sense, although I have never read a really convincing argument in its support.

In the early stages of fever, the increase in body temperature is achieved both by elevating heat production and by reducing heat loss. The animal both shivers and reduces blood flow to the extremities so that its ears and feet may feel cold even though the body temperature is elevated. When the body temperature has increased to the new set-point of the thermostat, the extremities, especially the ears, may now feel hot but the animal may continue to shiver, or otherwise sustain an elevated metabolic rate, to maintain the elevated body temperature. Fever is usually accompanied by inappetence and excessive loss of water, electrolytes and nitrogen in the urine. These factors, in combination, cause a rapid loss of body condition. In fever, the animal may feel (amongst other things) too hot or too cold, weak, depressed. thirsty but nauseated by food. I am also convinced that animals suffer headaches. One cannot be sure but horses and sheep press their heads against cool stone walls in circumstances such as increased pressure within the cerebro-spinal fluid that are known to be associated with severe headaches in man.

Table 5.2 Examples of the use of medicines and nursing for relief of the symptoms of sickness in animals.

Symptom	'Medical' remedy	'Nursing' remedy
Fever	Antipyretics	Thermal comfort
Pain	Analgesics Anti-inflammatory drugs	Physical comfort Rest Reduce stress at site of damage
Inappetence	'Tonics' Restore homeostasis	Reduce pain if present Oral titillation
Dullness	Unnecessary?	Rest
Fluid loss	Intravenous rehydration	Oral rehydration
Dyspnoea	Anti-inflammatory drugs Bronchial dilators	Air quality

When fever is caused by infection, it is logical to use antibiotics to remove the source of infection. It may sometimes be necessary to treat fever *per se* by the use of antipyretic drugs. More often, it may be both cheaper and kinder to reduce the distress associated with fever by appropriate nursing. In very rare cases, the body temperature may be elevated so high as to constitute a threat to life. In these cases, it may be necessary to cool the animal down with cold water. What is far more common is the problem of the farm animal such as the calf or young pig with a moderate but persistent fever. The box that provided adequate thermal comfort for the healthy animal now feels cold and the animal shivers continuously in an effort to maintain the elevated set-point for body temperature. This will not only accelerate the rate of loss of body condition but can become exhausting. The fevered animal will therefore benefit from a rug, a bed of deep straw, an infrared lamp or any other means designed to reduce heat loss and so permit the animal to maintain its elevated body temperature with minimal distress.

I have already dealt at some length with the problem of chronic pain and its relief by analgesic or anti-inflammatory drugs. However, the most effective approach to the relief of pain can often be through appropriate nursing. Thus the cow with laminitis will be less uncomfortable on deep straw in a loosebox than on concrete in a cubicle, not just because it hurts less when she stands up, but because she can lie down for longer without becoming cramped. The same principle applies to the cow whose udder is hot and swollen with mastitis. Antibiotics will treat the disorder by reducing the source of infection but application of cold water to the udder and regular stripping of milk from the infected quarter will both help to reduce the pain. These things are so obvious that they are often overlooked. Other forms of chronic pain associated, for example, with limb damage or even pleurisy, may only become severe when the animal is forced to move. Once again, good nursing should ensure that animals can rest in as much comfort as possible, with minimal disturbance for as long as is necessary.

Inappetence and anorexia in animals are governed by the same mechanisms that control hunger and appetite in the healthy individual. An animal may refuse food if:

(1) it hurts to eat;
(2) its gut is already distended by gas or undigested material;
(3) chemicals circulating within the blood signal satiety or nausea.

Eating is obviously a painful process if there is pain in the mouth from teeth that are infected or overgrown so that they cut into the tissues of the cheek. Less obviously, an animal with sore feet may be reluctant to eat if it has to walk to a feeding area and compete with others. When an animal is fevered or poisoned by toxins arising from bacteria or cell damage, the concentration of certain chemicals in the blood, especially amino acids, rises in a way rather similar to that following a protein meal. At the same time stress hormones from the adrenal cortex shift the balance of metabolism away from anabolic processes like growth and lactation, which involve the uptake and storage of nutrients, towards catabolism, involving the release of glucose and amino acids into the blood as substrates to support elevated metabolic rate and healing. All these factors will tend to reduce appetite. The animal that becomes toxaemic through poisoning, infection or severe metabolic crisis will experience damage to the liver and other tissues involved in metabolizing the products of digestion and breakdown of body tissues. In these circumstances the animal may stop eating altogether because it cannot even process the end products of its own tissue metabolism, let alone the end products of digestion. The sick animal elects not to eat for the same reason as that which governs most of its behaviour; because it senses that the action will make it feel worse rather than better.

Acute inappetence during acute disease is therefore an adaptive mechanism which need not be discouraged. Prolonged inappetence presents a rather more difficult problem. All animals that fail to eat for sustained periods will experience severe and possibly life-threatening loss of condition. Moreover, the tissues of the gut progressively lose their capacity to digest food. This problem is particularly severe in herbivores like the cow and horse which rely on a large population of microorganisms to predigest the fibre in plant cell walls, since these microorganisms die of starvation. Thus the appetite of an animal may remain depressed after the primary disease has passed. The first priority for the inappetent, convalescent animal is not to rebuild lost body tissue but to restore energy and electrolyte balance. Thus the first meals should be small, as tasty as possible and based on easily digestible carbohydrates. Once the convalescent but thin animal loses the sense of nausea associated with eating it will become very hungry indeed, driven by the demand for substrates from the recovering tissues. This, too, is entirely normal and should be encouraged.

Dullness and depression are natural consequences of fever, toxaemia, inappetence, dehydration or weakness. They may be considered an adaptive response and it makes more sense to allow a sick animal to be dull and depressed in reasonable comfort than to disturb it in a vain effort to improve its morale. It is, however, important to distinguish between depression as an adaptive response to one or more of the above, and inactivity caused by pain or paralysis since these may require prompt and specialist treatment.

One of the most severe and distressing problems faced by the sick animal is dehydration caused by loss of body water and electrolytes, particularly following prolonged diarrhoea and/or vomiting. We can be sure that dehydrated animals will feel weak. We can also reasonably assume that they will experience other symptoms which we associate with dehydration. Since these constitute most of the symptoms of a hangover, we may assume them to be a source of suffering. The most practical way to replace body fluids is through the mouth provided that what goes into the stomach does not further aggravate the problem by provoking further vomiting or diarrhoea. In these circumstances the animal cannot be sustained by water alone but requires a solution containing glucose, to provide energy that can be absorbed without the need for predigestion, sodium to restore extracellular fluid volume, potassium to restore intracellular fluid, and buffers such as bicarbonate to correct metabolic acidosis. Rehydration mixtures of this sort have during the last thirty years saved the lives of millions of children and other young animals with diarrhoea that would otherwise have died from dehydration. The remedy is so simple and based on such long-standing knowledge of physiology that it could have been adopted at least fifty years sooner.

On admission to the Royal College of Veterinary Surgeons, the new graduate vows 'to ensure the welfare of all animals committed to my care'. Since the welfare of an animal is determined both by its fitness and by how it feels, the veterinary surgeon has the responsibility not only to preserve and restore fitness but also to help an animal to feel better when it is sick. I repeat, being ill and feeling sick are not the same thing. The veterinary surgeon with undiagnosed flu-like symptoms tucked up in bed by a loving spouse and with whisky to hand probably feels that his or her welfare is being served rather better than if he or she were at work. The fevered, pneumonic calf, shivering in the corner of a damp, draughty barn, feels rotten and will be in no way comforted by the fact that the condition has been diagnosed by a trained veterinary surgeon and treated with antibiotics. To ensure the welfare of a sick animal it is not enough to treat the disease. One must also attend to the symptoms.

Death and dying

Death, I repeat, is not a welfare problem for the animal that is dead. Death of a mother will present real problems of survival for her offspring if they are unable to look after themselves. Death or separation of the offspring during the rearing period will also induce a temporary sense of distress in the rearing parent in most species of mammals and birds even though the immediate consequence for the parent may be an easier life. It can be said without recourse to anthropomorphism that many species appear to care at least as much for the survival of their dependent offspring as for themselves. It is, once again, the genetic imperative.

A much more difficult question is what, if anything, do non-human animals feel when they observe the death of another, unrelated member of their species. Clearly, if a flock of sheep are being savaged by a pack of dogs, each sheep will fear for its own safety and the sight and smell of blood and death of other sheep may contribute to that sense of fear. There is, however, a strong argument that it is more humane to kill farmed deer by shooting them in the field when they come up to eat at a feeding trough than to subject them to the prolonged stresses of the journey to and experience within the abattoir. The procedure is undeniably more humane for the animal that is killed instantaneously by a clean shot from a rifle with a silencer while enjoying an untroubled meal. Moreover, observers report that red deer appear to be untroubled by the sight of their neighbours at the trough crashing to the ground and continue to eat as if nothing untoward had happened. It is necessary to distinguish between

(1) a sense of fear, in the presence of death or a killer, as a motivating force for personal survival;
(2) a sense of anxiety generated by isolation from the reasurring presence of other animals, usually of the same species;
(3) a sense of loss generated by the absence of a companion;
(4) fear of the concept of death itself.

The next chapter will consider the concepts of fear, anxiety and companionship. An animal may experience a sense of fear, anxiety or loss in circumstances surrounding the death of another, but this does not necessarily imply that it has an existential fear of the concept of personal death as an end to existence. This abstract concept may be one of the very few fundamental sources of distress that is unique to man, or at the most, man and a very small group of species that might include some of the higher primates and, just possibly, elephants. For most species, it is, I believe, reasonable and humane to consider the welfare implications of death for those animals that survive in the context of only the first three of the four questions listed above.

The process of dying is more serious since it is likely to involve feelings of pain or sickness and fear. Dying, like pain and fear, is a subjective experience but, unlike pain and fear, not one which we can effectively communicate, even to our own species. Thus any attempt to enter the mind of a dying animal is, to say the least, tricky. However, I believe the problem is as open to cool, rational analysis as any other, even if some of the answers are unavailable. The paths to death are many and various but the number of ways of actually dying are rather few. Death is caused by an irreversible loss of brain function when

(1) the blood supply is cut off because the heart stops or the blood vessels are cut;
(2) the brain is starved of oxygen because the animal stops breathing or is denied oxygen;
(3) the brain cells are poisoned or inactivated (e.g. by anaesthetic);
(4) the brain is mechanically destroyed or severely concussed.

Animals either die (usually slowly) following a progressive deterioration of body function triggered by infection, neoplasia or the simple processes of ageing, or they are killed (usually quickly) as the result of an injury, whether accidental or deliberately caused by another animal such as man. The main questions that face us as humans are:

● 'When is it right to kill an animal or, alternatively, leave it to die or be killed by a species other than man?'
● 'What methods should we use to kill those animals we choose to kill?'

The natural, relatively slow death of an animal from disease or old age is likely to involve feelings of sickness, pain and probably fear, maybe not of death itself, but fear or anxiety generated by the animal's awareness that it is losing control of its own destiny. For those animals in the wild, out of the direct control of man, this is their problem, not ours. When animals are within our more direct dominion, we decide when to 'slaughter' if it is a farm animal, 'cull' if it is a protected wild animal, or 'put it to sleep' if it is a pet. In each case the animal gets killed. If longevity is not an essential component of animal welfare then it is not cruel to kill an animal humanely at any age. The corollary to this argument is that it can be cruel to keep an animal alive when its quality of life has deteriorated to the point that it suffers chronic pain or sickness and has no realistic expectation of recovery. Inevitably, however, our decision as to when that point has been reached will not be made in isolation but balanced against our perception of that animal's value to us, be it a chronically lame, emaciated cow who can still contribute milk and perhaps one more calf, or a chronically lame, incontinent dog whom we love and who still appears to experience some joy in our presence. Once again, this is a matter for Part III.

When killing is to be done, 'it were well it were done quickly'. English law requires animals to be 'slaughtered instantaneously or rendered instantaneously insensible to pain until death supervenes'. The intention of this law is to eliminate pain from the killing process. However, as I have indicated already, the law does not take into account the fear and other stresses that an animal may experience within the abattoir *en route* to the killing point. Exemptions to this law permit Halal and Shekita methods of ritual slaughter, in which the throat of the animal is slit without prior stunning. Defenders of these practices claim that the single incision is not painful. Although this is another judgement passed on the basis of total ignorance it may not be too far from the truth, given what is known about the lack of acute pain associated with sudden severe injury in man. However, fear, not pain is the major problem for an animal conscious of choking to death in its own blood. I shall consider ways of improving welfare for farm animals during transport from the farm and within the abattoir in Chapters 8 and 9. I shall conclude this chapter by stating that the main problem faced by all animals within slaughterhouses is not pain but fear and that the difference between conventional and ritual slaughter is one of relatively minor degree. The welfare of animals in slaughterhouses would be improved if existing law designed only to eliminate pain at the moment of death were replaced by a law designed to minimize all stresses associated with handling, transport, lairage and stunning. Such a clause might read 'at the place of slaughter animals must be handled, rendered unconscious and killed in such a way as to minimize pain and suffering'. This would encourage the development of integrated systems designed to reduce, and in some cases circumvent, the multiplicity of stresses experienced by farm animals on their last day of life.

6 Friends, Foes, Fears and Stress

'The time to lick your wounds is when danger has passed.'

Jeffrey Gray, *The Psychology of Fear and Stress*

It was never ordained that animals should love one another. The whole, successful business of Darwinian evolution has been based on the principle of survival of the fittest which requires that self-interest is paramount and conflict inevitable. It may not be attractive but it works. Simple extrapolation of Darwinian principles to man generates the Malthusian situation wherein the masses are condemned to poverty and squalor by limited resources, uncontrolled reproduction and an inadequate culling policy due to the lack of an effective predator species. While this situation does apply in too much of the world, we know that man, by the humane application of his intellect and acquired power, can create stable societies which permit him to display humanity to his brother man and other fellow mortals. Furthermore, societies in which altruism is possible become societies in which people wish to live. In other words, human altruism to brother man and other animals can succeed in advanced societies because it improves both the quality of our own lives and our chances for survival. Altruism now obeys Darwinian rules – i.e. it serves self-interest.

The utility of altruism is not a particularly profound concept but it is too profound for most animal species whose approach to self-interest is rather less subtle. When animals have to fend for themselves, their self-interest may be served by solitude (except at mating time) or by life in stable social groups. It will certainly involve conflict of interests between other animals competing for the same resource or the same mate. In addressing the question 'How do animals feel about their social life?' we must assume that animals will (nearly) always attempt to 'use' other animals to ensure personal survival or improve the quality of their own existence within a personal, and entirely selfish spectrum of pain to pleasure. Within these simple terms of reference animals may identify a few other individuals, usually but not invariably of the same species, as 'friends' who contribute a sense of security or companionship. They will identify a far greater number, both within and across species, as 'foes', whether as competitors or as a threat to survival. Finally, many carnivorous species, including humans, will view other species simply as food. Faced by such competition and threat, one of the senses most essential to survival becomes the sense of fear.

When man elects to domesticate an animal, he contracts, at least, to provide security of food supply and security from predation, until he is ready to become the predator. This undoubtedly relieves the animal of some of the stresses of a free-living existence but can introduce a new set of social problems. There will be conflict between animals of the same species as they establish hierarchies or 'pecking orders'. Moreover, the animal that grows up in the protected but abnormally unedifying environment of the farm, laboratory cage or city apartment may, as I have discussed earlier, fail to learn the distinction between threats that are real or merely apparent and so develop a chronic anxiety neurosis.

Animal conflict

I shall in this section consider only social conflict between individuals within species; animals who are sharing the same space, competing for the same resource and who will know something of each other's minds. The hunter and hunted will obviously know something of each other's strategy but their interactions are not social.

Table 6.1 Categories and examples of conflict between individuals within species.

Category	Examples
Aggression	
Threat display	Competing males, information gathering
Fighting	Males maintaining harems or leks
Killing	Cannibalism, fratricide in raptor birds
'Mindless' assault	Feather pecking, tail biting
Non-aggressive scrambling	Competition for food at a trough
Mutual avoidance	Territorial marking
Meddling with others	'Dogs in the manger'
Manipulating others	Cuckoos, female seals

Table 6.1, which categorizes types of conflict that may occur between individuals within species, has been drawn largely from Huntingford and Turner, *Animal Conflict* (1987). In a typical conflict situation, one individual initiates or threatens an attack and the other fights back, runs away or signals submission. This brief encounter has involved aggression, although maybe only from one party. Ethologists usually call such encounters 'agonistic behaviour' defined as 'a system of behaviour patterns having the common function of adaptation to situations involving physical conflict' (Scott and Fredericson, 1951). This definition makes the important point that in most normal situations, agonistic behaviour is adaptive, in that it can improve the

Darwinian fitness of a species and so favour its survival. It can also embrace all possible strategies for dealing with conflict situations listed in Table 6.1, many of which do not involve an element of direct aggression.

One of the most common and most successful forms of agonistic behaviour involves the ritualization of aggression into displays of threat and submission in which neither party gets hurt. This is seen amongst competing males throughout the animal kingdom. We can observe these rituals most easily in the dog or in ourselves. The dominant dog will approach with its tail and ears erect, its hackles up and its lips parted in a snarl. The submissive dog will have its ears laid flat, its tail between its legs, and its lips parted in an ingratiating smile (Fig. 6.1). If this does not appear to be submissive enough, it may roll onto its back, expose its unprotected belly and urinate. This extreme form of ritualized aggression and submission will occur when each individual knows his relative place in the hierarchy. Before this point has been established, individuals *may* fight but are more likely to proceed through an escalating series of postures and threats designed to convey the information that *I am bigger and stronger than you*. Once this information has been conveyed and the point agreed by both parties, it will cease to matter very much to either (i.e. it will not be a source of prolonged suffering) provided that both parties have the environmental space and resources to coexist. The rituals have succeeded in avoiding future conflict. An even more effective means of avoiding conflict, where space is available, is mutual avoidance based on scent marking of territory. This ritual is used, for example, by wolves as a highly effective method for establishing territory. It is also much used by, and a source of great interest to, domestic male dogs. Such rituals are designed essentially to avoid conflict and problems may only arise when the motivation for a quiet life is overridden by greater forces such as overcrowding, starvation or sexual desire.

Overt fighting between individuals within a species, as distinct from

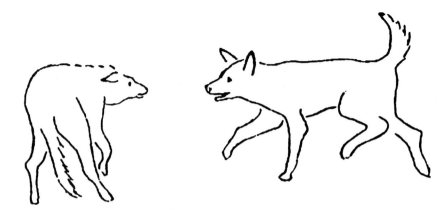

Fig. 6.1 Signs of aggression and submission in the dog.

threatening, pushing, wrestling or 'play-fighting' occurs naturally in the breeding season between males, especially in those species in which the males (e.g. stags, bulls, elephant seals) attempt to maintain harems. Although this extreme form of aggression may lead to severe injury or death, the evolutionary advantages are obvious; the fittest survive. The male that fights or furiously rushes around to defend his mating ground or invade that of another may suffer fear, pain or exhaustion but it has been his choice. Clearly the motivation to mate overrides these potential sources of distress. It is probably fruitless to contemplate the question 'how much do animals *enjoy* sex' but there is every reason to conclude that within these fighting males, the motivation towards sexual reward within the simple utilitarian pain-pleasure spectrum is powerful enough to override a number of sensations that would, in less exciting circumstances, be seen as highly aversive.

The behaviour of females within animal harems is every bit as adaptive and rather more cool. It is, of course, to the genetic advantage of a female to mate with the fittest male, especially if his only contribution to the prospects for survival of his offspring are the quality of his genes (i.e. he will not contribute to parental care). When a male is defending a large area of territory it could be argued that females remain passively within that territory. However, in some species of deer (kobs) and birds the males defend relatively small mating areas or 'leks' which females elect to enter. In doing so they are probably motivated both by their choice of mate and the desire to escape the unwilling attentions of others. There is some evidence that female elephant seals will encourage males to fight and mate with the winner. This is an elegant example of animals gaining a social advantage by the deliberate manipulation of others (Table 6.1).

Perhaps the most extreme form of agonistic behaviour within a species is the fratricide that occurs between chicks in some species of raptor bird such as the black eagle. The older, larger chick will kill its sibling to increase its own chances of survival. A cuckoo chick laid in the nest of a thrush will also eject the natural offspring. This is, of course, not fratricide but another example of one species manipulating the behaviour of another to ensure its own survival. Both of these behaviour patterns may, however, be considered as purely instinctive.

Conflict between animals for food may be aggressive, non-aggressive, or simply bloody-minded. When a flock of sheep rush to a trough at the sight of the shepherd arriving with a bag of pellets, their behaviour may be described as non-aggressive scrambling. Individuals are unlikely to experience fear or pain during this scramble, unless by accident, but those that fail to compete may well suffer hunger. Animals who are not motivated to eat at the time may, nevertheless, prevent others from getting access to the food source. This is commonly seen in cattle, pigs and even farmed salmon when individuals have to share a common feeder. In folk lore it is personified by the dog in the manger, barking furiously to deny a horse access to food that it, the dog, cannot eat.

A final and, in the context of this book, highly important form of agonistic behaviour is what I can only call 'mindless' aggression. This includes most feather pecking in hens and tail biting in pigs. Adult hens will, in certain circumstances, peck first at the feathers of other birds. As the skin of the pecked birds becomes inflamed or starts to bleed, this increases the motivation of other birds to peck at the site. The pecked individuals thus get pecked more frequently, injured more severely and may die of injury, infection or shock, whereupon they will probably be eaten by the other birds. Similarly young pigs, in certain circumstances, may begin first to suck, then nibble, then bite the tails of a few individuals and this can, once again, lead to severe injury and infection.

Both these problems are associated with farming systems where a large number of animals are reared together and tend therefore to be viewed as problems caused by the system itself. The traditional way to avoid these problems has been to trim the beaks of hens or dock the tails of pigs. Since we must assume that the feather-pecked hen or tail-bitten pig will suffer chronic pain, it can be argued that these mutilations are acceptable on welfare grounds since the benefit justifies the cost. If it could be shown that pigs 'miss' their tails (which I think is highly unlikely), or that the amputated tails are a source of chronic pain, or that the act of tail-biting is a sign of stress in the biter (rather than an antisocial source of pleasure) then the cost-benefit equation would change. We know from the studies of Gentle (1990) that hens can experience chronic pain from their trimmed beaks, which is presumably the reason that they cease to use them for anything beyond the essential tasks of eating and drinking. This is sufficient reason to enquire whether feather-pecking may be controlled by other, more humane methods.

The question 'Why do hens peck one another?' has received a great deal of study but has not yet generated the sort of answers that can be used to solve the problem. Hens are clearly motivated to establish a 'pecking order' or dominance hierarchy. This is an adaptive form of aggressive agonistic behaviour which should, in a satisfactory environment lead to a stable social community and so avoid further conflict. However, if the hens are so crowded that they cannot escape pecking, or so numerous that they cannot remember their place in the pecking order, then the environment may be said to be at fault. The problem is not, however, that simple. For the hen, the beak is a major tool for investigating the environment so that they peck at all sorts of things, motivated not only by the desire to feed, or acquire nest material, but also by curiosity or simply mindless instinct. An object may be pecked because of its colour, or because it is revealed by a shaft of sunlight and that object may happen to be another hen. Such behaviour is non-aggressive but equally it is non-adaptive, since it carries no obvious advantage to the pecker and clearly reduces the overall fitness of the flock. It is easier to control the problem posed by such 'mindless' feather pecking when hens are kept in small groups in battery cages in buildings without windows than when they are kept in large colonies in barns or with access to free-range, partly because of population numbers and partly through control of lighting.

This presents one of the classical dilemmas in farm animal welfare. If hens in flocks of commercial size are to be protected from suffering due to feather pecking they must either be confined in small groups in controlled environment houses (though not necessarily in the conventional battery cage) or beak-trimmed before they are given the freedom to live in colonies in enriched environments. In the more 'natural' circumstances of 6-12 hens in a back yard, feather-pecking may still occur, even to the point of cannibalism. However, such hens can be recognized as individuals and rescued by their owner.

The origins of tail-biting in pigs are also unclear but this, too, is almost certainly not aggressive in intent. Many cases may be attributed, in the first instance to frustration of the motivation to suck in the early-weaned pig, exacerbated by boredom or restlessness associated with chronic discomfort (if, for example, the pig house is cold or draughty). The incidence of tail-biting is lower when pigs are housed on straw than on concrete, presumably because the pigs are both more comfortable and can gain oral satisfaction from rooting. On the other hand, partial amputation of the tail does not guarantee protection from tail-biting. I would not recommend a ban on tail-docking of pigs as an abuse of welfare because, in present circumstances, it could do more harm than good. I do, however, believe that tail-biting is a symptom of an unsatisfactory husbandry system which implies that tail-docking is a crude and ineffective solution to a problem that can be addressed by other, more humane means.

The nature of fear

Fear, like pain, is a complex and highly subjective emotion that cannot properly be encapsulated within a single-sentence definition. Fear is a conscious, rational and emotional response to a perceived threat that acts as a powerful motivator to action designed, where possible, to evade that threat. It is also an educational experience, since the memory of previous threats, action taken in response to those threats and the consequences ('was it as bad or worse than anticipated?') will obviously determine whether the experience will be more or less fearful next time around. In attempting to understand the nature of fear in animals we should not necessarily assume that they feel fear in the same way as we do. We can, however, begin by analysing the origins and expressions of fear in ourselves and then proceed to compare these sensations and reactions with the physiology and behaviour of animals in similar circumstances. My main source of reference for this section is Jeffrey Gray, *The Psychology of Fear and Stress* (1987). In Fig. 6.2 I attempt to illustrate some of the essential properties of fear that may be common to man and sentient animals.

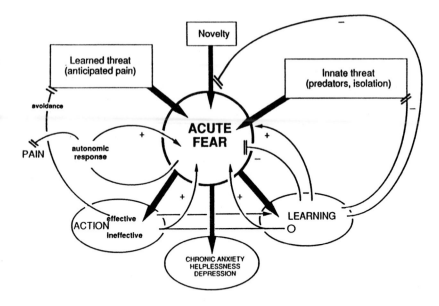

Fig. 6.2 Origins of fear and responses to fear in animals.

The things that frighten man may be divided into five categories:

(1) novelty: strange objects, sudden movements;
(2) innate fears: isolation, fear of the dark, snakes, spiders;
(3) fears learned by experience: anticipated pain, ridicule;
(4) signs of fear in others;
(5) fear of the future: assault, age, death.

Robert Burns recognized the fundamental difference between the nature of fear in man and animals.

> '...thou art blest, compared wi' me!
> the present only touches thee:
> But Och! I backward cast my e'e,
> on prospects drear.
> An' forward tho' I canna see,
> I guess and fear!'

To be more prosaic, I believe that non-human animals do not suffer chronic, existential fears of inevitable future distress, such as ageing, incapacity and death. They are also spared the anxiety which we may feel when we read or hear of threats of which we have no personal experience. There is good evidence to show that threats where the risk is very low (like mugging) or negligible (like a nuclear holocaust or death from 'mad cow disease') tend to induce a higher degree of anxiety in man than threats where the risk is real and close to home, like health risks from smoking or traffic accidents. Fear of death from 'mad cow disease' does depend upon literacy, and the media who prosper by fanning the fires of human fear, but it is, in essence, an expression of the first, most primitive of the fears listed above, namely the fear of the unknown.

At birth, of course, nothing is known and all is novelty. As I have indicated earlier, birds, mammals and human babies appear to be born with little sense of fear but a large amount of curiosity. This motivates the young animal to explore the environment, usually under the protection of a parent. The animal not only learns what does and does not constitute a threat but also progressively reduces the probability that it will encounter a truly novel experience. With increasing age, this innate sense of curiosity is progressively replaced by an innate sense of anxiety, so that an animal becomes increasingly cautious when faced by the unknown. This obviously increases its chances of survival. However, if it does not get the opportunity to experience the normal sights, sounds and smells of, for example, a farm or a city street while it is young, it is more likely to experience fear when faced by these novel experiences in later life and these acute fears may lead to chronic anxiety neuroses.

The second category of threats relates to innate fears. Humans and chimpanzees are frightened by snakes and in both cases this fear is innate; it occurs in individuals who have no direct experience of, or information concerning, the consequences of getting bitten. Certain species, such as the sheep, are innately frightened by isolation. These fears are intrinsic to the genetic makeup of the individual or species. The expression of this genetic fear may not be present at birth but develops during the process of maturation. We may assume that most prey species have an innate fear of their predator species. It is possible to identify and take recordings from single sensory nerves in the brainstem of sheep which identify objects and images of objects within broad categories, like food. For example, the sight of hay, or a bowl of sheep nuts, or a picture of a bowl of sheep nuts will, at some stage in the process of interpreting sensory images, be transmitted as a single item of information (namely food) and subsequently refined in the context of other incoming signals and, of course, memory. Another set of sensory nerves groups dogs and men (or pictures of dogs and men) into a single category, which may reasonably be called that of predator. The conclusion that most animal species have, for sound Darwinian reasons, evolved an innate fear of man as predator is reinforced by exceptions such as the penguin whose experience of man has been too short, and insufficiently threatening, for such a sense to evolve. Extending this argument, we may assume that animals are unlikely, as yet, to have evolved an innate fear of machines. They may fear them as novel objects or on the basis of previous experience. However, there is good evidence that broiler chickens express less fear when 'harvested' into travelling crates by machine than when the same operation is carried out by men.

The third category of fear arises as the result of a learned threat, i.e. it is acquired by experience. The dog that has had an unpleasant experience in a veterinary surgery will display fear when it is taken back. This is an example of the greatest and most primitive of learned fears, the anticipation of pain. The dog that is taken back to boarding kennels prior to the annual family holiday may display a rather more advanced form of learned fear in anticipation of desertion and isolation.

The final category of fear common to man and sentient animals is that engendered by the sight, sound or smell of fear in others of the same species. This sense is presumably largely innate and depends on the recognition of cues which may be species-specific. Young animals may learn to avoid danger by associating specific experiences, which did them no actual harm, with the expression of fear in their parents. The expression of fear, whether by posture, facial expression, sound, smell or action, clearly has survival value for the species.

To return to Fig. 6.2, an animal may experience an acute sense of fear when faced by an innate or learned threat, or simply by the unknown. This acute sense of fear will motivate the animal to action designed to reduce the threat, if possible – by running away, for example, from a predator. The fear will also become a learning experience. The animal will remember the source of the threat, what action it took, and what happened next. If the action was successful in avoiding the threat, or if the fear induced by the threat proved to be unfounded since no harm was done, then the animal will feel less fear when the experience recurs. The impala that repeatedly escapes without injury from the charge of the leopard, or the fox that repeatedly escapes without injury from the hounds may become less fearful, although equally cautious, in situations where it perceives itself to be at risk.

Fear also induces autonomic, hormone-mediated responses in animals and man such as sweating and an increased heart rate. There is an inadequate circular argument which postulates that these reflex, autonomic responses are themselves the source of the conscious sensation of fear. Although this is clearly not the whole truth, these autonomic responses to the original threat can create an element of positive feedback which heightens the acute sense of fear and so increases the animal's motivation to do something about it. Fear also triggers the release of endorphins in the central nervous system which reduce the immediate sensation of pain. The advantage of this is obvious. In the words of Jeffrey Gray (1987) 'the time to lick your wounds is when danger has passed'.

All aspects of acute fear and response to threat discussed thus far can be said to be adaptive and therefore a 'good thing'. There are circumstances, however, where the animal may be unable to exploit its acute sense of fear to resolve the threat. This may occur when:

(1) the action taken by the animal fails to remove the threat or the consequent pain;
(2) the animal cannot take effective action, because it is confined or overcrowded;

(3)   the animal is uncertain whether the perceived threat (the conditioning stimulus) will or will not lead to pain, or uncertain what action to take to avoid that pain.

The dog that is regularly whipped by its drunken owner will experience increasing fear as it learns that it can neither escape nor prevent the assault by a display of submission. The sow that is regularly attacked by other sows will experience more fear when all are confined in a pen than free-ranging in a wood. The laboratory rat that is required to perform actions in response to a signal such as a red or green light, either for reward or to escape punishment, will display increasing signs of fear and autonomic indications of chronic stress, such as increased adrenal activity, if it is uncertain whether the signal it sees or the action it takes will lead to a food reward or an electric shock. If an animal is repeatedly exposed to any of these situations in which it cannot take action to resolve its fear, or is prevented from taking action, or does not know what action to take, then acute fear may proceed through chronic anxiety to the condition called *learned helplessness* by animal psychologists but which corresponds closely to chronic pathological depression in man. In these circumstances animals and humans lose appetite, body condition, curiosity and the motivation to control their immediate environment. Whereas acute fear, in moderation, may be healthy and instructive, chronic anxiety or depression must be considered a profound form of suffering.

Stress and the general adaptation syndrome

Stress is a portmanteau word which crops up regularly in discussions of problems of animal welfare within phrases such as 'weaning stress' or 'transport stress'. The first, obvious problem is that the word stress, like the word disease, lacks specificity. It signifies that the animal has been presented with some sort of challenge to its welfare but it does not indicate the nature of the challenge and so gives no pointers as to how it might be resolved. It is also false to assume that exposure to stress necessarily causes suffering; the animal may adapt its behaviour or its physiology in such a way as to remove or, at least, accommodate the stress without incurring much more than a mild inconvenience. There is a third, semantic problem which is that the word is commonly used both to describe the stimulus (e.g. cold) and the response (e.g. hypothermia). All in all, it is a word that I tend to avoid wherever possible unless I can incorporate it into a more comprehensive analysis of a problem. Faced, for example, by the question 'Is it stressful to wean piglets from their mother at three weeks of age?' I would identify, at least, the following potential problems:

(1)   an abrupt change in diet, possibly leading to hunger, indigestion or food allergies;

(2)   a move from warm, bedded accomodation to a cold cage;

(3) exposure, and reduced immunity to microorganisms associated (especially) with gastrointestinal infection;
(4) withdrawal of the mother's contribution to security and education;
(5) fear of novelty or aggression from exposure to pigs from other litters.

It should be apparent that this analysis of what is meant by the phrase 'weaning stress' has followed the logic of the five freedoms.

The word stress can, however, be used in a specific sense, to define the 'general adaptation syndrome', an expression first used by Hans Selye to describe common features of the response of animals to a wide range of physical, or psychological stimuli which he called 'stressors'. The response of an animal exposed to a physical stressor such as cold, or a psychological stressor such as fear, will first be one of *alarm*, then proceed towards *adaptation*. However, if the intensity or duration of the stressor exceeds the capacity of the animal to adapt, the response will proceed to the third stage, that of *exhaustion* (Fig. 6.3).

In the initial *alarm* phase, the animal will increase secretion of hormones from the adrenal cortex (e.g. cortisol) and medulla (e.g. adrenaline). These hormones are designed to condition the animal for immediate action by switching the flow of blood and nutrients from long-term goals like growth towards immediate problems like fight or flight. Since increased secretion of adrenocortical hormones, typically cortisol, is a constant feature of the alarm response, concentrations of cortisol in the blood or saliva of animals are regularly used as a so-called 'objective' index of stress. However, this approach not only fails to differentiate between physiological and psychological stimuli to the alarm response (e.g. cold and fear respectively) but it can also fail to distinguish between alarm as a potential source of suffering, and excitement as a potential source of pleasure.

Some years ago I examined a thesis which described a study of 'transport stress' in veal calves. An early experiment demonstrated a significant elevation in plasma cortisol concentration in these calves during transportation and this was taken to indicate that the calves were stressed (and suffered) while in transit. However, a subsequent experiment revealed an even greater elevation in cortisol concentration when the calves received their twice-daily feeds of milk replacer. This was attributed to the excitement (and pleasure) of feeding. Now both these conclusions are entirely reasonable. However, suppose the animals on experiment had been pet dogs which appear to derive great excitement from a ride in a car, especially if they anticipate that it will lead to a walk in the country. In this case we would interpret the increases in cortisol concentration as indicating that a ride in a car was almost as exciting as a good meal. If we now attempt to interpret the calf data without prejudice, we have to accept the possibility that the veal calves found a ride in a lorry to be almost as exciting as a good feed. The moral of this rather silly story is that in this and many other examples in the stress literature, cortisol concentrations do not

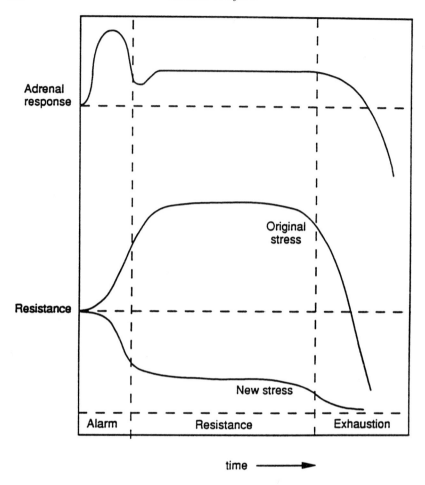

Fig. 6.3 The general adaptation syndrome.

represent an objective indicator of stress, but are being interpreteted *a posteriori* in an attempt to impart a gloss of apparent scientific respectability on impressions that may be entirely subjective.

Obviously stresses such as hunger, cold, pain and fear are associated with changes in the secretion rates and concentrations of hormones and other chemical transmitters in the blood and central nervous system. There is no doubt that a judicious selection of measurements of compounds such as corticosteroids, endorphins and vasoactive polypeptides, can contribute to the interpretation of the nature and intensity of a particular physiological or psychological stress but only when these are considered in association with a range of other distinct approaches based, for example, on observations of behaviour, motivation and aversion, responses to drugs etc. according to the 'triangulation' approach that I described in Chapter 5.

The *alarm* reaction describes, in essence, a rapid change in physiological state in response to an acute stressor. If the stressor persists or recurs at frequent intervals, the alarm response will proceed to that of *adaptation*, whereby the animal will accommodate the stressor but at some continued physiological or metabolic cost (Fig. 6.3). If an animal is chronically exposed to cold, it must sustain an increased metabolic rate in order to preserve homeothermy (see Fig. 4.1). This will be regulated, in part, by increased secretion of adrenal hormones and will, inevitably, divert nutrients from synthetic processes like growth or reproduction to meet the increased demand for energy to sustain heat production. In this simple example, the animal has achieved its primary objective, maintenance of homeothermy, but at some cost to its performance (e.g. growth, reproduction). The extent to which its welfare may be compromised during this adaptation phase will depend on:

(1) whether, after adaptation, the perceived intensity of cold or sensations related to cold (e.g. hunger) are sufficient to induce suffering;
(2) whether the animal can sustain fitness in the face of the chronic challenge from the stressor.

One category of synthetic processes that may be suppressed during both the alarm and adaptation phases of the general adaptation syndrome is the synthesis of cells and proteins of the immune system. An animal may successfully cope with the chronic stress of cold but display a suppressed immune response to subsequent infection and so be more susceptible to disease.

This is not the place for a detailed examination of the complex physiological and immunological responses to stressors such as cold or undernutrition. It is, however, important to consider the extent to which the general adaptation syndrome may be triggered by, and used as an indicator of, psychological stress. Christian (1970) conducted a classic series of experiments to investigate the responses of wild and laboratory strains of male mice to overcrowding induced simply by increasing the number of animals per cage. In both strains, increasing population density increased adrenal weights but reduced body weights and the weights of the thymus (associated, simplistically with the immune response), the testes and accessory sex glands. In these and other similar experiments the chronic stress of overcrowding reduced both fertility and life expectancy. It was, in effect, acting as a population regulator. The extent of stress experienced by an individual appears to be related not only to the number of agonistic encounters that it experiences but also to its place in the pecking order. The subordinate animal, or the animal that submits following an agonistic encounter because it is not defending its home territory appears to be the more stressed (according to its adrenal response) even if it repeatedly escapes without injury. This is clear experimental proof that a chronic psychological stressor can impair welfare both by inducing suffering and by compromising sustained fitness.

When man rears animals for strictly commercial purposes, whether on the farm or in the laboratory, he is motivated by economic pressures to stock them as densely as possible. The first constraint against overstocking in most normal circumstances is that of infectious disease. As stocking density increases so too does the opportunity for transmission of infectious disease. This may affect health and welfare at stocking densities below that likely to induce social stresses. However, when man is able to control infectious disease in densely stocked animals by use of vaccines (e.g. broiler chickens and laying hens) or antibiotics (e.g. growing pigs), or by rearing minimal-disease strains in protected environments (e.g. pigs or laboratory rats and mice), then the intensity of social stress may become sufficient to cause suffering to the animals.

Social stress may or may not be associated with a reduction in performance of the population and an economic loss to their owner. One of the standard arguments in favour of intensive farming systems is usually expressed as 'If they weren't happy they wouldn't grow so well'. This claim shares the faults of all attempts to encapsulate problems of animal welfare within a single sentence. It can also distort the truth. For example, the optimal productivity of a house full of broiler chickens is achieved at stocking densities and growth rates that cause ill-health and suffering to (at least) some of the individual birds. Reducing stocking density and growth rate would increase the fitness of the individual birds but reduce output and thus the income of the farmer. In this example optimal welfare clearly does not equate with optimal productivity. On the other hand, any critique of the welfare of animals in intensive systems that fails to demonstrate a reduction in health, growth rate or reproductive success in a significant proportion of the population will be weakened by its failure to provide evidence of these classic symptoms of stress.

Although the general adaptation syndrome is, by definition, non-specific, it does indicate that an animal is faced by a challenge to its welfare, and measurements such as cortisol concentrations, in association – for example – with measures of the effectiveness of the immune system, can give an indication of the intensity of the challenge. It cannot, in the absence of other information, diagnose the nature of the challenge (e.g. hunger, cold, pain, fear, crowding, etc.) so cannot indicate exactly how it should be resolved.

One feature of the lack of specificity inherent in the general adaptation syndrome is of profound importance in the context of animal welfare, namely the fact that the effects of different stressors appear to be additive. In an elegantly designed factorial experiment Stanley Curtis exposed growing chickens to a variety of potential stressors (e.g. protein deficiency, cold, infection, crowding, noise, repeated handling, etc.) and measured growth rates and adrenal and immune responses characteristic of the general adaptation syndrome. Analysis of the results of this factorial experiment first identified that some stimuli such as noise, did not constitute a chronic stress.

It also demonstrated that the effects of physiological stimuli (such as cold) and psychological stimuli (such as crowding) were additive. This is consistent with the multidimensional nature of MacFarland's model (Fig. 2.2) of the problems that an animal has to resolve if it is to stay within the limits of its capacity to avoid, or adapt to stressors without suffering. It also reinforces, yet again, my constant argument that animal welfare must not be defined in terms of single stimuli but interpreted in terms of the animals' ability to cope with all sensations that may determine suffering and all stimuli that may determine sustained fitness.

The company of their kind

It is a truth universally acknowledged within the literature and legislation on animal welfare that animals should be given 'the company of their own kind' so that they may have the (fourth) freedom to express normal social behaviour. It may seem churlish to question a freedom that appears so self-evident but it is in the nature of social intercourse where man differs most widely from that of the other animals. This is not least because man's actions are motivated and his feelings influenced to a unique degree by his awareness of the concepts of self and non-self, strategic advantage and morality. In addressing the questions 'When and why do animals need the company of other animals?' it is more than ever necessary to keep the argument simple and avoid anthropomorphism.

Keeping things very simple indeed, I list five reasons why an animal may need the company of another animal (not necessarily of its own kind, or species) and why it might suffer in its absence:

(1)   for sexual intercourse;
(2)   for security;
(3)   for cooperation, e.g. in provision of food or shelter;
(4)   for education;
(5)   for pleasure.

All these five reasons why a sentient, non-human animal should need the company of another animal are based on the principle of self-interest, i.e. each animal attempts to use all other animals to promote its own sense of well-being and/or promote the sustained fitness of itself and the inheritors of its genes. (The analysis of motivation is so much easier when it does not have to invoke morality!)

The motivation to sexual intercourse is primitive, powerful and, at the time, will override other powerful primitive emotions such as hunger and fear. It is also a primary source of animal conflict, especially between competing males, and a potential source of future suffering, especially for mothers and offspring faced by overcrowding and starvation. Man has recognized that full freedom of sexual expression is undesirable both for his/

her own species and for those animals within his/her dominion. It is, however, important to enquire whether a particular class of animal will *suffer* as a consequence of sexual denial, simply as a subset of the general question, central to the whole of this book, namely 'Can the cost of sexual denial be justified by the benefit to the animal itself, to the population of animals within that species, and to man?'

Since man usually controls populations of wild animals by selective culling rather than selective breeding, this question has most relevance to our treatment of farm animals and pets. Females are not motivated to sexual intercourse unless they are 'on heat', i.e. influenced by internal signals from sex hormones around the time of ovulation. In most species of pet and farm animal, adult males have the potential to be motivated to mate at any time but, in general, need to be aroused by the presence of a female in heat. To a large extent, out of sight (or out of smell), is out of mind. The female in heat, or the male in the presence of a female in heat, will display extreme signs of frustration if denied the opportunity to mate. The stimuli are both external and internal; i.e the presence of a potential mate and the drive from the sex hormones. If the external stimulus is absent the frustration may exist but at a much lower intensity. Removal of the internal stimulus by castration or ovariectomy massively reduces the motivation to mate (although it may not always eliminate it; gelded horses sometimes continue to copulate). If neutering an animal reduces its level of frustration and has no other untoward effects, then it is reasonable to argue that it can be used not only to control breeding for the convenience of man but also, in some circumstances, as a humane approach to improve the overall quality of life for animals – for example, a few sex-mad male dogs and most female cats (see Chapter 10).

Most gregarious species of animals need other members of their species for security and so will suffer fear of isolated. Sheep, for example, will almost always attempt to stay in close contact with the flock, especially when faced by a perceived predator such as a sheepdog. Having been somewhat dismissive earlier about the interpretation of measurements of plasma cortisol concentrations, I am now obliged to point out that cortisol levels in sheep have been shown to be elevated more by the act of isolation than by the sight of another sheep being killed and bled out. The company of an animal's own kind is, for many species, essential to freedom from fear. Solitary species such as the tiger are obvious exceptions to this rule. However, man has tended to domesticate herding species like cattle or sheep, or those with extended families like the wolf or dog. Such animals need the presence of companions if they are to avoid suffering and promote their self-interest.

Examples of cooperation designed to promote personal well-being and sustained fitness of the population are seen throughout the animal kingdom. Within insect populations such as ants and bees the cooperation is instinctive. The cohabitation of some species, e.g. grazing animals with birds such as oxpeckers and cattle egrets can also be said to be cooperative, but this too is an unwitting symbiosis. In the context of animal mind and animal suffering we should only consider those circumstances where animals make a conscious decision to cooperate and may suffer if this cooperation is denied. The most striking examples of conscious cooperation are those seen in species which select mates and stay together, sometimes for life, so that they may cooperatively rear their offspring. Such cooperation is normal behaviour for most species of birds but most unusual among the mammals, being restricted to man and a few other species that tend to form extended family groups, like New World primates (e.g. cottontop tamarins) and some carnivores such as lions, wolves and wild dogs. In all these examples the cooperation involves both the protection of the family and the sharing of food. Such cooperation is reinforced by bonding behaviour which may, without incurring accusations of anthropomophism, be called displays of affection. Furthermore, loss of the chosen mate appears to provoke distress.

For most of the mammals, however, there is very little evidence for cooperation, even in the most gregarious of species. This applies to most farm animals such as horses, cattle, sheep, pigs, and pets such as cats, rats, guinea pigs. Domesticated dogs seldom cooperate with each other, although they have descended from a cooperative species. They will, however, cooperate with man as guide dogs or sheepdogs, for example, feral dogs revert to hunting in packs.

One of the prime reasons why animals need the presence of others of their species is so that they may learn from them. Clearly, young birds and mammals learn from their parents and this education improves their ability to sustain their wellbeing. They will learn not only primitive skills like foraging, hunting and how to avoid danger, but also social skills designed to smooth their interactions with other members of their own species. There is good experimental evidence to show that pigeons have the ability to learn classical operant conditioning procedures, like pressing bars to obtain food, by observation of trained demonstrators or even video images of trained demonstrators. There is also some evidence that birds such as pigeons and hens learn faster when they recognize the demonstrator to be above them in the pecking order. This could be taken to imply an advanced state of social awareness, i.e. birds placing more value on the actions of dominant than submissive birds.. It could equally occur because the observers spend more time watching dominant birds in the interests of their own comfort and security.

The capacity of different species and different individuals to learn from one another or to interpret complex or abstract symbols is one of the most useful indicators of the complexity of their minds. In the context of the present argument it is only necessary to point out that animals are more likely to suffer if they are denied the opportunity for education in youth and much of this education is likely to come from other members of their species. To give just two examples: lambs that are orphaned at birth and artifically reared often neglect their own offspring. Puppies that have been isolated from contact with other dogs during a critical 'socialization' period between weaning at eight weeks and completion of a vaccination programme against distemper etc. at 14 weeks often fail to develop the typically cheerful approach of the dog to its social life and become neurotically aggressive or shy.

One of the most effective forms of education for a young animal is play. Pedantic behaviourists may claim that the role of play in young animals is entirely educational but it requires a very strange and stern mind to conclude that puppies, kittens or lambs at play are not having fun. This conclusion brings me neatly to the last category of possible reasons why an animal may need the company of others and suffer from their absence. Staying cool, I would define this as the motivation of one animal to favour the company of another selected individual to enhance its own pleasure. If this behaviour is to be successful on a sustained basis it is likely that this pleasure will have to be mutual. There can be no doubt that some animals form and sustain social bonds for reasons that are not linked to the sexual need to mate or rear offspring nor, to any great degree, to the need for security, but simply because they appear to enjoy each others company. In brief, some animals can form friendships. Before hard-headed scientists accuse me of hopelessly sentimental anthropomorphism, I shall add quickly that I think this motivation for social behaviour is rare. Most non-sexual bonds between pairs or small groups of animals can be attributed to primitive needs, like security, and much play, in young animals, is primarily directed towards personal satisfaction – the individuality of the playmates does not really matter. However, horses and especially donkeys appear to form close bonds with favoured individuals (i.e. friendships) and suffer if these bonds are broken.

Dogs are very special. I suggest that they are perhaps the only animal species that actually forms friendships with (or loves) man. All other species that we have domesticated, whether to eat, ride, flaunt or love, have adapted to human contact in a way simply and coolly designed to favour their own well-being. Thus they will work for man, or do a variety of more or less pointless tricks for a utilitarian reward like food or to avoid punishment. The dog is, I believe, the only animal species that will run itself ragged simply to give pleasure; to induce an expression of satisfaction in its human master. Once again, this is interpreted by behaviourists as an extended form of infantile behaviour in a species that, in the wild, formed extended family groups with a well-defined hierarchal structure. That is as may be but it cannot be denied that this intensity of affection uniquely exposes the dog to the possibility of both suffering and pleasure.

Part III
Advocacy:
What We Can Do For Them

Constructive approaches to the problem of man's dominion over the animals

'Until he extends the circle of his compassion to all living things,
man will not himself find peace.'

Albert Schweitzer

7 The Workers: Farm Animals

'Knock, knock! Who's there in the name of Beelzebub?
Here's a farmer that hanged himself on the expectation of plenty.'

William Shakespeare, *Macbeth*

The dissertation on animal welfare now proceeds from analysis to advocacy. In Part II, I examined the sensations, moods and experiences that affect how animals feel and so determine the quality of their lives. In Part III, I shall consider what we can and should do to be fair to those animals over whom we have dominion; in other words, how we can best reconcile what we want from other animals with a proper and effective concern for their quality of life. In a comprehensive analysis of potential welfare problems faced by the animals within our dominion, each species would require its own book. I shall therefore be deliberately selective, concentrating on those problems and those species which, I believe, require the most urgent attention.

Some recapitulation is necessary at this stage. The welfare of any animal is determined by the state of its mind and body; how it feels within a spectrum that ranges from suffering to pleasure and its ability to sustain physical and mental fitness. If an animal is to achieve a sense of mental wellbeing, its physical and social environment should allow it to act to avoid hunger, thirst, heat, cold, pain, sickness, fear, frustration, exhaustion, etc. before the intensity of these potential sources of suffering becomes too severe. If it is to sustain physical fitness, then imposed methods of breeding, feeding, housing and any artificial manipulations should not be allowed to compromise its ability to live its allotted, maybe brief, life span without suffering from physical problems such as chronic pain, hunger or exhaustion.

Much of Part III deals with the current welfare state of the animals we raise for food and offers specific proposals as to how we might improve their welfare within the realistic constraints of commercial agriculture. This emphasis reflects not only the intensity of the physiological demands and environmental constraints imposed on individual farm animals but also the sheer scale of the problem. The number of animals killed for human food consumption is huge and, like most huge numbers, difficult to grasp. Perhaps the best way to personalize the magnitude of the livestock industry is to point out that in a lifetime of 70 years, the average British citizen will consume some 550 poultry, 36 pigs, 36 sheep and 8 oxen plus 10 000 eggs and dairy products (milk, butter, cheese, etc.) equivalent to 18 tonnes of milk. For a population of 60 million, meat consumption alone equates to an annual slaughter of 470 million poultry, 31 million pigs, 31 million sheep and 7 million cattle. To bring the importance of farm animals to the whole welfare debate into even sharper focus, I would add that for each British citizen who lives to 70 years, thanks, in part, to scientific advances in nutrition and medicine, the number of mice sacrificed in scientific experiments is two!

Food animals as a commodity

Farm animals are conventionally described as livestock. The very expression 'live stock', which I shall adopt with some regret, implies that we view both food of animal origin and the animals that provide that food as a commodies. Like all commodities, the food and the animals are taken for granted when plentiful and cheap but become highly valued when in short supply. Although the number of practising vegetarians or vegans in the developed world is large and growing, it is an inescapable fact of life that the great majority of humans who can afford to do so, prefer to eat diets which include meat, eggs and dairy products, so that the rich nations consume far more of such foods than the poor. A typical British supermarket contains a seductively wide choice of food products of animal origin. Consumers entering the supermarket to buy meat, eggs or dairy products, primarily to meet their essential need for food, will select individual products within the wide range of commodities available according to some or all of the following criteria:

(1) expectation of a good meal: (i.e. perception of eating quality of food based on appearance and past experience);
(2) perceived value for money (i.e. cost relative to competing products);
(3) convenience (e.g. ease of storage and cooking);
(4) health considerations (e.g. risks of obesity, food poisoning, cardio-vascular disease);
(5) animal welfare considerations.

The first question to ask in this context is 'To what extent do animal welfare considerations affect consumer choice?' In the last thirty years, since the publication of Ruth Harrison's seminal book *Animal Machines*, there has been a steady increase in public concern for the welfare standards of farm animals. The most severe criticism has been directed at the most intensive forms of production, namely egg production from hens in battery cages, and meat production from pigs, broiler chickens and veal calves. Production of beef and lamb has received much less criticism, mainly because it presents a more natural image of animals in fields eating grass. These welfare concerns have been expressed most vigorously in Western Europe yet, within the same last thirty years, *per capita* consumption of meat in Western Europe has remained relatively static. There has been a decline in the consumption of red meats such as beef and lamb, but this has been matched by an increase in consumption of pig and, especially, poultry meat. *The systems of meat production that attract most criticism on welfare grounds are those that attract most custom in the supermarket.* The main reasons for the relative increase in consumption of pig and poultry meat are that these products have progressively become seen to offer better value than beef or lamb. They are cheaper. They are perceived to be healthier, largely because they are lower in fat, and they are attractively and conveniently presented in such a way as to offer the reliable promise of a quick, tasty meal. These real incentives to select chicken or pork in preference to beef or lamb are overriding any tendency to reject these products for reasons relating to animal welfare. White veal is a special case which I shall discuss in Chapter 9.

There is, of course, no such thing as the standard consumer. Many readers of this book may already try to incorporate a proper concern for farm animal welfare into their food buying habits. Supermarkets and other food stores do sell a range of products from animals on the basis of a quality assurance that they have been reared in conditions superior to the minimal welfare standards prescribed by law and outlined in the UK Codes of Welfare for Livestock. Audrey Eyton in her book, *The Kind Food Guide*, gives details of these products and where they may be purchased. The Royal Society for the Prevention of Cruelty to Animals (RSPCA) has recently introduced 'Freedom Foods', which offers the assurance that producers have agreed:

(1) to operate according to improved standards of welfare for animals on the farm, in transit and at the point of slaughter;
(2) to accept regular inspections to ensure that these standards are maintained.

Such schemes are based on a realistic approach to improving farm animal welfare. They do not fall into the trap of 'impossibilism', i.e. seeking too much and ending up with nothing. Unfortunately, they are catering for a small minority. None of the 'high welfare' product lines has yet, to my knowledge, sustained a market penetration in excess of 10%, and most fall very far short of this modest target. Perhaps the most intensively criticized of all forms of food production from animals, namely egg production from laying hens in battery cages still accounts for over 90% of all egg consumption in the UK. Short-term 'blips' in consumption of battery eggs have not been linked to welfare concerns but to transient and frequently misguided health scares, e.g. fear of infection by *salmonella*, or the assumed dangers of dietary cholesterol. These fears tend to reduce overall egg consumption but promote a short-lived, relative increase in the consumption of free-range eggs on the even more misguided assumption that such eggs are somehow healthier.

We cannot escape the conclusion that the majority remain content to eat battery eggs and broiler chickens, more so than beef or lamb, which indicates that while their concern for animal welfare may be real it is not paramount. I repeat, the systems that arouse most concern on welfare grounds, namely pig and poultry production, are those that are achieving the greatest success in the market by meeting consumer demands for eating quality, convenience and value for money.

The farm animal welfare movement has generated a great deal of anguish among a great number of consumers (and farmers!) but it has not, as yet, had any significant influence on the quality of life for the vast majority of animals reared for food. The number of people who take the extreme position and become vegan, or at least vegetarian for humanitarian reasons has increased and may continue to increase and this will reduce the number of animals raised for food. This will have no direct impact on the welfare of those that are still being reared for meat. However, the vegetarian argument can affect animal welfare indirectly by persuading meat eaters to think. My favourite vegetarian, hearing that I was preparing a paper on the ethics of meat eating (Webster, 1994), suggested 'That should be brief. There are none. You can only do it if you don't think about it at all.' I don't agree, but she has a point. My own position is that the exploitation of animals, for any reason, can only be justified if we think very hard about about what we are doing and how they, the animals, feel about it. This is why I believe that real improvements in welfare for the majority of farm animals are most likely to come from pressure exerted by the minority who are prepared to eat food of animal origin but demand higher standards of both quality and welfare for their meat, milk and eggs. At present, this minority is small, often poorly informed and dangerously vulnerable to con-men. They may, however, be *right* and that is something to build on.

If we are to achieve significant improvements in animal welfare within commercial, largely intensive systems of livestock production we need, first, to examine, without prejudice, how and why livestock farming has got to the point where it is today; why, for example, intensification has been so commercially successful and what are the special welfare problems faced by animals in modern husbandry systems. We can then explore general strategies and specific proposals designed to achieve realistic improvements in animal welfare by one or more of the following means:

(1) improvements to husbandry systems that are economically competitive within a consumer-led economy;
(2) education of the consumer to demand improved production standards based on a perception of welfare that is as close as possible to that of the animals themselves;
(3) legislation to achieve improved minimum standards for animal welfare when these cannot be achieved through the operation of the free market.

Costs and benefits in livestock production

In a free market there are consumers who use products (or 'goods') and there are resources from which products are made. The successful product within a competing set (e.g. alternative foods) is that which the consumer prefers and this, in essence, means that which is seen to provide most benefit, measured in terms of nutrition, taste or fashion, relative to its cost. The successful producer within a competing set (e.g. farmers) is the one who provides best value for money to the consumer at least cost to himself. In a capitalist society, farmers must compete with each other for consumer demand. Inevitably some producers will profit at the expense of others who will fail and go out of farming. This operation of the principle of survival of the fittest benefits the consumer because the producers that survive are those who can offer better (i.e. higher benefit:cost ratio) goods. According to the classic, capitalist, Adam Smith argument, the invisible hand of the market has operated for the general good, in both the economic and moral sense of the word, because everybody is a consumer, including the farmer who benefits from competition to supply the goods that he, too, has to buy. However, the restricted morality of this generic economic argument breaks down when applied to the business of livestock production since this involves a third party, namely the sentient animals involved in the enterprise, who are not consumers and therefore have no mechanism for achieving their needs through the operation of market forces.

Fortunately, no civilized or moral society operates strictly according to the principle of free market economics. There are laws such as the abolition of slavery to protect individuals from unacceptable exploitation and suffering. The intent of anti-slavery legislation was, I believe, entirely altruistic, although it is fair to argue that it has served the interests of the free market since free men can become bigger and better consumers than slaves. There are also laws to protect sentient animals from 'unnecessary suffering' for reasons that may genuinely be called altruistic. The difficulties with such law and practice lie only in defining unnecessary suffering, i.e. in deciding where lines should be drawn. Here, as elsewhere, my argument and advocacy will not be based on absolutes but on analysis of cost:benefit ratios, where costs and benefits are considered in relation to the consumer, the farmer, the sustainability of the land and, of course, the welfare of the animals we rear to provide us with commodities such as food and clothing.

Figure 7.1 illustrates, in very general terms, the principles that relate increasing productivity to cost and benefit for the farmer and for his animals. Since the figure relates to all forms of livestock production, extensive and intensive, meat, milk or eggs, the units on both axes must be arbitrary. The farmer must meet two types of cost: fixed and variable. Variable costs are broadly those involved in the rearing of each animal, e.g. feeding and stock replacement, and must set against income from the sale of goods from each animal to define gross profit margin. Fixed costs are for overheads such as housing, labour and debt repayment, which must be paid at the same rate, independent of marginal changes in output or gross profit margins. Figure 7.1(a) shows variable costs increasing at an accelerating rate with increasing productivity. This is largely determined by the cost of feed since the more

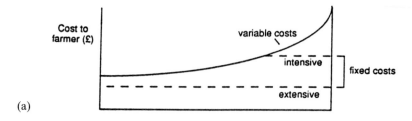

(a)

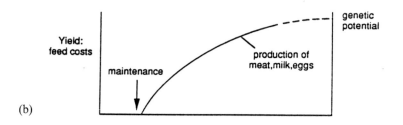

(b)

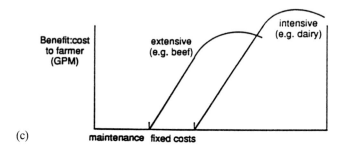

(c)

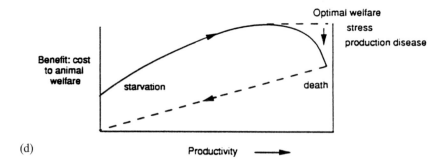

(d)

Fig. 7.1 The costs and benefits of increasing productivity to farmers and their animals.

productive animal not only requires more food, it usually requires higher quality and therefore more expensive food. Fixed costs are shown as two horizontal lines. They are usually low for extensive systems (such as beef production from cattle on range) where the animals largely fend for themselves, and high for systems which require expensive buildings, machinery and labour, such as dairy production.

An animal will not begin to yield an output of saleable product such as lean meat, milk or eggs until it is fed in excess of maintenance. Thereafter, the efficiency of production, namely the ratio of output to feed and other variable costs increases sharply as the increasing yield (e.g. of milk) offsets the cost of maintenance (Fig 7.1(b)). The output of milk, lean tissue growth, etc. has a theoretical maximum which is determined by the genetic potential, of the animal. Moreover, as animals approach their genetic potential output of saleable product relative to input of food tends to decline as the animal partitions an increasing proportion of nutrients into its own body fat reserves relative to saleable products like lean meat, milk, or eggs.

Figure 7.1(c) illustrates the effect of increasing productivity on the ratio of benefit:cost for the farmer. These curves are derived from the first two sets describing costs and output relative to feed costs. The farmer makes no profit at all until he has first met the fixed costs of his farm and the maintenance costs of his animals. Thereafter the ratio of benefit:cost rises sharply with increasing productivity. Eventually this curve turns over and starts to decrease because costs increase with increasing productivity at an accelerating rate but output at a decelerating rate. These curves also show that when fixed costs are relatively low, as in extensive systems, optimal benefit:cost for the farmer can be achieved at a relatively low level of output. The farmer, for example, who overfeeds his beef suckler cows on expensive concentrates, is wasting money since this extra feed will simply make the cows fat; it will not increase their annual output of saleable product above one calf per year. On the other hand, when fixed costs are high, as in dairy production or intensive pig or poultry production in expensive, controlled environment buildings, the farmer is compelled to operate at a higher level of productivity (i.e. he must work his animals harder) in order to make any profit at all. In these circumstances, optimal efficiency of production is likely to be achieved at a point very close to the genetic limit of the animals.

The argument, so far, assumes that all animals are operating not only as machines, but as machines that will not break down, however fast they are driven. The bottom curve, Fig.7.1(d) illustrates the effect of increasing productivity on the welfare of the animals and is based largely on the approach of John McInerney (1993). Low levels of productivity in farm animals are likely to be associated with low levels of welfare. Feed is poor and housing is poor because both farmer and animals live in poverty. Increasing productivity will, at first, bring benefits to the animals through improvements, for example, to nutrition and environment. The impetus to increase the productivity of breeding sheep by doubling their production from one to two lambs per year has undoubtedly improved the welfare of ewes which are now adequately fed and housed over winter rather than left out hungry on the hills. There comes a point however, above which increasing productivity begins to reduce welfare

(1)   by reducing 'fitness' (e.g. increasing the probability of metabolic or skeletal disorders);
(2)   by reducing quality of life (e.g. due to problems of overcrowding, aggression, chronic pain).

Eventually, in McInerney's model the stress of increasing productivity kills the animal and productivity returns to zero.

When taken together the family of curves in Figure 7.1 becomes a model of the effects of increasing productivity on the welfare of farmers and their animals. As illustrated, it is simple but generic. In subsequent chapters I shall apply these principles to examine benefit:cost ratios in specific circumstances, e.g. for broiler chicken production (Chapter 8) and suggest compromises between the valid needs of the consumer, the farmer and the animal. The most important general conclusion that emerges from Figure 7.1 is that the best way is the middle way. In any debate on animal welfare, someone will invariably claim that extensive systems are necessarily good and intensive systems bad for animal welfare. It should be clear from Figure 7.1 that this claim is not just over-simplistic but fundamentally wrong. It is, however, fair to claim that the greater the amount of capital invested by the farmer, especially into intensive systems, the harder the animals must work to repay that investment.

The impetus for intensification

Having considered theoretical aspects of the relationship between productivity and benefit:cost ratios for the farmer and his animals, I shall now examine some of the practical reasons that led to the intensification of livestock production and discuss, still in general terms, the implications of intensification for quality of life and sustained fitness of the animals, the farmers and the environment. Within traditional, family-scale farming systems, most ruminants destined for meat production were largely expected to look after themselves by foraging for grass and other roughage. These were extensive, low fixed-cost enterprises. The farmer and his family would, however, cut, carry and conserve food for the house cow because they obtained more value from her milk, as food or money. Pigs and poultry were the scavengers who ate food that would otherwise have gone to waste. The young pigs intended for the table or for sale as cured ham were housed in styes and fed on house and farm swill to ensure that they fattened as quickly and as cost-effectively as possible. Breeding sows and chickens would usually be given the run of at least part of the farm, since this enabled them to forage for some of their own food and reduced the cost and labour of housing, bedding and manure disposal. The traditional farmer who allowed pigs and chickens free range on his farm was not being inherently kinder than the modern factory farmer, he was simply adopting the strategy most appropriate to his own circumstances.

These simple principles formed the basis for livestock production from the beginning of agriculture almost to the present day. There have been greater changes in the last 60 years than occurred in all the previous history of agriculture. The greatest pace of change was during a period of about 20 years from the 1950s to the 1970s. The main economic forces driving the intensification of livestock production were:

(1) improved mechanization of agriculture, permitting the bulk movement of feed and manure;
(2) increased profitability of livestock production, based (in some cases) on direct or indirect subsidies, thus permitting capital investment in buildings and equipment;
(3) increasing consumer incomes leading to (i) increased demand for meat, eggs and dairy products and (ii) increased costs of labour relative to costs of feed, fuel, housing and equipment;
(4) increased investment in agricultural research leading to (i) increased efficiency of production in healthy animals and (ii) improved disease control through development of vaccines, antibiotics, etc., thereby enabling animals to be housed at a high stocking density.

In short, livestock farmers were presented with the opportunity to expand production to meet an unprecedented rise in demand and, at the same time, reduce production costs by taking animals off the land and enclosing them in buildings containing machinery to supply their food and remove their excreta. Having made the strategic decision to house his animals, the farmer was then compelled to stock them as densely as possible, not only to maximize output relative to the cost of buildings and equipment but also to minimize feed costs by minimizing the amount of energy expended by the animals in activity and keeping warm (see Fig. 4.2).

Intensification of pig and poultry systems improved the availability and reduced the cost of the products and consumers responded by buying more eggs, poultry and pig meat. The invisible hand of the market wrote clearly that these were better products. It is fashionable to proclaim that meat from the supermarket does not taste as good as meat bought at the farm gate or that battery eggs do not have the taste of those from hens on free range but such dinner table talk belies our actions. The nature of taste preferences is too complex a subject to discuss here but suffice it to say that most alleged differences in taste between 'factory-farm' and free-range products are either non-existent or very small indeed. In practice, they have minimal influence on our buying habits. Whatever we may think as individuals, it is an inescapable economic truth that the 'best' product is simply that which most people wish to buy when they are given a free choice.

Intensification and sustainability of livestock production

Agriculture exists primarily to provide food for man. We eat food to acquire nutrients and the nutrient we need the most is energy. The primal source of energy for the earth is the sun and agriculture exists to convert solar energy into food for man and other animals. Traditional systems of livestock production depended on solar energy to grow the crops and the work (energy expenditure) of man and animals to harvest them. These systems were not necessarily sustainable. Individual communities frequently exhausted their local resources and died out or moved on. Modern subsistence farming in Africa is not preserving the environment any better than industrialized agriculture in the developed world. However, the prime mover for the agricultural revolution of the last 60 years has been the massive increase in the use of fossil fuels both to drive the machines that harvest, process and transport crops and to increase crop yields through the use of artificial fertilizers. Fossil fuels such as oil and gas represent, of course, the solar energy conserved by plants in previous milennia. Since the prime function of agriculture is to provide a sustained source of food energy to man and the only primary source of energy income to agriculture is the sun, the use of fossil fuels in agriculture is equivalent to spending acquired capital rather than current income and this is, by definition, unsustainable, unless that capital expenditure can be repaid by increased output.

The efficiency and sustainability of agricultural systems is another huge topic which can only be touched on here. For an elegant exposition of the efficiency of energy use in agriculture, I recommend Pimentel and Pimentel, *Food, Energy and Society* (1979). I raise the issue in this context because much blanket condemnation of modern livestock production tends to throw criticisms of animal welfare, environmental sustainability, and other hate objects such as 'big business' into the same pot. The argument usually proceeds along the following lines:

(1)   modern, intensive, 'factory' farming is unsustainable because it is so dependent on the use of fossil fuels;
(2)   factory farming of, for example, pigs and poultry is immoral because it uses vast resources of grain that could have been used to feed man;
(3)   intensive factory farming is cruel to animals.

Now all these accusations contain important elements of truth but they cannot, in truth, be used as slogans to condemn intensive systems out of hand and call for a return to traditional, i.e. extensive, ways. I have already indicated (Fig. 7.1.) that the relationship between intensification and welfare cannot be described in simple linear terms; i.e. more intensive does not automatically imply worse. The relationship between intensification, fossil fuel use and sustainability is also far too complex to be dismissed by a slogan or soundbite.

Table 7.1 uses the logic pioneered by Pimentel and Pimentel to summarize the essentials of energy exchange in four different modern, commercial livestock systems, egg production from battery hens, intensive pig production, intensive dairy production and extensive production of beef from suckler cows on open range. It is a gross oversimplification of many complex assumptions but it still needs some explanation.

Each hen is assumed to produce 300 eggs per year, each breeding sow 1300 kg pigmeat (total weight of carcasses) from 22 piglets per year, each dairy cow 6000 litres of milk and each range cow 290 kg carcass weight from one calf per year. The next two lines indicate the proportions of gross energy that are consumed as food by the 'productive' and 'support' animals. The 'productive' animals are those actually yielding food, e.g. the hens in lay, the cows in milk and the slaughter generations of fattening pigs and calves. The 'support' animals are the breeding generation of sows, hens and beef cattle, plus hens before the point of lay and dairy heifers before the time of first calving. The proportion of food consumed by the support generations in pig production (i.e. the breeding sows and boars) is less than 20%. It is even smaller (about 12%) for breeders of broiler chickens. For beef cattle and sheep, which have only one or two offspring per year, the proportion of food energy consumed by the 'support' animals is about 42% and 75% respectively. The figure is larger for sheep than cattle because lambs, typically, are killed at 3-4 months of age; only the breeding generation needs to be fed over winter.

Table 7.1 calculates the yield of food for man relative both to the amount of food energy consumed by the animals and the amount of fossil fuel energy used by the system. Food for man is expressed both as kilojoules (kJ) of food

Table 7.1 Efficiency of energy use in animal systems.

	Hen	Sow	Dairy cow	Beef cow
Primary yield/year	300 eggs	1300 kg	6000 l	290 kg
Gross energy (kJ/MJ)				
to 'productive' animals	790	830	720	580
to 'support' animals	210	170	280	420
Yield of food for man				
kJ/MJ feed	140	182	170	37
g protein/MJ feed	2.31	1.09	1.72	0.16
kJ/MJ fuel	210	328	136	550
g protein/MJ fuel	3.46	2.55	1.36	2.37
'Complementary' food intake	0.2	0.25	0.85	0.8
Net yield, food for man				
kJ/kJ ME	0.25	0.35	1.76	0.35
g protein/MJ ME	4.1	2.1	17.6	1.5
g protein/g feed protein	0.37	0.19	1.6	0.14

energy, since that is the most important nutrient and as grams (g) protein for man/Megajoule (MJ) food energy for animals, since we tend to argue that we eat foods of animal origin not for energy but because we need the protein. In fact this argument is spurious. Except in a few exceptional circumstances, we do not actually *need* the animal protein; we eat meat, milk and dairy products simply because we like them. Be that as it may, the most intensive systems of animal production – eggs, pigmeat and dairying – all return similar yields of 14% to 18% of food energy entering the system. According to these calculations pig production is marginally superior in terms of energy yield but is least efficient in terms of protein yield. The efficiency of conversion of food energy for animals to food energy for man from beef cattle and sheep on extensive range is very low (less than 4%).

Perhaps the most alarming set of numbers in Table 7.1 are those which reveal that none of the systems of livestock production, intensive or extensive, achieve anything close to equivalence of food energy yield relative to consumption of energy from fossil fuels. In these examples, dairy production is the least efficient (136 kJ/MJ fuel). This can be attributed both to the high use of fossil fuels in collection and storage of milk and in the manufacture of inorganic fertilizer for grass and maize crops. Extensive meat production from range cows with calves finished on feedlot is more efficient in terms of fossil fuel consumption but even this only achieves an output of 550kJ/MJ fossil fuel use (or 0.55kJ beef/kJ fuel). None of the modern systems of livestock production, whether intensive or extensive is sustainable in its current form because it is failing to supply sufficient energy to repay that taken from capital reserves. I should emphasize that the 'squandering' of fuel reserves on farms is modest compared to that which occurs beyond the farm gate to meet alleged consumer demand for attractive packaging, processing and the transportation and refrigeration necessary to provide goods all over the world at any season. The only point I wish to make in this context is that extensive systems are much less efficient than intensive systems in overall use of plant energy and not much more efficient in the use of fossil fuel energy. The most extensive systems of all systems of animal farming, e.g. meat and work from native cattle in Africa are the least efficient in relation to land use and the food needs of man. They use very little fossil fuels but yields of food energy are very small and only just exceed the energy expended by man and animals in producing the food (see Pimentel and Pimentel, 1979). Subsistence agriculture is simply not consistent with the quality of life that we have come to expect for ourselves and it is arrogant nonsense to claim that it is the best (because it is the traditional) solution for the poor of the world. All rational analysis of the evidence points to the conclusion that calls to return to extensive (near subsistence) systems of agriculture in order to save the planet are romantic but wrong.

All rational analyses also force one to the conclusion, however, that current systems of agriculture in general and livestock production in particular are ultimately unsustainable. I do not envisage (for the foreseeable future) an apocalyptic scenario where fossil fuels have been entirely exhausted but there will come a time in the not-too-distant future when their increasing scarcity will make them prohibitively expensive for use in the production of a commodity such as food. As fossil fuels become more expensive there will be an increasing incentive to use cultivatable land to grow biomass for fuel. This inevitably implies less land for animal production and higher fuel costs, both of which will favour more intensive systems of livestock production since there will still be those who can afford to buy meat, milk and eggs.

The strongest argument in favour of livestock farming is that based on the capacity of animals to consume food sources that are complementary to, rather than compete with, the needs of man. These include grasses and forages which man cannot eat or crop residues and those parts of plants grown for human consumption which we cannot or elect not to eat and therefore feed to animals rather than allow them to go to waste. Table 7.1 shows that whereas pigs and hens can only obtain 25% and 20% of their food from such complementary sources, ruminants can perform at high efficiency on forages and crop residues so that only 20% of their feed need come from ingredients such as cereals which we could eat ourselves. This applies not only to dairy cattle but also, to the surprise of some, to beef production from range cattle (e.g. in the USA) where the slaughter generation are fed large quantities of cereals on feedlot. This is because most of the time, most of the animals, i.e. cows and unweaned calves, are not on feedlot but on open range eating grasses.

When output is expressed as net yield of food for man relative to intake of food in a form that man could eat himself, we discover that the dairy cow can generate 76% more food energy for man than she consumes. This makes her a very valuable animal indeed. Beef production from range cattle still remains very inefficient (by this measure) but the overall efficiency of the enterprise is greatly increased when beef is produced (as it is in the UK) as a byproduct of the dairy industry. Pig and poultry production appears to compete largely for the same food source as man but the criteria used in Table 7.1 neglect to consider the food which we could eat but don't. I have several times made the point that in traditional farming systems pigs and poultry were scavengers of our waste. It is quite possible to operate the scavenging principle on a modern commercial scale, either by processing crop residues to increase their nutritive value for pigs and poultry, or by operating piggeries in association with supermarkets to salvage food that overruns its 'sell-by' date.

This analysis of the efficiency and sustainability of livestock production systems has been based almost entirely on examination of input:output relationships, using energy as a common currency whose value (unlike money) can be measured in absolute terms. It has not been my intention to analyse the role of food animals in the ecosystem in detail, merely to illustrate that such analysis is at least as complex as the analysis of what constitutes animal welfare. The moral of this is that while moral outrage is easy (and therapeutic), the practical application of morality to our exploitation of the animals and the land is less easy and should be approached with caution. To illustrate this point I would like briefly to address a fashionable canard, namely the destruction of the Brazilian rainforest allegedly to produce the North American hamburger (see Rifkin, *Beyond Beef*, 1993).

There can be no doubt that the rainforest is being stripped at an immoral and unsustainable rate. It is also a fact that beef cattle are grazing the cleared land. However, the beef output from these animals makes a miniscule contribution to North American beef consumption (less than 2%). What is even more interesting is that it also makes a small contribution (15%) to the wealth of the land owners who are stripping the forest (Hecht,1993). Those who are plundering the rainforest are doing so, not for immediate cash income from cattle, but to acquire wealth by investing in land which will increase in cash value. The cattle are being used in the same way as cattle were used in the early American West. When man owns or is surrounded by more land than he can work for himself, cattle become an easy, and sometimes romantic, way of managing land surplus to immediate requirements. They do not generate much in the way of immediate income for the owners or wealth for the community relative to the amount of land in use but they are a cheaper way of keeping down the vegetation than employing people to cut the grass. Exactly the same principle applies to Scottish landowners who 'conserve' for grouse moorland rendered vacant (of people) by the Highland clearances. The inequities of land ownership are a proper subject for anger but one should not necessarily blame the hamburger.

How hard do animals work?

The basic natural laws that determine the efficiency of livestock production systems (Fig. 7.1) dictate that farmers should work their animals hard and show that the more intensive the system, the harder the work necessary to achieve optimal efficiency. Since this book is all about marginal costs and benefits rather than absolutes of right and wrong, it is necessary to ask 'How hard *do* farm animals work and are there circumstances where, in striving for the biological and economic limits to productivity, we may exceed the reasonable bounds of humanity?' Table 7.2 compares food energy intakes and work rates in a range of mammals and birds using the convention of expressing all energy exchanges per unit of metabolic body size (i.e. as kJ energy intake or expenditure per kg body weight$^{0.75}$ per day). The use of this term makes possible valid comparisons of energy exchanges in animals of different body size . Thus the metabolic rates of an adult rat living in a laboratory cage and an adult man dividing his life between home and office, are the same. Each consumes 520 kJ metabolizable energy (ME) per kg$^{0.75}$ per day, uses it all for work and burns it all off as heat, thereby maintaining energy balance, and neither gains nor loses weight. The work of the largely sedentary man and rat mainly involves maintenance of the integrity of the body; relatively little can be attributed to physical exercise, but it is work none the less.

Let us now consider the work involved in physical labour. A British miner in the 1940s when there was relatively little mechanization (but lots of mines) expended 625 kJ/kg$^{0.75}$ per day, only 20% more than the sedentary clerk, which suggests both that labour down the mines was not especially arduous and that he did little or no work in the home. Some of the highest work rates (800kJ/kg$^{0.75}$ per day) were seen in traditional foresters. This work load is similar to that of ruminants such as Eland foraging for maintenance on the African plains. The most extreme forms of hard labour in animals have been recorded in birds during migration or during the time that they are seeking food for their young (1580 kJ/kg$^{0.75}$ per day). One class of human can compare with this work rate, namely those supreme human masochists, the cyclists in the *Tour de France* (1510 kJ/kg$^{0.75}$ per day). Both birds and cyclists are working at about three times 'maintenance', although in each case this extreme intensity of effort only persists for a few weeks.

The work (energy cost) of growth is relatively modest, even in the most extreme examples of rapid growth as seen in pigs and poultry (800 and 600 kJ/kg$^{0.75}$ per day respectively). Rapid growth in poultry does create welfare problems caused by skeletal disorders in birds outgrowing their strength but it is not, in the strict sense of the word, hard work. However, a typical dairy cow yielding 35 litres of milk a day has a metabolic rate of 1020 kJ/kg$^{0.75}$ per day, and an ME intake of 1860 kJ/kg$^{0.75}$ per day, i.e. she has to sustain a work rate twice that of maintenance and process nearly four times the amount of food required for maintenance. The work rate of a dairy cow is only exceeded in these examples by the song birds and those cycling masochists. Neither group sustains this work rate for months on end and no group matches the dairy cow in terms of ME intake.

Animal breeders have, of course, given more attention to selection for milk yield in the dairy cow than any other class of farm animal. Peak yields in excess of 55 l/day are not uncommon. This requires a work rate of 1300kJ/kg$^{0.75}$ per day which is not quite as severe as that of the racing cyclist and is something most of us could achieve, for example, by jogging 6 to 8 hours per day. It is however necessary to point out that peak milk yields (35 l/day) in the typical UK dairy cow are not that different from other species of lactating mother such as a sow with 12 piglets, a Labrador bitch with eight puppies or a dairy goat with a yield of 1.2 l/day (Table 7.2). The work rate of the lactating woman with one child is modest by these standards but it still compares with heavy manual labour such as coal mining. Lactation is very hard work for all species. However, as we shall see in Chapter 8 the most abnormal features of the work required of the dairy cow (and goat) are not just the intensity of the metabolic load but the length of time it must be sustained. Moreover, the main welfare problems are not necessarily related to productivity *per se* but to forms of nutrition, housing and management that are

Table 7.2 A comparison of metabolizable energy intakes and energy expenditures ($kJ/kg^{0.75}$ per day) associated with different activities in some mammals and birds (from Webster, 1992).

Work	Species	Energy exchanges ME intake	Heat
Maintenance	White rat	520	520
	Man, clerk	520	520
Labour	Miner	625	625
	Endurance cyclist	985	1510
	Herbivores on range	700	700
	Birds feeding young	1580	1580
Growth	Pig (20 kg)	1200	800
	Broiler fowl (2 kg)	1000	600
Lactation	Dairy cow (35 l/day)	1860	1020
	Sow (12 piglets)	1680	900
	Woman (1 child)	720	590

inadequate for the high performance animals that we have created by selective breeding.

The acceptable limits to productivity

One assumption central to my argument throughout this chapter has been that as livestock systems approach the biological or economic limits of productivity, the animals within these systems are likely to suffer a deterioration in their welfare. Once again, it is possible to use the logic of the five freedoms to identify, in general terms, possible contributors to poor welfare through ill-health or mental suffering that may be linked directly to feeding, breeding and housing to achieve maximum possible productivity:

(1) hunger, malnutrition or metabolic disease due to a failure to supply nutrients appropriate to the genetic or physiological potential of the animal;
(2) chronic discomfort through overcrowding, inadequate bedding, loss of condition following malnutrition, etc.;
(3) chronic pain or restricted movement due to distortion of body shape and/or improper housing and bedding;
(4) increased susceptibility to infectious disease due to overcrowding, poor hygiene or immunosuppression caused by metabolic exhaustion;
(5) lack of behavioural expression in barren environments;
(6) metabolic or physical exhaustion caused by the stress of prolonged high production.

These potential sources of poor health and welfare can be interdependent and additive. For example, the large, genetically superior dairy cow consuming a ration based largely on grass silage may suffer both from hunger and pain, or at least chronic discomfort, in a cubicle house partly because the quality of feed has been inadequate to meet her nutrient requirements for lactation and she has lost condition, partly because the wet silage has contributed to poor hygiene and predisposed to foot lameness, and partly because genetic selection has created a cow too big for the cubicles. Similarly, heavy strains of broiler chicken may suffer pain for the last third of their short lives primarily because they have been selected for very rapid growth, but the problem (for them, not the farmer) has been compounded by the fact that they have been given free access from birth to highly nutritious food and kept in the light for 23 hours per day.

I shall be dealing with specific welfare problems of the farm animals in the next two chapters. For the moment, I hope to have made it abundantly clear that while I acknowledge the soundness of most of the reasons for intensification of livestock production, I also believe that there are serious welfare problems built into the structure of these systems and that some of these problems should not be allowed to continue. In short, I believe that change is essential. The most successful forms of change are those which evolve spontaneously. The classic example is natural selection where changes occur by chance and success is determined by necessity. Successful, planned political change depends on an ability to forecast the future and this is notoriously difficult. Some improvements to animal welfare have arisen and will continue to arise by a process akin to natural selection, but only where these are consistent with improved efficiency of production or, at least, the operation of the free market. The most obvious examples of such changes are improvements in animal health attributable to advances in nutrition or to the control of infectious disease. However, some of the most important concerns relate to problems where the welfare cost to the animal does not impair its productivity as an individual or the overall productivity of the unit. Examples include psychological problems such as fear, boredom, frustration, and physical problems such as chronic discomfort or pain, especially in breeding females. In this case, it is unrealistic to expect welfare to improve spontaneously. The problem for us is essentially a moral one which can only be resolved by political means, since politics should be the public expression of popular morality. However, since we are not dealing in absolutes, the biggest problem is deciding just where, in law, to draw the line.

Thus improvements to farm animal welfare will develop naturally in response to advances in research, development or commercial practice only when these also succeed in improving the product, i.e. the quality or price of meat, milk or eggs. Improvements in the quality of life for farm animals which are unrelated to the quality of their products will only be achieved if consumers make the moral decision that this is what they want. I shall develop this theme in more depth in the final chapter, 'Right thought and right action'. For the moment, it is necessary only to state that this can be achieved by:

(1) a radical shift in consumer choice towards high welfare products.
(2) legislation (in response to consumer pressure) to enforce improved minimum standards for welfare.

In both cases, the consumer, who is not directly involved in the business of production, is seeking to interfere with natural forces. This is, I believe a perfectly moral and proper thing to do but it needs to be done with extreme caution, bearing in mind the following principles:

(1) While it is unnecessary to guarantee that an enforced change will always make things better, it is necessary to guarantee that the change will not, in some circumstances, make things worse.
(2) Any change imposed by legislation must be enforced fairly within the economic community since the law will become an ass if it forces those who obey it out of business.
(3) 'If it ain't bust, don't fix it.'

We have, at present, laws to define minimum welfare standards for farm animals in intensive husbandry systems, although most constitute no more than a cynical acceptance of the *status quo*, There is, for example, legislation to 'protect' the welfare of laying hens in battery cages by providing each bird with 450 cm^2 floor space for the duration of its adult life. (The pages of this book are each 360 cm^2 in area. A laying hen is offered 1.25 times as much.) This law is designed simply for the protection of exsisting producers. Good law should however be made by the people for the people and can, in a democracy, be changed in response to pressure from the people. Although improvements to farm animal welfare should not be designed in such a way as to put those few who obey it out of business it is possible to improve animal welfare through legislation, even if this increases the costs of production, provided that this legislation is properly enforced and applies to all producers. This is much easier said than done but it is an issue that I shall address repeatedly throughout Part III.

Ultimately, improvements to farm animal welfare are not going to be achieved by people who pass laws or people like me who write books, but by the farmers who look after the animals. When the animal welfare movement first gathered pace, it was strongly resisted by farmers who viewed its early advocates as a bunch of 'know-nothing do-gooders' out to make life difficult for the farmer, who knew what was best for his animals. However, farming opinion has been steadily changing for the better, partly because farmers have been alarmed by pressure from the public and from the media, partly because the more rational farmers and welfarists have stopped throwing rocks at one another from their entrenched positions and started to communicate, and partly (and by no means least) because farmers have discovered that increasing productivity in a static market does not equate to increasing wealth.

In the year between leaving school and entering university (1956–7) I worked on a mixed farm of 100 ha, which achieved most of its income from a herd of 32 dairy cows, plus a little from the produce of about 500 laying hens and 12 breeding sows. This enabled the farmer to put three children through public school, hunt two days a week in season, actually *work* on the farm only at hay and harvest time and drink a bottle of whisky a day. I am not applauding his life style, merely describing it to illustrate the fact that increasing output through intensification of animal production has not necessarily enriched the lives of farmers. Intensification of (especially) pig and poultry production has been of great benefit to the consumer but has forced both farmers and their animals to work ever harder or face the prospect of being culled. Over the same period, the image of the farmer has changed from that of the jolly red-faced man beaming from the cover of the books we read as children to that of the mean, rapacious profiteer, bespoiling the environment and condemning his animals to a life that is nasty, brutish and short. Now it is not much fun to be addressed as a mean rapacious profiteer even when it is true, but when one is having to struggle ever harder to make ends meet, this image can be a source of real distress and must contribute to the abnormally high proportion of farmers who commit suicide, not, as Macbeth's porter would have it 'on the expectation of plenty', more often on the realization that their farming careers could be summed up as working all hours of the day until the money ran out. Central to my advocacy for improved standards of farm animal welfare is the premise that farming is an honourable profession. My aim is therefore to improve the quality of life for all sentient animals on the farm, and that includes the farmer and his or her family. I would also argue that since it is the consumer who has benefited most from the intensification of animal production, it is the consumer who will have to concede the most in order to ensure that farm animals get a fair deal. If their lives are to have more value, we shall have to value them more highly.

8 Pigs and Poultry

'Diligent human care for the welfare of such animals as are confined in a few advanced zoological parks can act as a touchstone for the welfare standards of these managed animals.'

Edward Carpenter, *Animals and Ethics*

The expression 'Factory farming' is an emotive but nonetheless accurate title for systems of intensive livestock production where the animals have been removed entirely from the land and housed in large controlled environment buildings containing machinery to supply their physical needs and remove their waste products. The two aspects of intensification that cause most concern on grounds of animal welfare are:

(1) working animals at the limits of productivity;
(2) overcrowding animals in barren environments.

This chapter considers welfare aspects of pigs and poultry production, where these aspects of intensification have been taken to an extreme degree and so incurred the most wrath from the animal welfare advocates. It is necessary at the outset to recapitulate briefly the main reasons why intensification of pig and poultry production has been so successful, in a strictly commercial sense. These were considered in more detail in Chapter 4.

(1) ease of handling and storage of dry, cereal-based feeds;
(2) reduction in feed costs through control of air temperature;
(3) improved control of infectious disease in densely stocked buildings by (i) vaccination, (ii) antibiotics and (iii) supply and maintenance of minimal disease stock.

The successful application of factory farming methods to pig and poultry production brought down the price of eggs, pig and chicken meat, standardized the product and the public responded by buying more. I repeat, *the products that arouse most concern on welfare grounds are those which the public has increasingly preferred to buy*. I shall now examine, in some detail the main welfare problems faced by pigs and poultry in commercial production systems and propose a series of priorities for change designed to improve welfare in ways that are consistent with good, economically sound husbandry.

The welfare of pigs

A typical commercial breeding sow will be mated for the first time at approximately 220 days of age and give birth to her first litter of about 10 piglets after a pregnancy lasting 114 days. She may successfully rear nine of these piglets until they are weaned at 20–28 days. She will return to oestrus and be remated about 5–10 days later to repeat the whole procedure at intervals of approximately 140 days, thereby producing 23 weaned piglets per year. For most of her adult life she will be pregnant and live in the company of other pregnant, dry (non-lactating) sows. This will be interspersed by periods of approximately one month when she will be in accommodation designed to ensure successful farrowing and nursing of her piglets. The cycle will continue until her productivity falters, whereupon she will be culled. For most sows this will occur sometime between her second and eighth litters. The welfare of sow will be determined by:

(1) how she feels at the time, which will be determined largely by the environment to which she is exposed and the ration she is given to eat.
(2) her capacity to achieve sustained fitness which will be determined in part by the environment to which she is exposed but also by her breeding and the physiological demands imposed upon her constitution.

Accommodation for dry sows

At the time of going to press, the three most common commercial husbandry systems for dry sows are:

(1) individual sow stalls, with or without tethers;
(2) covered yards with individual feeding stalls or electronically operated feeders;
(3) outdoors with individual arks.

Table 8.1 presents an outline analysis of the pros and cons of these alternative husbandry systems according to the logic of the five freedoms. As in Table 1.1, the words and short phrases that appear in the table are, for reasons of space, oversimplistic and intended only as keys to subsequent discussion.

In all three systems the farmer will provide the sows with sufficient nutrients to meet the demands of maintenance and pregnancy for obvious, sound commercial reasons. In these circumstances the sows may experience metabolic hunger but no more than that felt by an adult human on a diet designed to maintain (not lose) body weight. It is unreasonable to claim that the intensity of this hunger is sufficient to cause suffering. However, the systems differ widely in the extent to which they permit the sows oral satisfaction. The sow outdoors that can root in the earth in the expectation of an occasional reward in the form of a worm or some such morsel will derive far greater satisfaction than the sow on concrete in an individual stall with no

Table 8.1 Outline analysis of the welfare of dry sows in different husbandry systems.

	Sow stalls	Covered yards	Outdoor arks
Hunger, nutrients	Usually adequate	Usually adequate	Usually adequate
Oral satisfaction	Severely frustrated	Usually adequate	Usually good
Comfort, thermal	Some cold stress	Good	Heat, sun, cold
Physical	Poor	Good	Usually good
Pain and injury	Leg injuries, bedsores	Wounds from fights(?)	Usually good
Sickness	Kidney infections(?)	Good	Good
Normal behaviour	Severely restricted	Good	Good
Fear and stress	Frustration	Fighting(?)	Usually good

opportunity to work for any satisfactory reward. However, an outdoor sow equipped with a nose ring to deter it (through pain) from rooting in the ground may be even more frustrated than the enstalled sow because the reward is ever, tantalizingly, present.

Sows that are housed in yards derive considerable oral satisfaction from rooting and eating straw. However, a deep, clean bed of straw may be unavailable or unacceptably expensive. Jim Bruce at the Centre for Rural Buildings of the Scottish Agriculture College has developed a 'straw-flow' system whereby sows or growing pigs can remove straw from a container at the higher end of a sloping pen, eat some, and progressively tread the rest down towards a manure channel at the opposite end. This innovation is an excellent example of a low-cost, functional solution to a welfare problem based on a proper understanding of pig motivation.

The covered, dry, well-bedded straw yard undoubtedly ranks first in terms of thermal and physical comfort. The sow compelled to stand and lie on concrete in an individual stall, whether constrained by the dimensions of the stall or by a tether, lacks the physical comfort of a bed when she wants to rest and the opportunity to stretch her limbs with a little gentle exercise. The heat lost from a sow lying on concrete at air temperatures below 15°C is sufficient to cause systemic and local cold stress. Systemic cold stress will increase the sow's feed requirement or cause her to lose condition. Local cold stress, leading to reduced blood flow, may contribute to or exacerbate injuries to skin and limbs.

Sows out of doors will frequently be exposed to the stresses of cold, rain, heat and the risk of sunburn. Arks offer only partial protection, especially from heat stress. However, much can be done to reduce the intensity of these stresses, by providing shade and wallows during the summer, for example, and ensuring that arks are well bedded and on well-drained land during the winter. The objective is not to create a stress-free environment but one in which the animals can cope, preferably through their own constructive action.

For outdoor sows the risk of pain and injury (other than sunburn) is very low. Sows in stalls on concrete have a higher incidence of injuries to feet, inflammatory swellings of joints and abrasions to their skin. If these superficial abrasions become infected the infection may track down to damaged joints, set up a septic arthritis and cause severe, chronic pain. Tethers around the neck or chest can also cause chronic skin damage. These problems can be avoided if the stalls are provided with adequate bedding. Sows in stalls are also prone to develop 'dog-sitting' behaviour, i.e. sit on their haunches. This may be because they become uncomfortable both standing and lying (and cannot, of course, go for a walk). Dog-sitting may be unnatural for a sow but it is not inherently a sign of stress, rather a sensible solution to a problem of discomfort. However, sows dog-sitting on wet, unhygienic floors are prone to ascending infections of the urinary tract leading to kidney disease which is both distressing and life-threatening.

The main welfare problem for dry sows living in covered straw yards is the threat of fear, injury and pain from fighting. Sows are aggressive creatures and have considerable ability to cause damage. Out of doors, aggression is seldom a problem because sows have the space to avoid or defuse agonistic encounters. In yards, problems occur typically when sows are mixed or in association with feeding. There are three basic approaches to this problem. Traditionally, sows in yards have been provided with individual feeding stalls. This is effective but expensive. Recent years have seen the development of electronically-controlled feeding stations which admit sows once or twice daily to receive their allocated ration (Fig. 8.1). The sow is secure within the feeding stall but potentially at risk from aggression on the way in and the way

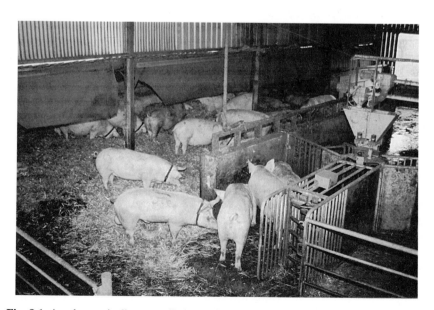

Fig. 8.1 An electronically controlled sow-feeding stall.

out. Some of the first units to install electronically controlled sow feeders experienced severe problems of aggression. However, with improvements to design and management designed to achieve stress-free entry and exit, these feeders are starting to make a very successful 'high-tech' contribution to improved sow welfare.

A simpler, cheaper solution is to scatter pellets of feed over as wide an area of the straw yard as possible. This carries the double advantages of ensuring that the sows are dispersed and will devote much of their day to foraging. Farmers who use this system ensure me that not a pellet is overlooked. One drawback to the system is that it does not allow the farmer to adjust each sow's ration according to her body condition. This is an important consideration for sows in the period immediately after weaning but by mid-pregnancy most sows should be in similar condition and require similar amounts of food.

Farrowing and nursery accommodation

The pig gives birth to large litters. Average litter sizes are about 10 to 12 for Western breeds of pigs rising to 16 for the Chinese Meishan breed. Within such a species it is entirely normal (i.e. consistent with natural selection) for some members of each litter, usually the weakest runt or dilly pig, to die before weaning. Farmers, however, for reasons that are both commercial and honourable, try to reduce mortality in young piglets to the absolute minimum. To this end, it is normal to move sows into a farrowing crate prior to giving birth and keep them so confined until the piglets are weaned three to four weeks later. It is also common to use drugs to induce farrowing during the normal working week. The conventional farrowing crate (Fig. 8.2) restrains the sow so that she can do no more than stand up and lie down. The piglets can move freely either side of the crate and enter a creep area usually heated by a lamp where they can rest in thermal comfort and may get their first exposure to food other than milk.

The main objective of the farrowing crate is to prevent the sow from crushing any of her piglets when she lies down and by this criterion it must be counted a success. However, it is undeniably even more uncomfortable than a dry sow stall and severely restricts the opportunity for social contact between sow and piglets. Moreover, the sow that is confined in a crate during the period prior to farrowing is unable to satisfy her powerful motivation to build a nest (Fig. 4.3). These real costs to the welfare of the sow must be set against the potential benefits to the welfare and survival of her piglets. These benefits are sometimes exaggerated on both welfare and commercial grounds, since such farrowing accommodation is expensive. When sows are allowed to farrow in arks out of doors, the only protection for the piglets is a rail around the walls and some bedding. Recent records from the Meat and Livestock Commission (MLC Pig Yearbooks) reveal little, if any difference

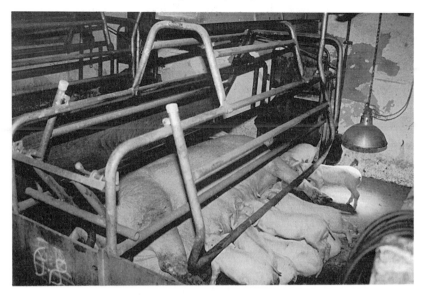

Fig. 8.2 A farrowing crate for sows.

in piglet mortality from birth to weaning in (the better) indoor and outdoor systems. In one survey, deaths from crushing were 0.7 piglets per sow per year more outdoors than indoors with farrowing crates but this was exactly offset by reduced deaths from disease. The reason for this is partly genetic. Sows destined for outdoor units are selected for maternal ability. They are not only more careful with their piglets but more agile and less likely to come crashing down on their offspring. If sows selected for indoor units were moved outside, one would expect piglet mortality to be higher.

There have been several attempts to design farrowing and nursing accommodation that better suit the welfare needs of both sow and piglets. An alternative approach to improving the welfare of the sow and her piglets is not simply to tinker with the farrowing accommodation but to re-examine from first principles what it is that the farmer is trying to achieve. The farrowing crate is certainly not designed to assist farrowing. The sow is uncomfortable, frustrated and compelled to drop her piglets on the same spot she drops her faeces. The crate exists almost solely to protect piglets from crushing. In practice, this is only likely to occur in the first 48 hours of life. Thereafter the crate is, arguably, superfluous, although some farmers cross-foster piglets at a later age to even up litter numbers and this is accomplished more easily when the sow is confined. In most circumstances however, the crate could be removed when the piglets were two or three days old, or the sow and piglets moved to lower-cost nursery accommodation.

This is a specific example of a highly important generic argument. The effects of the farrowing crate on the welfare of the sow and piglet are not only inherently complex but should not be considered in isolation from other, economic aspects of the housing and management of a herd of breeding pigs. The pros and cons of farrowing need to be considered in the context of the overall system of husbandry. If, for example, the accommodation for the sow and her piglets were redesigned on the basis that the sow occupied a maternity suite for approximately five days, then proceeded with her piglets to nursery accommodation, the maternity suite could incorporate an existing or improved design of farrowing crate. In either case, the overall cost of this specialist accommodation could be reduced because it could be used for about four times as many sows, and the sows would benefit because they would be severely confined for less than one week rather than four. It would then be necessary to examine the potential to reduce the costs of accommodation both before and immediately after weaning (see below). An overall reduction in the cost of accommodation for sows and young piglets, or a shift in the distribution of these costs, can, in theory, increase the optimal time for weaning piglets from three to five weeks of age. I am not necessarily offering this as the new, best way to rear piglets, only illustrating by example how a systems approach to problems of animal welfare can be used to direct research and development towards husbandry practices that can be of benefit to both parties – producer and pig.

Growing pigs

Under natural conditions, a sow would complete the process of weaning her piglets on to solid food by about 12 weeks of age. The preferred age for weaning piglets in commercial herds has, over the last 40 years dropped, first from eight to five weeks, and has now settled at three weeks of age. This development has primarily been to maximize the number of piglets reared per sow per year, but also to reduce the costs of sustaining the metabolic needs of the sow during lactation. In Chapter 6 I listed the most important potential stresses for piglets at the time of weaning:

(1) an abrupt change in diet, possibly leading to hunger, indigestion or food allergies;
(2) a move from warm, bedded accommodation to a cold cage;
(3) exposure, and reduced immunity to microorganisms associated, especially, with gastrointestinal infection;
(4) withdrawal of the mother's contribution to security and education;
(5) fear of novelty or aggression from exposure to pigs from other litters.

The risks to piglets from all but the last of these potential stresses increase as the age at weaning is reduced. The abrupt change of diet at 21 days almost invariably causes some damage to the epithelial lining of the small intestine. On its own, this is unlikely to cause obvious signs of distress, disease or loss of performance. However, it does predispose the piglet to enteric infection from opportunist organisms such as *Escherichia coli*. For this reason it is 'normal' to include antibiotics in diets for early-weaned pigs. This is an example of the routine use of antibiotics to mask a deliberate abuse of one of the fundamental principles of good husbandry, namely the need to ensure that the system itself does not cause the animals to suffer harm. If, of course, antibiotics are not used, early-weaned piglets are likely to suffer more.

It is customary to house piglets weaned at 21 days of age in cages or 'flat decks' in controlled environment buildings at an initial air temperature of 28–30°C. Behavioural problems such as tail-biting can begin to develop at this time, attributable in part to the barren environment and in part to the frustration of sucking behaviour. Piglets weaned at 5–6 weeks of age can be housed in simpler accommodation such as kennels or covered yards, insulated and enriched by the presence of straw.

The main welfare problems for pigs during the latter stages of growth are overcrowding, discomfort, pain, injuries and inflammation (e.g. bursitis) in limbs associated with being compelled to lie on concrete, pain and injury from aggressive encounters while feeding, and pain from mindless mutilations like tail-biting. The MAFF Code of Recommendations for the Welfare for Pigs lays down minimum housing standards for growing pigs. These do not require, but strongly recommend, the use of bedding such as straw both to improve comfort and to enrich the behavioural repertoire of the animals. Once again, Bruce's 'straw-flow' system offers an attractive compromise that yields a high benefit to the welfare of the pigs at low cost to the farmer.

Handling, transport and slaughter

Whenever animals have to be handled or transported on the farm, from farm to farm, to and within the abattoir, the basic aim must be to minimize both the intensity and duration of any stresses. Most of the principles and practices necessary for the humane handling and transport of animals are discussed in detail in a new book, *Livestock Handling and Transport* by Temple Grandin (1994). The potential welfare problems for pigs in transit are well understood and need not be discussed in detail here. They may be summarized very briefly as follows:

(1) hunger and thirst on prolonged journeys;
(2) thermal stress, especially heat stress due the pig's limited ability to regulate heat loss by evaporation;
(3) motion stresses leading to injury, physical exhaustion or nausea and vomiting;
(4) fear, pain and injury attributable to the actions of other pigs or human handlers.

Most unstressed pigs in novel environments are motivated more by curiosity than by fear. This means that they will, even in the abattoir, usually move at reasonable speed in the direction desired by their handlers provided that the path forward is clear, unthreatening, easy to negotiate and they are not distracted. It follows that pigs can usually be moved with relative ease, given a combination of good handling facilities and good sense based on humanity and experience. The pig that is goaded up a steep ramp into a dark lorry finds the path unclear and difficult to negotiate and its state of mind is not improved by threats and assaults from its handlers. This type of situation, which is all too common, arises from the lack of both good facilities and good sense and becomes a source of unnecessary stress to all parties.

The welfare of pigs at the point of slaughter is a cause for real concern. For most pigs in the UK, slaughter is a two-stage process; stunning followed by sticking. The animals are first stunned (but not killed), usually by electric shock and then 'stuck' and bled out, i.e. killed by having their throats cut. The legal requirement for the stunning procedure is 'to render the animals instantaneously insensible to pain until death supervenes'. However, a survey of electrical stunning procedures in commercial abattoirs in the UK during the period 1988–90 revealed that nearly 20% of pigs were either improperly stunned in the first place or were showing signs of recovery before they bled to death (*Meat Manufacturing & Marketing*, 1993). Part of this problem could be attributed to bad practice. This can be remedied (and, in many cases, has been remedied) with advice and pressure from the veterinary surgeon responsible for control of animal welfare within the abattoir. However, the system itself is inherently flawed. When pigs are allowed to move in groups and of their own volition to the stunning point, it is necessary, for safety reasons, that the slaughterman who moves among the pigs operates the stunning tongs at a relatively low voltage (90–120 v) which may fail to stun some pigs, particularly if the tongs are not properly applied, and will almost certainly fail to *kill* any of the pigs, so that some may start to recover before they have been bled out.

There are two ways to overcome this fundamental flaw in the stunning process. One is to apply a high enough voltage to ensure that all the pigs are killed instantaneously. This is consistent with meat quality. It is not necessary for the animal's heart to be beating during the bleeding out process. However, high voltage electrical stunning has to be combined with a conveyor system that delivers the pigs to the stunning point in such a way that they are practically unable to move at the time that the tongs are applied (see Grandin, 1994). The second alternative is to use gaseous stunning. To date, this has involved lowering the pigs into a pit containing a high concentration of carbon dioxide in air. Since carbon dioxide is heavier than air it remains in the pit. The pigs lose consciousness in less than a minute but do show signs of distress before this occurs. Moreover, sticking and bleeding out needs to be done quickly because the pigs recover quickly on removal from the stunning chamber. The best of the existing stunning systems based on carbon dioxide undoubtedly cause more distress at the point of stunning than the best of the high voltage electrical stunning systems. However, the aim is to minimize all the stresses likely to be experienced by pigs in the abattoir and the best of the carbon dioxide systems do permit free, minimally-stressed movement of pigs right up to the point that they enter the gas chamber.

The very phrase 'gas chamber' has a chilling ring. However, the principle of gas stunning has great potential to improve the humanity of the slaughter process for both pigs and poultry. Mohan Raj at Bristol has developed methods of stunning and killing pigs and poultry based on exposing them to gas mixtures containing carbon dioxide and the inert gas argon which replaces oxygen. Animals exposed to these mixtures lose consciousness without showing any signs of distress. Mohan Raj has also studied the aversion of pigs and poultry repeatedly exposed to stunning concentrations of carbon dioxide and to carbon dioxide/argon mixtures. The animals are reluctant to enter the straight mixture of carbon dioxide and air, and remember this aversion, but pigs, for example, will willingly enter and reenter the carbon dioxide/argon mix for the reward of an apple and lose consciousness in mid-chew. They simply lose consciousness (and, in the abattoir, die) without being aware that anything untoward has occurred. This sort of compassionate but non-squeamish research may not be immediately attractive to the passionate advocates of animal welfare but it is the sort of knowledge we need if we are to achieve real improvements in the treatment of farm animals.

The welfare of poultry

Broiler chickens and turkeys

The typical modern commercial broiler chicken is reared in large groups (5000 to 50 000 birds per flock) on litter and with near continuous lighting, (23 hours on:1 hour off) to reach a slaughter weight of 1.8 to 3.0 kg at an age of 42 days. This spectacular rate of production has been achieved in part by advances in nutrition and building design but mainly by intense genetic selection for absolute growth rate in muscle (especially the more attractive white breast muscle) to the virtual exclusion of all other traits that may affect fitness. Similarly, the turkey has been intensely selected to produce very large breasted birds that will typically be slaughtered at ages from 16 to 24 weeks and weights from 8 to 20 kg. The birds are reared in groups on litter, either in a controlled environment house or a naturally ventilated barn. Despite the intensive rearing conditions, most serious infections of broiler chickens and turkeys can be controlled by the use of low-cost live vaccines, good site hygiene and other therapeutic measures (which do not include the routine use of therapeutic antibiotics). The birds have ample access to water and a nutritionally balanced diet. They are protected from heat or cold and, if the litter is well managed, they have a comfortable bed. Mortality rates from infectious diseases are very low. Stocking densities are very high towards the end of the rearing period. The recommended maximum stocking density for broiler chickens is 34 kg of bird mass per m². This corresponds to about 750 cm² of floor space per 2.5 kg bird. At this stocking density healthy birds can continue to find feed and water. Moreover, problems of aggression such as feather pecking and cannibalism are practically unknown in broiler chickens. Turkeys, however, are prone to fighting and cannibalism and debeaking is common practice.

In the early days of the welfare debate most of the criticism of intensive husbandry systems was directed at the extent to which they restricted natural maintenance behaviour or, in the words of the Brambell Committee (1965), denied animals the freedom to 'stand up, lie down, turn round, groom themselves and stretch their limbs'. Intensive systems for growing broiler chickens and turkeys in colonies and on deep litter largely escaped criticism according to this (restricted) definition of welfare and, it must be said, these systems appear to meet most of the five freedoms as defined for use throughout this book and by the UK Farm Animal Welfare Council (FAWC). However, both systems fail badly to meet one of the two fundamental criteria for good welfare, namely the need to achieve sustained fitness.

Genetic selection of broiler chickens for rapid growth and gross hypertrophy of the breast muscle has created serious problems of 'leg weakness' in the heavy, fastest growing strains. 'Leg weakness' is a euphemism used to describe but not diagnose a long and depressing list of pathological conditions of bones (e.g. tibial dyschondroplasia), joints (e.g. septic arthritis), tendons (e.g. perosis) and skin (e.g. hock burn). For more details see the FAWC Report on the Welfare of Broiler Chickens (1992). Similar problems are seen in the heavy strains of turkeys. Kestin *et al.* (1993) have demonstrated that the incidence of leg weakness sufficient to cause moderate to severe impairment of leg movement in broiler chickens reaches approximately 25% in heavy strains by the time of slaughter at 42 days of age but is below 5% in strains less intensively selected for rapid growth which may reach slaughter weights between 70 to 90 days of age. I must emphasize that the pathology and pathogenesis of these leg disorders is complex and multifactorial but most of the conditions can be attributed, in simple terms, to birds that have grown too heavy for their limbs and/or become so distorted in shape as to impose unnatural stresses on their joints.

As I indicated in Chapter 5, we do not yet have unequivocal evidence that these disorders of bone and joint are associated with chronic pain, largely because, as yet, we know so little of the neurobiology and pharmacology of pain in birds. However, on the balance of the evidence we must conclude that *approximately one quarter of the heavy strains of broiler chicken and turkey are in chronic pain for approximately one third of their lives.* Given that poultrymeat consumption in the UK exceeds one million tonnes per annum, this must constitute, in both magnitude and severity, the single most severe, systematic example of man's inhumanity to another sentient animal.

The laying hen

In Chapter 1, I compared the welfare of the laying hen in a battery cage and in commercial 'free range' flock as a first illustration of the application of the logic of the five freedoms to the evaluation of animal welfare in different husbandry systems (Table 1.1). To restate the argument in brief, the hen has been domesticated from the jungle fowl which lived in small groups and spent the day foraging on the ground, protected by the undergrowth from attack from the air, and roosted at night on the low branches of trees in reasonable security from attack from the ground. Within these small groups, birds could also develop stable pecking orders so that while intraspecies aggression was a reality, it was not a serious problem.

In commercial units based on the conventional battery cage, laying hens are stocked so densely as, in effect, to fill up all the available space. The cages are entirely barren. The hens will be expected to lay an egg a day for a period of about 50 weeks by which time they will be described, with brutal realism, as 'spent'. The welfare problems of the caged layer have been described many times and at length (see Fraser and Broom, 1990). Very briefly:

(1) *Nutrition:* generally satisfactory, but the incidence of osteoporosis implies that calcium, phosphorus and vitamin D nutrition are not ideal.
(2) (a) *Thermal comfort:* satisfactory.
(2) (b) *Physical comfort:* hens do not require cushions (unless incubating eggs), damage to feet and feathers has been severe but can be reduced by improvements to cage design.
(3) (a) *Pain and injury:* bone weakness and fractures consequent upon osteoporosis.
(3) (b) *Infectious disease:* generally satisfactory.
(4) *Normal behaviour:* severely restricted, especially nesting and dust-bathing.
(5) *Fear and stress:* probably no major problems.

The most serious welfare problems for the caged layer are the frustration of normal behaviour and the lack of sustained fitness. Studies of motivation in hens, using the economic demand theory of Dawkins (1983) reveal that hens are extremely powerfully motivated to seek a nesting area in which to lay their eggs. Hens will also work to achieve increased space *per se*, up to an area of 900 cm^2. They will use dust or other forms of litter for grooming when it is provided but are less inclined to work for it than to enter a nest box. These studies need to be interpreted with some caution. Hens *may* be less strongly motivated to enter a dust bathing area than a nest box. Alternatively it may be that the drive to dust bathing (in a hen without external parasites) is external whereas the drive to lay the egg in the 'right place' is internal. In other words, when the dust bath (but not the nest box) is out of sight, it is also out of mind.

In my opinion, the battery cage, *in its current form*, does not meet acceptable minimum standards for the welfare of the laying hen. A detailed consideration of improvements to cage design is beyond the scope of this book (but see Sherwin, 1994). However, I believe the three essential features of an acceptable cage containing four to six birds are:

(1) a suitable nesting site;
(2) a perch, to improve fitness of feet and legs and discourage the birds from roosting in the nest boxes;
(3) 900 cm^2 space per bird (additional to that within the nest boxes).

One of the 'natural' features of cage systems is that the birds are kept in small groups. Alternative husbandry systems for laying hens which keep birds in large colonies whether indoors on the ground or in a tiered aviary or with access to free range out of doors are all faced by real problems of intraspecies aggression, mob hysteria and the consequent fear and stress experienced by birds that are unable to maintain personal control of their physical and social environment. Mortality rates of birds in large, commercial colony systems are usually greater than for hens in cages and most of these deaths can be attributed to problems of aggression, fear or stress rather than to infectious disease. Moreover, in some large free range units half the birds elect to stay permanently within the house, which rather invalidates the whole point of the exercise. While I am absolutely convinced that a dozen hens free-ranging in a traditional farmyard with access to good food, and the shelter and security of barns and strawstacks enjoy a life style that is close to being ideal, I interpret the large amount of available evidence to conclude that, when all five freedoms are taken into consideration, the welfare of laying hens in large, commercial colony systems is at least as bad as that of hens in the conventional battery cage.

Handling, transport and slaughter

One of the great, brutal truths of the animal welfare story is that we care for animals in direct proportion to their value to us. This value may be defined by economics, sentiment or fashion. We will, for example, give more care to how we transport an expensive racehorse or a well-loved dog than a spent hen. As I write this section, there is a flurry of public concern over the transport of sheep by air from Australia to Singapore, *en route* to Halal slaughter in the Arab states. Now this trade does raise serious welfare problems relating to the duration of the journey, the quality of the environment and stockmanship *en route* and the process of ritual slaughter at the end, problems that could all be avoided by killing the animals as close as possible to their farms of origin and exporting the carcasses. There is, however, nothing inherently stressful about being on an aircraft or, in good weather, on board ship. Humans pay good money to do it all the time. Any problems must be defined by the nature of acute and chronic stresses that may, or may not, occur in association with the journey. These are:

(1)   fear and pain associated with handling and mixing;
(2)   thermal or motion stresses during the journey;
(3)   hunger, thirst and exhaustion;
(4)   risks of infection.

   The problem for poultry is that life is cheap and, for spent hens, very cheap. Thus the trade is prepared to accept a very low incidence of broiler birds found dead on arrival at the abattoir but a considerably higher incidence among spent hens. Poultry are removed off the floor or from cages by handlers who are faced by such large numbers and have to work so fast that they cannot reasonably be expected to treat each individual with tender care. Some studies have revealed that removal of spent hens from battery cages was likely to break at least one bone per bird. However, recognition of this problem has led to improvements in handling procedures and cage front design. On the journey, the birds are packed tightly into travelling crates and transported on lorries where the control of temperature and ventilation is minimal, depending largely on the use of curtains and the speed of the vehicle. Our studies with an artificial chicken, 'Gloria' (Fig. 8.3) and her descendants, have revealed severe problems of both heat and cold stress for birds in transit. Indeed, for most commercial vehicles there are almost no environmental circumstances where the birds will be thermally comfortable

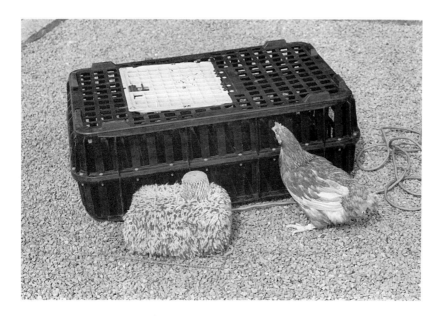

Fig. 8.3 Gloria, an artificial chicken for measuring thermal stresses on birds in transit.

both when the vehicle is at rest and in motion. They are either comfortable while in motion and too hot while stationary, or comfortable while stationary and too cold while in motion. (Incidentally, the official name for our artificial chicken is 'stress integrator, chickens in transit', which abbreviates naturally to SIC transit; hence 'Gloria'.)

Thermal stress is undoubtedly the major killer of poultry in transit. Unlike hunger and thirst, the stress begins at once, although the extent of hypo- or hyperthermia increases with time. Pain associated with motion of the vehicle in broilers with 'leg weakness' and layers with broken bones, is the next most important welfare problem, followed by fear. Poultry display extended periods of tonic immobility following transport. In hens but not broilers, this appears to be related to the length of the journey. There can be no doubt that the length of the journey contributes to the stress and the potential lethality of transport but most of the abuses can be attributed to the unsatisfactory nature of the environment within the vehicles. If the quality of the environment were as good as that on the farm unit, then maximum permissible journey lengths would only need to be defined according to the birds' requirements for food and water.

The procedure for slaughter of nearly all chickens and most turkeys is to suspend the birds upside down on shackles around their legs then transport them to an apparatus desgned for electrical stunning and subsequent sticking, with a man down line from the sticking point to kill any bird that has been improperly handled by the machinery. As with pigs, the humanity of this process is determined largely by how well it is operated and supervized. However, certain welfare abuses are intrinsic to the system. Suspending birds upside down on shackles must induce some degree of fear. More seriously, this procedure must seriously exacerbate the intensity of pain in chickens and especially the heavier turkeys with chronic leg disorders. The stunning process cannot guarantee 100% efficiency. Finally, the whole stressful procedure takes time. Gas stunning with a carbon dioxide/argon mixture is as effective and humane for poultry as it is for pigs. Moreover, the method of gas stunning (and killing) is compatible with killing birds in their transport crates thereby circumventing all the stresses involved in handling and shackling within the abattoir. In principle the approach could be taken even further. Spent hens, for example, could be humanely killed by carbon dioxide and argon while still in their battery cages, thereby circumventing all the stresses associated with handling and transport. There are inherent problems of this approach, relating to public health and meat quality but there are no absolute reasons why these may not be overcome.

Priorities for change

Change for the good will occur by natural evolution if it is consistent with natural selection. In the specific context of the production of a commodity such as food from animals, this means that change will occur naturally only if it is consistent with the operation of the free market. Current pig and poultry systems meet the needs of almost all the market. This is because the majority of consumers value the eggs, poultry and pigmeat primarily according to their cheapness and consistency. These are sound criteria but they do not always dominate consumer behaviour. If people purchased motor cars only according to these criteria the streets would be full of Ladas. It is tempting to suggest that the standard broiler chicken is the Lada of the meat trade. If the public valued their food the way they value their motor cars, the market would be wide open for high quality products, one essential criterion of quality being an assurance as to the quality of life of the animals.

One conclusion that should be obvious from this chapter is that many of the highest priorities for change to improve pig and poultry welfare are not likely to bring about a simultaneous increase in productivity. Thus it is unrealistic to expect them to evolve through the operation of the free market. This implies that they can only be achieved either through a radical change in the public perception of quality of the product, which can only be achieved through education, or by legislation to enforce or encourage higher welfare standards. I have already stressed that legislation designed to interfere with market forces is tricky, particularly when it attempts to embrace something as complex as the quality of life of a sentient animal. I repeat, therefore, the principles and cautions outlined in the previous chapter:

(1) it is unnecessary to guarantee that an enforced change will always make things better, but necessary to guarantee that the change will not, in some realistic circumstances, make things worse;
(2) any change imposed by legislation must be enforced fairly within the economic community.

With these cautions very much in mind, let us consider what might be done, by the application of new knowledge, by education, or by legislation to improve the welfare of pigs and poultry. In most cases legislation is too crude an instrument to define the quality of life for a farm animal but, in the case of the laying hen, I believe that there is sufficient evidence to support legislation to provide caged hens with a recognizable nesting area, a suitable perch and $900 \, cm^2$ free space per bird. Such legislation would not be entirely satisfactory to the birds, still less satisfactory to the most passionate advocates of animal rights but would constitute an unequivocal improvement on the *status quo*, subject to the guarantee that the new law would remain unchanged for at least the next 10 years. The poultry industry can play to almost any set of rules, properly enforced. What it cannot be asked to accept is constant shifts in our definition of acceptability. The legislation does not have to define ideal standards, although it must not create more problems than it solves. This could arise if there was an absolute ban on keeping small groups of hens in cages of any form, since commercial producers could not then protect their hens from the welfare problems associated with large colony systems.

Legislation does not have to be proscriptive (e.g. a ban on the battery cage). It is also possible to legislate for the common good by fine-tuning market forces. The reason why the battery cage has become so dominant is that no other system can compete economically as a mass producer of eggs. It is neither necessary nor realistic for legislation to attempt to define optimal environmental standards for hens; it is sufficient, and more conducive to new thinking to encourage producers to improve welfare by whatever means they think best. If egg producers were presented with new legislation setting minimum standards for caged layers based on the proposals I have listed above they would have the option of buying new cages or developing alternative systems since the legislation would remove or greatly reduce, the current commercial advantage of the cage system.

All attempts, such as those within the Council of Europe, to devise legislation to improve the welfare of the laying hen have, so far, been obsessed with the need to define minimum standards for cage design. There is, however, a much more attractive way to achieve the same objective, namely improved living standards for the laying hen. This is to devise financial incentives and penalties designed to shift the economic balance in favour of alternative systems such as a subsidy for producers who kept birds on free range with flock sizes no larger than 200 birds. There need be no limit to the number of flocks maintained on any one farm. The standard response of Eurogovernments to such a suggestion is that legislation by financial incentive is impossible since there is no new money. That objection can be easily dismissed. There is no need for new money. In 1993, 42% of income to farmers within the European Union came from government grants and subsidies using taxpayers' money. At present, many subsidies, such as those for extensification and set-aside are dictated almost entirely by the need to avoid overproduction. There is some emphasis on the maintenance of environmental quality and living standards for the small farmer but, at present no example of subsidy directly designed to improve quality of life for the animals. One of the main aims of subsidy is to maintain the quality of life on the land, and this should imply quality of life for both farmers and their animals. I suggest most strongly that matters of animal welfare should be central to any discussion as to the best use of agricultural subsidy.

I have already indentified the problems of leg weakness and chronic pain in heavy strains of broilers and turkeys as my top priority for change. The problem is, in fact, readily soluble by relaxing selection for rapid growth and/ or by reducing nutrient supply during early development. However, both these things slow down production and therefore increase costs, and producers will not do this unless they are compelled to do so or can market 'high welfare' birds at a reasonable profit. Most supermarkets now stock free range broilers. This, in itself, is not a sufficient guarantee of freedom from chronic pain since heavy strains show a high incidence of leg weakness in all forms of accommodation. It is necessary to read the small print before buying quality-assured, high welfare products. However, if the small print indicates that the birds are not killed until they are at least 70 days of age this means that they are of the slower growing, fitter strains. Personally, I almost never eat broiler chicken unless it is of a light, slow growing strain, free range and usually corn fed. By so doing, I eat smaller portions of a better tasting bird, the heavier strain of broiler being, in my opinion, little more than an edible plate, all flavour to be added retrospectively. By such means I satisfy the needs of my conscience, my health (by eating relatively less meat and more vegetables) and my palate. To this consumer, this chicken has real added value.

As the public becomes more aware of the realities of poultry production the more likely they are to put pressure on producers to improve production methods by choosing high welfare products in the shops. It would, however, be unrealistic to expect major changes in buying habits in the short term and the problems of leg weakness are severe and require radical action now. The FAWC report on the welfare of broiler chickens (1992) states:

> 'The Council considers that the current level of leg problems in broilers is unacceptable. We recommend that steps should be taken to ensure that there is a significant reduction in the number and severity of leg problems. It will be the responsibility of the industry to achieve this objective and the Council intends to look at this aspect of broiler production again in five years' time, when significant improvements should be apparent. If no reduction in leg problems is found, we may recommend the introduction of legislation to ensure the required improvements.'

This is quite a strong statement for a quasi-governmental body, although the industry needs to do considerably better than achieve 'no reduction in leg problems'. It is too soon to say how effective this recommendation will prove to be but it is fair to say that the broiler breeders are acting upon it*.

Before leaving the issue of leg weakness in broilers I should point out that there is nothing inherently inhumane in producing a finished bird at 42 days of age. If, through genetic selection, improved nutrition or control of lighting the poultry industry can produce a bird ready for slaughter in 42 days or 30 days or less, I shall have no objection provided that they can clearly demonstrate that the birds do not suffer during the course of their short lives. On the basis of current evidence the onus is on the industry to prove absence of suffering, rather than on the scientist or welfarist to prove that it exists.

At present, there is extreme public pressure to amend legislation relating to animal transport. Some of the arguments confound welfare with chauvinism, but much of the concern is well-founded. The Commission of the European

---

Footnote to second impression: The broiler industry has responded to public criticism encapsulated by the FAWC 1992 report. Tests for leg disorders similar to that developed by Kestin now form part of quality assurance schemes in commercial broiler flocks and the problem of leg weakness is undoubtedly less severe than it was 6 years ago. This has been achieved in small part by genetic selection but more by changes to management; in particular, by restricting artificial day length so that birds do not overeat in the first two weeks of life. There are two positive messages here. First, one of the greatest of welfare problems has a simple solution. Second, public opinion has worked!

Communities (CEC) have prepared a new proposal for a Council Directive (COM (93) 330) on the protection of animals during transport. In the explanatory memorandum they recognize that many problems are not due to transport *per se* but the quality of the environment within the vehicles. However, the specific proposals relate only to minimum space allowances, maximum travel times and minimum resting times between journeys. Unless there is provision to feed and water animals on the vehicles, maximum travel times for poultry, including that for loading and unloading will become six hours for broilers and pullets, eight hours for ducks and twelve hours for other poultry. Maximum travel times for pigs between stops for food and water will become 12 hours.

These proposals address only those stresses which are primarily a function of journey length, e.g. hunger and thirst, and imply differences within and between species which are unsupported by evidence and inconsistent with Codes of Welfare requirements for feeding and watering within animal houses. The proposed constraints on the length of journeys for poultry reflect the real concern that poultry are more likely to be severely stressed (or killed) during transport than other farm species. However, the main stresses on birds in transit are not primarily the problems of long journeys, thirst, hunger and exhaustion, but fear, pain in damaged limbs and, especially, heat and cold stress. The proposal to limit journey times (inclusive of loading and unloading) to six hours for broilers and pullets may save some lives in badly designed vehicles, although deaths in transit are far commoner in low value 'spent' hens and they can be transported for 12 hours. It will undoubtedly create real problems for the industry and could create welfare problems for the birds if the loading process is rushed to comply with the law. As a constructive solution to this dilemma, I suggest that these proposals for maximum journey time be retained, but propose exemptions for hauliers whose vehicles are able to ensure proper standards of thermal and physical comfort for the birds both while at rest and in motion. This is another specific example of a generic theme. What I propose is legislation which carries elements of both carrot and stick. If it led to significant and widespread improvements in vehicle design it would do far more to improve the welfare of poultry (and pigs) in transit than administratively tidy but intellectually timid legislation based on journey times alone.

The central tenet of existing slaughter legislation is that 'animals must be slaughtered instantaneously or rendered instantaneously insensible to pain until death supervenes'. However, pain at the point of slaughter is not the only welfare problem and a quick stun is not ideal if it is only achieved after the animal has had a frightening or distressing journey to the stunning point, goaded along a dark corridor or suspended upside down on shackles. The objective of legislation and good practice must be to minimize *all* stresses associated with handling, transport, lairage and stunning. The welfare of pigs and poultry could be improved by appropriate gaseous stunning and killing of animals, especially if this procedure were used to minimize handling, e.g.

gassing animals while still on farm or in their transit pens or cages. This would need new legislation in relation both to welfare and public health. If the existing phrase 'animals must be rendered instantaneously insensible to pain' were replaced by a more flexible clause such as 'at the place of slaughter animals must be handled, rendered unconscious and killed in such a way as to minimize pain and suffering'. this would encourage the development of integrated systems designed to reduce, and in some cases circumvent, the multiplicity of stresses experienced by pigs and poultry during their last day of life.

Legislation can be an effective route towards improved procedures for handling of animals in transit and at the point of slaughter since these procedures are relatively straightforward. It is far less easy to devise legislation to improve husbandry systems on the farm since, in this case, one has to take into account all possible effects of an imposed change in husbandry on everything that contributes to the animals' quality of life. In the examples I have given so far, I believe that my proposed minimum standards for battery cages would constitute a significant improvement in the quality of life for the caged layer. Moreover, I believe it would create no new problems, such as an increase in feather pecking, although this needs to be tested by trials on a commercial scale. On the other hand, I repeat my belief that a simple ban on the battery cage, in any form, would do more harm than good by exposing birds in commercial flocks to the known perils of large colony systems.

The situation becomes even more complicated when we consider possible legislation to improve welfare standards for pigs. The UK government, but not yet the rest of the European Community, has agreed to impose a ban on the housing of dry sows in individual unbedded stalls, with or without tethers, with effect from the year 1999. I am satisfied that there is sufficient evidence to justify this proposal. I would not argue the case, as many do, simply on the basis of abnormal stereotypic behaviour such as bar-chewing. However, when all the evidence, including chronic discomfort, pain and injury, is taken into account, then I am satisfied that the case for a ban on the semi-permanent housing of dry sows in unbedded stalls becomes overwhelming.

Any legislation to ban sow stalls, however, must ensure that it will not, in some circumstances, do more harm than good. Some proposals that appeared in early drafts for Euro-legislation have been ludicrous, such as the suggestion that dry sows could be housed in stalls provided that they were released for one hour per day. The well-meant intention was presumably to allow the sows the opportunity for exercise and social contact. It would not, I fear, have been a very happy hour. The main objections from the pig industry to a total ban on sow stalls are:

(1)   If sows that are currently stalled and fed individually have to be housed in groups, it would be difficult, (i) to avoid fighting and (ii) to ensure that each sow is individually fed to maintain optimal condition.

(2)   If all the sows currently housed in stalls and on concrete were housed in straw yards, there would not be enough straw to go round.

These objections would carry more weight were it not for the fact that many pig farmers are managing perfectly well without stalls at present. Even when the sow stall was at its peak of popularity, it accounted for only about 55% of the UK herd of breeding sows. Currently, approximately 38% of dry sows are kept in stalls, 44% in yards and 18% in outdoor units. The recent expansion of outdoor units does, in some measure, reflect a desire to improve the welfare of the breeding sow. The survival and success of outdoor units also reveals that they can, on the right land, compete with intensive systems. In other words, the sow stall, unlike the battery cage, is not the only commercially viable option within current law. It may be the most economic option when the land is too wet and heavy for an outdoor unit or when the farm cannot produce sufficient straw bedding for sows in yards. However, plenty of farmers keep dry sows in good condition and free from aggression in straw yards, though it requires good stockmanship. Objections to a ban on sow stalls are based on a limited economic argument; alternatives to the sow stall are less economic only for those farmers who elected to use stalls because their land, and/or their crops, were not suited to alternative forms of pig production. One of the most powerful criticisms of intensive pig and poultry units is that they no longer farm the land in ways best suited to its climate and geography. A ban on sow stalls may persuade farmers who are not farming proper pig country to seek alternative enterprises. I see no good reason why the ban should cause a significant increase in the price of pig meat.

Most other aspects of pig welfare on the farm are more likely to be improved through research and development than by proscriptive legislation. This is mainly because questions such as the development of optimal systems for farrowing, nursing and weaning piglets are too complex to be addressed by the imposition of strict rules. It is most unlikely that there is a single best solution to this question and any legislation based upon a current Euro-compromise definition of best practice would be more likely to inhibit than encourage development. I am, however, optimistic that the welfare of pigs can and will get better through the application of new knowledge and understanding, humanely applied. During the last 50 years the livestock industry in the developed world, generously supported by government research, development and advisory services, has been hugely successful in producing all the food we need, with a steady improvement in real quality and a steady reduction in real cost. This is what the public wanted and they got it, in spades. Having more than satisfied its demand for good cheap food, public opinion now calls for improved standards of environmental quality and animal welfare. If that is what the public wants, then farmers (given proper support) can do that too.

9 Cattle and Other Ruminants

Milch cow: 'a cow yielding milk or kept for milking: a ready source of gain or money.'

Chambers English Dictionary

Ruminants are animals which evolved to graze and browse the grasses, herbs and leaves of the bush and the open plains. Man has derived enormous benefit from domesticating the ruminant and exploiting it as a source of food, clothing, work, fuel and fertilizer. In most circumstances in most parts of the world, he has found it expedient (i.e. cost-effective) to leave the animals to forage and ferment the grasses and other fibrous feeds for themselves rather than take them off the land and use machines to harvest all the bulky forage and spread all the bulky fertilizer. One outstanding exception to this general rule from the earliest days of agriculture has been the animal (cow, goat or buffalo) that provides milk and dairy products for the family and for sale. Chambers Dictionary defines *milch cow* as 'a cow yielding milk or kept for milking: a ready source of gain or money'. Because milch cows have always been able to generate wealth it has always been worthwhile for their owners (i) to cut, cart and store food for them and (ii) to care for them as individuals. The dairy cow has added quite as much value to the life of the Indian as the horse has to the life of the Englishman and the two races have responded accordingly by erecting taboos against the killing of such precious animals

These sound biological and economic principles have largely survived the mechanization and intensification of farming, although often in radically modified form. Many beef cattle and sheep are still farmed for much of their lives in 'natural', extensive fashion, and most dairy cattle are still treated as individuals with real value. This sense of value is strictly unsentimental. The word 'cattle' has the same Old French root as 'chattel' implying property for personal use. On the whole the farming of cattle and sheep has escaped public criticism, save for that directed at the rearing of calves entirely on milk substitute diets for the production of white veal. The criticism of white veal production is well founded. The lack of criticism of the welfare of cattle and other ruminants in other modern systems is less well founded and stems in part from the limited concept of animal welfare which equates it only with behavioural freedom. Before proceeding to consider specific welfare problems of ruminants it is necessary to restate and illustrate by example four of the themes central to my overall argument:

(1) Good welfare does not necessarily equate with extensive or 'natural' systems of husbandry.
(2) Behavioural freedom is only one of the five freedoms that define positive welfare.
(3) The severity of suffering experienced by an individual animal is defined both by its intensity and by its duration.
(4) The optimal present and future welfare of any animal requires a compromise between conflicting present and future needs.

Consider the welfare of a 'flying' flock of sheep: draft ewes brought down from the hill in middle age and sold to a farmer who neither knows nor cares much about sheep but wishes to get one more lamb crop from them at minimal cost. In this example the sheep are outwintered on poorly drained lowland pasture close to a housing estate. Using all five freedoms to analyse their welfare at the end of February, we discover that:

(1) the ewes are emaciated due to chronic underfeeding. This is immediately obvious on palpation of the lack of muscle and fat cover over the lumbar vertebrae but does not show under the fleece.
(2) the ewes regularly suffer cold stress during periods of wet weather because they are not only forced to stand in the rain but lie in the mud. As their body condition deteriorates so the severity of the cold stress is increased.
(3) half the ewes are in chronic pain from untreated foot rot.
(4) the ewes are regularly frightened (and some have been injured) by uncontrolled dogs from the housing estate.
   But,
(5) *the ewes have total freedom to engage in behaviour natural to their species.* In this example the classic manifestations of sheep behaviour are panic and flight.

This is, I admit, an extreme and hypothetical example (although by no means unknown). It does, however, illustrate my first two themes. The farming of sheep, and ruminants in general, has received far less public criticism than the factory farming of pigs and poultry, mainly because to the casual eye the systems appear to allow sheep and cattle more freedom to display their natural repertoire of behaviour. I would, however, hope to have convinced anyone who has read this far that the *intensity* of suffering experienced by the sheep in the above example is likely to be worse than that of the battery hen.

The overall severity of suffering must be considered in terms of both intensity and duration, and can be expressed as:

Severity of suffering $= f_1$ (intensity) $\times f_2$ (duration)

The intensity of suffering experienced by a cow undergoing Halal or Shekita slaughter and conscious of choking to death in its own blood is extremely severe, but the duration is brief. The intensity of suffering experienced by the hen in the battery cage is less severe than that involved in ritual slaughter. It is, however, an abuse of welfare that lasts an adult life-time. I would not wish to express in precise mathematical terms the relative importance of the intensity and duration functions f_1 and f_2 in these two examples. However, application of the principle persuades me that the overall severity of suffering experienced by a hen in a conventional battery cage greatly exceeds that experienced, for example, by a beef animal ritually slaughtered after a life at grass.

My fourth central theme, implicit in the concept of the five freedoms, is that action to achieve optimal welfare standards for animals must be based on compromise, not only between the needs of the farmer and his animals but also between the different contributors to animal welfare. Moreover, this compromise should be assessed not only in terms of the intensity of all possible sources of present suffering or pleasure but must also consider the future consequences of any action. Consider the welfare of young calves or puppies. They undoubtedly have a behavioural need (i.e. are powerfully motivated) to socialize and play. However, in many practical circumstances, calves or puppies that are given the freedom to mix in early life are at far greater risk of sickness or death from diseases such as, respectively, salmonellosis and canine distemper. To ensure their future welfare it is frequently necessary to restrict their behavioural freedom *for a while*. The short time isolation of a calf or puppy may be acceptable when it serves the long-term interests of the animal. The practice becomes unacceptable when the decision is made to isolate a veal calf in a crate or tether a dog to a kennel for much of its lifetime.

With these general points in mind let us consider the welfare of the animal that works harder for man than any other, namely the dairy cow.

Welfare of the dairy cow

The life of a typical European or North American suckler beef cow that produces one calf per year while living outdoors for most or all of the year is broadly similar to that of the wild ruminant on open range. She will feed her calf until it is weaned at a natural age of six to eight months. She will secrete milk at a maximum rate of perhaps 8–10 litres per day which the calf will drink in four to six meals per day. The total lactation yield of the cow may be less than 1000 litres and the maximum amount of milk contained in the udder at any time will be approximately two litres. A good European or North American dairy cow will typically be a black and white Holstein/Friesian who will also produce one calf per year, starting at two years of age. When she is at her peak (e.g. in her third lactation) she may produce between 6000 to 12 000 litres during a total lactation period of 10 months with a two-month 'rest' before she calves again and the process is repeated. Typical maximum daily yield will be between 30 to 40 litres although 57 litres (or 100 pint bottles) of milk per cow per day is not unknown on dairy units in regions like California or Israel which can supply not only the cows but also the nutrition to sustain such a yield. The milk will be removed by machine two or three times per day so that the maximum amount of milk contained within the udder at any one time may exceed 20 litres, ten times the likely maximum for a beef cow suckling her own calf.

The two processes are very different. Indeed, it may be argued that the dairy cow is exposed to more abnormal physiological demands than any other class of farm animal. Table 7.2, which compared food energy intakes and work rates in a range of mammals and birds revealed the intense metabolic demand of lactation in the dairy cow. Using a fanciful, but accurate analogy, I suggested that to achieve the daily work rate of the dairy cow, a man would have to jog for six to eight hours per day, every day.

Table 7.2 also illustrated the point that despite the efforts of breeders to select cows for greater and greater yields the peak milk yield and work rate of the typical dairy cow is not, in fact, so abnormal when compared on an interspecies basis with some litter-bearing species such as the sow and bitch. For most mammals, lactation is very hard work. The most abnormal feature of the work required of the dairy cow (and goat) is not so much the intensity of the metabolic load as the length of time it must be sustained.

In welfare terms, the good news for the highly productive milch cow is that, unlike, for example, the battery hen, she is a very valuable individual. A good British dairy cow should generate at least £1000 gross profit margin per year. The bad news is that, in order to convert this into net profit she has to be worked to the limits of her productivity to meet the high fixed costs of labour, housing and machinery plus other possible costs such as the purchase of milk quota (Fig. 7.1). These limits are defined by:

(1) the genetic and physiological potential of the mammary gland to synthesize and secrete milk;
(2) the capacity of the cow to forage for, consume, digest and metabolize nutrients required for maintenance, lactation and simultaneous pregnancy;
(3) the capacity of the dairy cow to meet the sustained metabolic demands of lactation without succumbing to exhaustion or production diseases.

In most practical circumstances, the capacity of the mammary gland to synthesize milk exceeds the capacity of the cow upstream to find, eat and digest enough food to supply the mammary gland with nutrients. As I have indicated earlier, there are a few places in the world such as California and Israel where herds of dairy cows, permanently housed in highly expensive accommodation and fed highly expensive balanced rations can sustain daily yields in excess of 50 litres and total lactation yields in excess of 15 000 litres. However, such circumstances, where milk production is close to the maximum possible rate of milk synthesis, are few and far between. A herd of

Holstein cows in the UK may not be that genetically inferior to the California Holstein but when grazed over summer and fed over winter on a diet consisting principally of grass silage, a herd average of 8000 litres per cow would be considered very good. Both the improved Holstein housed over winter in the UK and the unimproved African cow eating standing hay during the dry season could produce much more milk if the quality of their food was improved.

Health and welfare problems for the dairy cow may arise as a direct consequence of the intensity and duration of the metabolic demands of lactation or, more probably, as a consequence of conditions of feeding, housing and management inappropriate to the physiology of the animal bred for high yields. I compare the high-performance dairy cow to a high-performance racing car. When the car is right, the fuel is right and the maintenance is right, the performance can be spectacular. If the fuel is inadequate, the racing car (or dairy cow) will underperform and if the maintenance is inadequate they break!

The main welfare problems that may arise through breeding, feeding, housing, managing or otherwise manipulating cows for high productivity include:

(1) hunger or acute metabolic disease, due to an imbalance between nutrient supply and demand.
(2) chronic discomfort, through bad housing, loss of condition, etc.
(3) chronic pain or restricted movement due to distortion of body shape, bad housing or management.
(4) increased susceptibility to infectious or metabolic disease.
(5) metabolic or physical exhaustion after prolonged high production.

Metabolic hunger

The high genetic merit, lactating dairy cow is faced by an intense, sustained demand for nutrients to sustain the capacity of the mammary gland to synthesize milk. Her problem is to meet this demand for nutrients within the practical constraints determined by:

(1) the quantity and quality of the available food;
(2) the capacity of her digestive system to process the food into metabolizable nutrients;
(3) the time available for eating without seriously eroding her conflicting need to rest.

The typical UK cow overwintered on a ration consisting mainly of bulky, slowly digested grass silage may not only be unable to produce milk to her genetic potential but she may also feel, simultaneously, hungry, 'full up' and physically tired. She feels hungry for nutrients to support the high metabolic requirement for maintenance and lactation. She feels 'full up' because, to satisfy her metabolic hunger she has filled her rumen with slowly digestible bulk food (mainly silage). She feels physically tired, partly because of her high work load and partly because her motivation to eat conflicts with her motivation to rest.

Using the concept of MacFarland's egg (Fig. 2.2) to evaluate these effects, we may predict that the high performance cow attempting to meet her nutrient needs on a diet largely consisting of grass silage will chronically operate close to and may, on occasions, exceed the limits of her ability to accommodate these conflicting sensations and motivations without suffering. Selection of cows for ever higher yields may tend to exacerbate welfare problems of metabolic origin, associated with the impossibility of resolving the conflict between metabolic hunger and digestive overload, if the genetic 'improvement' is not accompanied by parallel improvements in nutrition. However, selection of cows for higher yields does tend to produce a superior cow, not just a superior udder; and one of the primary attributes of the superior cow is an improved ability to consume, digest and metabolize food.

On the other hand, procedures such as the regular injection of recombinant growth hormone (bovine somatotropin or BST) simply increase the capacity of the mammary gland to synthesize milk without adjusting the anatomical or physiological ability of the cow to process nutrients. In most practical circumstances, therefore, injections of BST are likely to intensify the cow's conflict between the problems of hunger, digestive overload and physical exhaustion and increase the risk that some cows will be made to suffer to meet these conflicting demands.

Lameness

One unequivocal source of suffering in dairy cows is that caused by the pain of lameness, especially from injuries to their feet. Surveys of cases of foot lameness treated by the farmer or his veterinary surgeon reveal an incidence of about 25% per year. The average working life of the dairy cow is four (one-year) lactations and inspection of the feet of cull cows at slaughter reveals evidence of past or present foot damage in nearly all animals. In other words the UK dairy industry is living with a painful, crippling disease with a morbidity rate close to 100%!

The most common place to see foot lameness in the UK is in dairy cows overwintered in cubicle houses rather than in straw yards. The most common time is shortly after calving. The problem is worse than it was 40 years ago mainly because most cows now live in cubicle houses rather than straw yards, a practice that developed in parallel with the conservation of grass as wet silage rather than dry hay. Wet silage produces wet faeces – too wet for most straw yard systems. Table 9.1 outlines some of the main factors involved in the complex aetiology of foot lameness (for further details see Blowey (1993)

Care of the Bovine Foot; Webster (1993) *Understanding the Dairy Cow*). Overfeeding starchy concentrates can create rumen acidosis, release of endotoxins and vascular damage to the feet, presenting as laminitis. To understand the pain of laminitis it helps to imagine crushing all your fingernails in the door then standing on your fingertips. Cows are more prone to foot injury if compelled to stand for long periods on concrete, especially if it is covered in wet, acid slurry. The risk is increased if the cows are fed wet grass silage, if the concrete floors are not scraped regularly, or if submissive individuals, such as newly calved heifers, are bullied out of cubicle accommodation and made to stand for long periods in the passageways. The appearance of clinical foot lameness shortly after calving is partly due to the changes in feeding and housing that occur at this time. However, there is new evidence that early, microscopic damage to the feet of heifers can begin four to six weeks before calving and these may get worse as a direct consequence of physiological changes occurring around the time of parturition (Kempson and Logue, 1993). At the University of Bristol farm our cows have for many years overwintered in cubicle accommodation. Nowadays, in order to minimize the risk of foot injury cows and heifers are housed on straw for at least four weeks before and after calving.

Table 9.1 Factors predisposing to lameness in dairy cows.

	Examples
Breeding	Hind leg conformation, foot colour
Nutrition	Direct: laminitis on starchy feeds
	Indirect: wet, acid slurry on grass silage
Housing	Poor cubicle design
	Hard, wet, slippery concrete
Management	Poor foot care
	Twice-daily milking
Behaviour	Prolonged standing of submissive cows
'Stress'	Physiological changes about the time of parturition

The most striking feature of foot lameness in dairy cows is that approximately 75% of cases occur in the abaxial (outer) claws of the hind feet. Since we may reasonably assume that effects of feeding and housing affect all four feet (and all eight claws) equally, the predisposition for the outer claw of the hind feet must be attributable to the conformation of the dairy cow. Figure 9.1 examines, from the back end, a typical adult Friesian dairy cow and a typical heifer (her daughter) pregnant with her first calf. The obvious difference between the two is the size of the udder. The second point of distinction is that whereas the hind legs of the heifer are straight up and down, those of the older cow have been distorted by distension of the udder so that

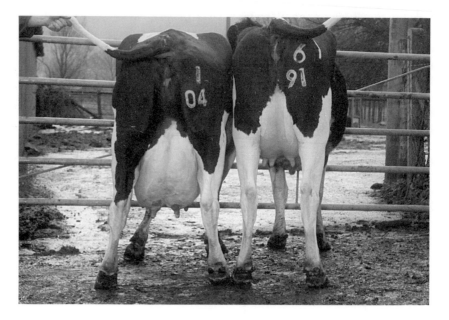

Fig. 9.1 Rear views of a mature Friesian cow and her heifer daughter.

the cow has become 'cow-hocked'. The stifle is displaced outwards and the hocks inwards thus throwing more weight onto the outer claw. (Stick a football between your thighs and try it!)

The rapid distension of the udder at the time of first calving and subsequent enlargement of the udder necessary to accommodate up to 20 litres between milkings undoubtedly predisposes to foot lameness by causing uneven load on the inner and outer claws. Cattle breeders (unlike broiler breeders) have always been careful not to select their cows on performance alone but also on the basis of conformation, paying particular attention to the shape of the udder and hind limbs so as to reduce the risk of lameness and mastitis. However, as always, there is a conflict of objectives. Cows with better (wider) udders tend to have worse (more cow-hocked) back legs. The main problem for the dairy cow is not the conformation it inherits at birth but the conformation it acquires as a result of the abnormal distension of the udder. For the conventional high-yielding cow in the conventional cubicle house, the most effective way to reduce the abnormal load on the outer claw of the hind foot is to trim the feet in such a way as to balance the weight load on both claws even though the cow is compelled to stand cow-hocked (see Blowey, 1993).

To summarize this section; lameness is perhaps the greatest of the current welfare problems for dairy cows because it is a source of chronic pain and the incidence is very high. The problem has got worse in recent years for reasons that are inherent to the production system, i.e. the popularity of grass silage and cubicle houses compounded by the increasing demand on the herdsman to look after more and more cows. However, the problem can be kept under control through the application of some classic principles of good husbandry and some new knowledge relating, for example, to foot trimming and management at calving time. Furthermore, lameness costs money and therefore improved welfare by reducing foot lameness is consistent with improved productivity. Thus the most effective route to the reduction of lameness in dairy cattle is through education to ensure the application of existing knowledge. I do not see a need for new legislation, nor, for that matter, a great deal of new research.

Milking and mastitis

A typical Holstein dairy cow may yield 15–25 litres at a single milking. The conventional, but abnormal process of twice-daily milking allows 10 times the normal amount of milk to accumulate in the udder. This undoubtedly reduces milk yield and may predispose both to mastitis and to lameness. When nutrient supply is not limiting (which is not very often) the peak yield is determined by physiological processes taking place within the mammary gland. These are ultimately determined by the genotype of the cow. However, milk yield can be increased by injecting hormones such as BST or, more naturally, by increasing the frequency of milking or, most naturally, by the stimulus of suckling a calf. Recent work from Israel has compared milk yields in early lactation in genetically high quality Holsteins fed a high quality diet on three treatments: (i) milked three times daily (39 l/d) (ii) six times daily (46 l/d) and (iii) combined thrice-daily suckling with thrice-daily milking (52 l/d). Milk yield was increased 18% by increasing milking frequency from three to six times daily and a further 11% by allowing the cow to continue to feed her calf. This experiment demonstrates clearly that, when nutrition is not limiting, the first constraint on the peak milk yield of the genetically superior Holstein is not the genetic and physiological potential of the mammary gland to synthesize milk but the artificial nature and infrequency of the stimulus to release milk.

Two other aspects of this study are of special interest in a welfare context. First, the production response to the adoption of a more frequent (more natural) milking practice was at least as great as that likely to result from the injection of BST. Second, these highly selected Holstein cows showed an increase in milk yield in response to the natural stimulus of suckling their own calves that was, in proportional terms, just as great as that seen in 'primitive' African cattle. In absolute terms it was, of course, far greater.

Mastitis is another of the great health and welfare problems for dairy cattle. The farmer who can keep the incidence of mastitis below 30 cases per 100 cows per year is doing very well. Incidences above 60% per year are all too common. The incidence of mastitis has probably got neither worse, nor better, in the last forty years despite, on the one hand, the intensification of dairy farming and, on the other, the advent of antibiotics. The two factors appear to have cancelled one another out. There have been several claims that increasing milk yield, whether by breeding, feeding or injections of BST, is linked to an increase in mastitis but the evidence is unconvincing. It is true to say that the greatest incidence of mastitis is at the time of peak yield and cows with a high milk flow *rate* may be more prone to pick up infection through the teat canal but there is little convincing evidence to link yield *per se* to factors such as reduced immuno-competence which would increase predisposition to mastitis or other infectious diseases.

There is, however, some evidence to suggest that the incidence of mastitis may be reduced by increasing the frequency of milking to four times daily. Reducing the quantity of milk stored in the cistern of the udder and the duration of storage may clear potential pathogens more quickly and reduce udder distension thereby reducing the risk of picking up organisms such as *Escherichia coli* via the teat canal. On the other hand, more frequent milking may possibly increase the risk of teat damage and increase opportunities for invasion by environmental pathogens after each milking. There is a real need for further research into the effects of frequent milking on the pathophysiology of mastitis.

The development of automatic milking systems using robots for placing the teat cups offers an exciting opportunity to rethink the husbandry of dairy cows in a way that could be consistent both with increased productivity and with improved health and welfare (Fig. 9.2). The cow that can, without having to queue, enter an automatic milking station of her own volition four to six times daily to be fed and/or milked as appropriate will certainly have the potential to produce more milk. She may also be less prone not only to mastitis but also to lameness because of the reduced distension of the udder. However, her demand for nutrients will increase and any welfare problems associated with an imbalance between nutrient supply and demand will become worse. Thus a robot that milked cows four to six times daily may reduce the stresses on the udder but it would only improve overall welfare if feeding and management were also modified to ensure;

(1) the diet was of sufficiently high quality to provide the extra nutrients required to meet the increased yield.
(2) the diet was balanced to achieve stable fermentation and so avoid the stresses of ruminal acidosis and laminitis.
(3) the ration was supplied in such a way that it could be eaten in not more than eight hours per day so as to avoid conflict between the cows' motivation to eat and their motivation to rest.

If these needs can be met then one of the most extreme symbols of the factory farm, the milking robot, may prove to be one of the most successful marriages between high technology and animal welfare.

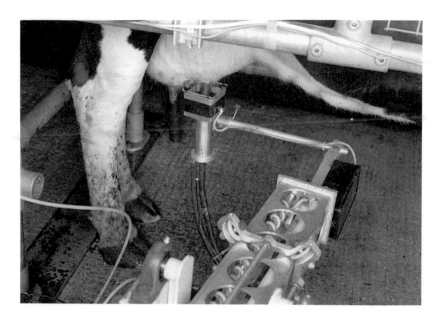

Fig. 9.2 A robot arm for milking dairy cows.

Metabolic diseases and exhaustion

Some of the most common health and welfare problems of the dairy cow are the metabolic or production diseases. In essence, these occur when the cow is unable to meet the acute or chronic metabolic demands of maintenance, pregnancy and lactation. In the most acute forms of production diseases such as milk fever or grass staggers, the cow simply runs out of calcium or magnesium respectively and, if untreated, will die in a matter of hours or minutes. Other diseases such as ketosis and the fatty liver syndrome are due to abnormal demands on energy, especially fat, metabolism. Good dairy farmers and their veterinary surgeons work hard to minimize these diseases for sound economic reasons, but it is an inescapable fact that their incidence is linked to the level of productivity we demand from the dairy cow.

Applying the rule that the severity of welfare problems is determined by their intensity and duration then the most serious problem is not the acute production disease (which will be treated) but the chronic problem faced by the cow who becomes progressively unable to meet the sustained physiological and metabolic demands of lactation and suffers a severe loss of body condition, perhaps a reduced resistance to infection and, almost certainly, a feeling of exhaustion. A significant proportion of dairy cows that are culled after only one to four lactations are very thin, probably infertile and/or chronically lame and it is difficult to escape the conclusion that such animals are 'worn out' by sustained hard work. Since a healthy beef cow may produce ten or more calves in a working lifetime no one can deny that such cows have been worn out at an unnaturally young age. Unlike the cow with acute milk fever or ketosis, the chronically exhausted cow does not present an immediate financial risk for the farmer, by dying or drastically reducing milk yield, and so will normally be expected to soldier on until she is culled at the end of her lactation.

Since I do not believe that a 'normal' life span is a necessary criterion of good welfare I have no objection to the principle of culling *per se*. It is obviously good husbandry to practise selective culling to achieve genetic improvement. However, I cannot accept that the health and welfare of dairy cows is satisfactory (whether considered nationally or on an individual farm) when a substantial proportion of young animals has to be culled for reasons that are associated with a degree of suffering that may last for several months. When these things do occur, it is more humane to cull sooner rather than later but our first objective should be to prevent them from occurring in the first place.

It should be clear that I believe too many dairy cows suffer from hunger, pain and exhaustion for reasons that can be attributed directly to the work load and life style to which they are exposed. However, I do not believe that these problems will be solved by public outrage or proscriptive legislation. This is partly because they are too complex for legislation but mainly because most dairy farmers actually do care for their cows and not just for financial reasons. If they did not they would have chosen an easier job. Both the dairy cow and the dairy farmer need our understanding. Understanding the dairy cow is a matter of heart and mind. We need to understand how she operates as a high performance machine and to recognize her as a sentient and highly engaging creature with the capacity to suffer. Her welfare depends on our knowledge, honesty and compassion; the knowledge to keep her fit, the honesty to acknowledge that a chronically lame or exhausted cow will suffer, even while she continues to make money, and the compassion to remove that suffering or, preferably, the source of it.

The dairy cow and her calf

The job of the dairy cow is to produce milk for human consumption so, in nearly all commercial herds, her calf is removed shortly after birth and reared artificially. Public debates on this issue tend to generate more heat than light, the opposing views being that 'nothing could be more cruel than to snatch a baby from its mother' or that 'it's perfectly acceptable because we've always done it'. Although (as always) I shall avoid such absolutist statements, I do accept that separation of the dairy cow from her unweaned calf does cause suffering. The problem (as always) needs to be addressed in cost:benefit terms. How may the cost to the animals be minimized? What is the benefit to mankind? Are there any circumstances in which the cost:benefit equation is so out of balance that the act may be said to constitute unnecessary suffering?

In a herd of suckler or wild cattle it is normal for the calf to feed from its mother for at least the first six months of life. However, cattle are a species that hide their young calves rather than keep them following permanently at foot. In other words, the strategy that cows have evolved to protect their calves is to leave them lying in the grass at a distance from the main herd and to return to them at infrequent intervals (four to six times per day) for suckling. As calves grow they tend to keep company with other calves during the day, although they usually return to lie with their mothers at night. It is therefore normal for the calf to be absent from its mother for hours on end. In dairy herds, the most common practice is to leave the calf with its mother for about 24 hours so that it will, in four to five feeds, drink enough colostrum to acquire the antibodies necessary to protect it from infectious diseases. Thereafter the calf is removed to rearing accommodation and fed rationed amounts of milk or commercial milk replacer plus highly digestible dry feed to stimulate early rumen development so that it can be weaned off any form of milk diet as early as four to five weeks of age. When calves are reared artificially it is in the interests of both farmer and calf to wean them onto solid food as soon as possible. The biggest source of economic loss is a dead calf and the main cause of death in the first weeks of life is enteric infection leading to diarrhoea or septicaemia. One of the best ways to avoid this problem is to ensure that calves do not drink too much milk (which would occur if calves were left with their dairy-type mothers) and to encourage the calves to adapt to dry feeds and so develop the rumen as quickly as possible.

In a few dairy herds, calves are reintroduced to their mothers twice daily and allowed to suck until they reach two to three weeks of age. This practice is especially popular with farmers who sell calves on to specialist rearing units at this age for the sound commercial reason that such calves usually look fitter than calves bucket-fed from the second day of life. This practice of housing a calf separately from its mother but reuniting them for feeding two or three times daily is quite similar to what occurs in the wild and appears to work to the satisfaction of both cow and calf, so long as it persists. A few farmers might just extend this practice for up to eight weeks. The problem is that that by two months, or even two weeks after the calf's birth, the cow and calf have formed a powerful emotional bond. Weaning at this time (the French word *sevrage* is more accurate) causes profound, prolonged distress to cow, calf and anybody else who happens to be in earshot. My personal view, shared by most dairy farmers, is that if it is not possible to keep a calf with its mother for six months, as in a suckler beef herd, then the least cruel act is to separate them as soon as possible after birth. Of course, the cow has innate maternal instincts and these are abused but the cow that was removed from her own mother at birth and is given no opportunity to bond with her own calf does not reinforce these powerful instincts by learned behaviour. She suffers, but not for long.

Any proposals to delay weaning to accommodate human sensibilities would, in present circumstances, be likely to do more harm than good. However, circumstances differ. As we have seen, not only the primitive African cow but also the improved Holstein produce more milk if allowed to suckle their calf as well as be milked by hand or machine. In Africa where the cow can forage for herself but feed for early-weaned calves is prohibitively expensive the most economic solution is to share the cow's milk between the needs of her calf and her owner. The needs of the calf are not in direct competition with those of the farmer since, overall, the cow can give more milk.

There are at least three good reasons to suggest that calves born to high-yielding dairy cows may, in future, be reared for longer on their mothers' milk:

(1)   When milk produced in excess of quota carries such a financial penalty as to make it a dead loss, it is better fed to calves.

(2)   The economic advantages of rearing calves on milk replacer rather than whole milk are, in part, artificial since they are supported by subsidies designed to offload skim milk and whey surplus to butter and cheese production.

(3)   The largest survey to date of diseases of calf rearing revealed that the incidence of infectious disease in calves reared on milk replacer was seven times that of calves reared on whole milk.

However, while it is likely that more calves will be fed on whole milk until the time that they are weaned onto solid food, it would not be in the interests of either calf or farmer to postpone this weaning beyond about six weeks of age. Thus, with some reluctance, I am forced to the conclusion that if the separation of calf and mother is to be done, 'it were well it were done quickly'.

New techniques in cattle breeding

Even though most dairy cows fail to perform to their genetic potential due to deficiencies in nutrition and management, genetically superior cows, by definition, produce more milk. Thus dairy farmers can improve the productivity of their herd, slowly but surely, by selection of superior individuals. To date this has been achieved largely by selection of semen from bulls whose superiority has been proven by the performance of their daughters. Moreover, superiority of the progeny is defined not only in terms of milk yield and composition but also according to conformation. These different criteria of superiority cannot all be achieved in the same individual and the farmer has, as always, to compromise. However, I repeat, dairy heifers (unlike broiler chickens) tend to be selected for physical fitness at least at the onset of their first lactation. The dairy cow suffers less from problems directly attributable to her genotype than from feeding and management systems that are inappropriate to the genotype.

In the UK genetic progress through conventional bull selection has, in recent years, been running at about one per cent per annum. Since there are no theoretical or practical reasons to suggest that dairy cows will approach selection limits in the foreseeable future this means that in 25 years a farmer could expect a 25% genetic improvement. This is very useful but it is slow. The rate of genetic improvement by selection of superior cows as well as bulls can now be increased by techniques based on multiple ovulation with embryo transfer (MOET). This involves some or all of the following procedures:

(1)   use of hormones to induce the superior cow to produce up to 20 embryos at a time rather than one;
(2)   collection of embryos, usually involving laparoscopy;
(3)   (possibly) multiplication of embryos by embryo splitting or nuclear transfer;
(4)   insertion of embryos in recipient cows, usually via the vagina and under local anaesthesia.

The commercial exploitation of new scientific knowledge that has made possible these new techniques poses ethical questions, many (but not all) of which concern the welfare of the animals involved. As always, we have to examine the costs and benefits, thus:

(1)   Will the animal suffer? If so, how much?
(2)   Who, if anyone will benefit? If so, how much?

In reviewing the impact of new biology on the welfare of farm animals, the UK Farm Animal Welfare Council (FAWC, 1993) stated 'We accept that scientific investigation aims to be impartial and without prejudice so that it is impossible to pronounce *a priori* how any particular piece of new knowledge will affect farm animals'. Nevertheless they recognized certain procedures that may have harmful consequences. These include 'the manipulation of body size, shape or reproductive capacity by breeding, nutrition, hormone therapy or gene insertion in such a way as to reduce mobility, increase the risk of pain, injury, metabolic disease, skeletal or obstetric problems, perinatal mortality or psychological distress'. This implies that the welfare implications of new biology should be defined not by the method used to manipulate the animal but by its consequences. Thus it was conventional selection procedures, not new technology, that crippled the heavy breeds of broiler fowl and FAWC has called for the industry to achieve a significant reduction in these conditions within five years. For the dairy cow, the main question at issue is not whether genetic selection is creating an abnormal cow but whether any of the special procedures involved in MOET, embryo splitting etc. may be a cause of suffering. The possibilities are:

(1) *Pain and/or fear associated with the procedure itself or its immediate consequences.* It is assumed for legal purposes that this problem can be overcome by use of appropriate anaesthesia. There is, however, good evidence that following procedures such as laparoscopy in man, pain may persist for some days. It is, at least, necessary to address this possibility in cattle and especially small ruminants such as sheep for whom laparoscopy is the method of choice for embryo insertion.

(2) *Problems at calving caused directly by unconventional breeding.* The most obvious risk is calves that are too large at birth. This can occur if there is a genetic mismatch between large calf and small foster cow. However, this is more likely to occur with beef than dairy cattle (see below). In addition an unexplained problem of severe oversize has emerged in calves from embryos transferred to recipient, or foster cows, especially after a prolonged period of culture *in vitro*. The birth weights of such calves can be from 20% to over 50% above normal, apparently because early life outside the uterus has disrupted the switches that control the normal course of pregnancy. With calves that big Caesarian section becomes the only alternative to a highly stressful or impossible delivery.

There will undoubtedly be legislation to control application of new science and technology to increase productivity or otherwise exploit animals for our advantage because the public demands it. In the UK, when animals used for science are exposed to any procedure which may cause pain, suffering distress or lasting harm (however slight, like taking a blood sample), those animals involved are protected by the Animals (Scientific Procedures) Act (ASPA) 1986. This applies a cost:benefit analysis which weighs the cost of any procedure to the animal against the likely benefit to mankind (or other animals). Obviously, the greater the cost, the greater the need for justification. For reasons that should be clear by now I happen to think this is a very sound law and I shall discuss it in much more detail in Chapter 12. When procedures such as multiple ovulation and embryo transfer were first investigated scientifically, both animals and operators were protected by ASPA (1986). One of the main benefits was deemed to be the acquisition of new, potentially useful knowledge. Now that the science has been done and embryo transfer in cattle is simply a commercial undertaking it is covered only by legislation which seeks to ensure that it is done competently (i.e. under the supervision of a veterinary surgeon). Nowhere does the legislation enquire whether the cost to the animal is justified by the benefit to anyone.

Since a cow is a cow whether used for science or commerce, there can be no ethical reason why she should not receive at least the same degree of protection from the law that we grant to the laboratory animal. When science makes it expedient for us to expose cows to some degree of non-therapeutic surgery to accelerate genetic progress, we need legislation that applies a cost:benefit analysis at least as rigorous at that applied by ASPA(1986) before the technique is pronounced acceptable for commercial exploitation.

We would then be faced by questions such as 'are the surgical procedures involved in multiple ovulation and embryo transfer justified by an increase in genetic gain of a herd of dairy cows from a current rate of 1% to 3%?'

My personal interpretation of this particular cost:benefit equation is that the procedure is acceptable as currently practised in cattle but should not be permitted for commercial purposes in sheep until a less severe technique can be developed than that currently based on laparoscopy. Another specific example of the general question 'How much does the animal suffer and what good will it do?' is, of course, the use of BST to increase milk yield. The discomfort associated with regular injections and the increased risk of problems such as mastitis may be small but they are real. The risk that a higher proportion of cows will complete their short lives in a state of chronic exhaustion is equally real and a far greater cause for concern. If cows for commerce had the same rights as rats for research then this cost would have to be assessed against the potential 'benefit' to society of a drug which consumers in the rich world do not want, those in the poor world cannot afford, a product which no dairy farmer actually needs and one which will drive some out of business. I rest this particular case.

Beef cattle

Approximately half the prime beef produced in the UK comes from calves born to dairy cows and reared artificially. The other half comes from calves born to suckler or range cows managed extensively and expected to produce and rear one calf per year. On the open, sparsely populated prairies and pampas of North and South America, the majority of beef comes from calves reared for six to twelve months on open range, then 'finished' on a high-cereal ration on feedlots over a period of about five months. Public criticism of beef production from range cows tends to be directed at mutilations such as branding and castration, where the intensity of suffering may be intense but brief, and the unnatural feeding of cereals and growth promoters to animals in feedlots. Otherwise, the practice is seen to be reasonably natural and therefore acceptable.

My greatest concern is for neither of these things but relates, as in the case of the dairy cow, to welfare problems arising from the need to maximize the productivity of the breeding female. Whereas the primary role of the dairy cow is to produce milk for sale, with her calf as a useful byproduct, the only crop from the beef cow is the beef produced by her calves, and eventually herself. To improve the output of beef per cow per year it is necessary to 'improve' the size of the calves, the shape of the calves or the number born at any one time. All these things can create problems for the beef cow. These include:

(1) obstetric problems caused by calves that are too large at birth;
(2) obstetric problems in cows with a misshapen birth canal;

(3)   recurrent pain from repeated, premeditated Caesarian sections;
(4)   problems after calving associated with twinning;
(5)   problems associated with the act of embryo transfer.

The ease of calving depends primarily on the size and shape of the calf relative to the size and shape of the birth canal. Since the main source of income to the suckler beef farm comes from the sale of weaned calves, the main aim in suckler beef production is to produce a calf that will be as large and meaty as possible at the time of weaning. This is achieved by selection for large, meaty bulls. The major breeding companies selling semen for artificial insemination do monitor the incidence of calving difficulties and withdraw bulls with special problems. However selection for large, muscular bulls inevitably tends to increase the risk of obstetric problems associated with calves that are overlarge at birth. One way to reduce the birth-weight of calves is to restrict food supply to the pregnant cows to ensure that they are thin, but not emaciated, at the time of calving.

Selection for 'beefiness' (a high muscle:bone ratio and a high proportion of meat in the expensive cuts around the rump) in the breeding cows can predispose to a reduction in the dimensions of the pelvic canal through which the calf must be delivered. This is seen most strikingly in animals which carry the recessive gene for 'double muscling'. such as Belgian Blue bull. The term is, in fact a misnomer. There are no extra muscles, all muscles, especially those in the hindquarters, are simply very large. The gene for double muscling would, in natural circumstances, be a lethal recessive because the dimensions of the pelvic canal are so reduced that most females are unable to give birth without recourse to Caesarian section.

Although the homozygous recessive carrying both alleles for double muscling is not a commercial proposition, the F1 hybrid born to a double muscled bull does grow normally and present a meatier carcass to the butcher than normal beef animals of the same breed. It can therefore be commercially expedient to breed double-muscled bulls to produce meaty F1 hybrids when crossed with normal beef cows. Since the normal cows should have normal pelvic dimensions, such a crossbreeding programme will not constitute unnecessary cruelty. However, in order to produce double-muscled bulls it is necessary to maintain a population of double-muscled cows, all of which will produce their calves by repeated, premeditated Caesarian section. This, in the opinion of FAWC, is an unacceptable practice since it involves a 'manipulation of body size, shape or reproductive capacity by breeding in such a way as to ... increase the risk of ... obstetric problems (and) perinatal mortality'.

Entrepeneurs wishing to exploit the apparent commercial benefits of double-muscling argue that giving birth by caesarian section under local anaethesia is likely to be less painful than a normal delivery. This may be so *at the time*, but it neglects the strong probability that some pain will outlast the duration of action of the anaesthetic (see Chapter 5). I would expect at least some cows submitted to repeated Caesarian sections to suffer chronic abdominal pain associated with internal scarring and possible adhesions.

The most effective way, in theory, to increase the productivity of the beef cow is to make her produce twins. Over the last 30 years there have been several attempts to put this theory into practice, either by the use of hormones to increase ovulation rate or by inserting two or more embryos collected from a superovulated donor cow. In commercial units, most of these schemes have failed, mainly because many cows that give birth to twins suffer from postparturient problems (such as a retained placenta) and may subsequently become infertile. A survey by Eddy and others (1988) of the full economic implications of natural twinning in dairy cattle revealed that for every cow that gave birth to twins rather than a single calf the farmer lost £75!

Although twinning, when considered in isolation, does not appear to be a commercial proposition, it assumes importance when considered in association with the technique of multiple ovulation and embryo transfer (MOET). It is common to insert two embryos into recipient cows, if only to increase the probability that at least one will implant. It is also likely to be cost-effective when the donor embryos are from high genetic merit cows and bulls and so have a high cash value relative to that of the foster mother. The transfer of embryos into recipient cows is governed by law and a Code of Practice which states that embryos should be inserted via the vagina and cervix, with local (epidural) anaesthesia and under the general supervision of (although not necessarily by) a veterinary surgeon. It can be argued that this practice is little different from the established practice of artificial insemination. In both cases a rigid catheter is passed through the cervix. The main difference is that it is much easier to pass the catheter into the uterus when the cow is in oestrus and the cervix is both relaxed and well lubricated.

These potential welfare problems for the beef cow all derive from the fact that she is faced with only two commercial options: to produce the largest, meatiest calf that she can reasonably be expected to deliver or go for meat herself. Since her own potential value as a beef carcass is quite high, beef producers are prepared to carry a higher incidence of obstetric and other problems at calving time than the dairy farmer, since calving problems for the dairy cow are likely to impair the income she generates from her subsequent lactation. In other words, the commercial strategy for suckler beef production has an in-built high risk of calving problems.

To summarize my position, I would say that only one of the 'unnatural' procedures used to increase the productivity of the breeding beef cow is absolutely unacceptable. This is the use of repeated, premeditated Caesarian section for the breeding of double-muscled (and possibly other heavily muscled) strains of beef animal. The procedures involved in the current practice of MOET in cattle, but not sheep and goats, should cause no more suffering at the time of implantation than other routine husbandry practices such as foot trimming and dehorning, although these are carried out for the benefit of the cattle. The greatest risk of welfare problems associated with MOET and other aspects of embryo culture *in vitro* are those likely to occur at the time of calving and it is these that should assume greatest importance under the umbrella of 'veterinary supervision'. My expectation, rather than my moral wish, is that MOET and related procedures will only prove to be cost-effective when used to promote rapid genetic improvement, especially when this involves the exportation of embryos. Real genetic improvement and long-distance transport of embryos rather than live animals both add weight to the benefit side of the cost:benefit equation. My other expectation is that many farmers will continue to be seduced by MOET salesmen and their veterinary colleagues into buying 'services' that will do neither them nor their cows any good.

Veal production

We come now to one of the most bizarre and, in my opinion, unequivocally cruel forms of livestock production, namely the rearing of calves in small wooden crates on liquid, iron-deficient diets for the production of white veal. Unlike the intensification of pig and poultry production, which evolved to meet a universal consumer demand for cheap food, the white veal industry has evolved to meet a minority demand for expensive luxury food. A typical veal production unit in, for example, Holland or France abuses all five freedoms:

(1) The calves are deprived of dry feed. This denies normal rumen development and predisposes to the development of hair balls which may cause chronic indigestion.
(2) In order to produce 'white' meat the intake of dietary iron is restricted to the point where some calves will become clinically anaemic.
(3) Calves are confined individually in wooden crates, 80–90 cm wide and cannot, in the latter stages of growth, turn round, groom themselves, adopt a normal sleeping position, or even, without difficulty, stand up and lie down.
(4) The incidence of infectious diseases such as diarrhoea and pneumonia are abnormally high and are kept under control only by the liberal and repeated use of antibiotics.
(5) Deprived of solid food, the calves develop stereotyped behaviour patterns such as tongue rolling, crate-licking or mutual tongue sucking.
(6) In most units the calves are kept in low light and out of the sight and sounds of farm activity.

This catalogue of abuse provokes the question 'How did a system so abnormal ever evolve in the first place?' Intensive veal units were developed in the 1950s to handle surpluses of male calves and skim-milk from the dairy industry. In some ways, this was no more than a huge scaling-up of a practice as old as agriculture which used surplus milk from the house cow to fatten her own calf for special occasions such as the return of the prodigal son. The biblical fatted calf would have been given little access to forage and cereals because they were needed for its mother. When killed at three months of age or less, its meat would have been very pale because cow's milk is naturally deficient in iron. The assumption that veal meat should be 'white' is not a recent affectation, simply an unthinking acceptance of our peasant heritage.

When, in the early 1980s Claire Saville, David Welchman and I began to question and investigate the practice of rearing calves for white veal, we were advised by the industry that this was a high-risk operation and any well-meaning attempts to improve welfare by offering calves solid food or allowing greater social contact would only make things worse by increasing the spread of disease. This argument derived some support from the relative failure of some commercial attempts to rear veal calves in groups, e.g. the 'Quantock' rearing systems in which calves were housed on straw and provided with teat dispensers delivering milk replacer *ad libitum*. Calves in this system undoubtedly had more behavioural freedom than those in crates but were even more prone to infectious disease. However, the main reason they failed to compete with calves in crates, bucket-fed controlled amounts of milk replacer twice daily, was an inferior food conversion efficiency; they drank more expensive milk, relative to their weight gains.

Table 9.2 A comparison of the performance, health and welfare of veal calves in different rearing systems.

	Crates	Quantock	Access
Growth	Uniform	Some 'poor doers'	Uniform
Food conversion ratio	1.5–1.6	1.6–1.8	1.5–1.6
Physical comfort	Bad	Good	Good
Infectious disease: enteric (%)	19	4	<5
respiratory (%)	9	18	<5
Behaviour: oral	Abnormal	Some problems	Normal
locomotor and social	Impossible	Normal	Normal

Table 9.2 attempts to combine the results of a broad survey of the performance, health and welfare of veal calves in commercial husbandry systems and a series of small-scale trials conducted by us at the University of Bristol in an attempt to devise from first principles an economically and morally acceptable way of rearing calves for veal. Since the numbers of animals involved in the survey and our trials are unbalanced, this table should be treated with some caution (for more detail see Webster, Saville and Welchman, 1986). We were, however, able to demonstrate that it is possible to rear veal calves in such a way as to combine good growth rates and food con-

version efficiency, good health and behavioural freedom *plus* meat that would be acceptable to the veal butcher.

We called our approach the Access system (Table 9.2 and Fig. 9.3). Calves wearing transponders were reared in groups of 14 to 20 in straw yards and given access to a computer-controlled feeding station which dispensed rationed amounts of milk replacer and a small amount of solid feed containing sufficient digestible fibre to stimulate rumen development. All the calves had to learn was that a teat would appear in one station if they were due for a milk feed but would not appear if they had already had enough; similarly for the solid ration. All calves acquired these basic computer skills within two days. The Access system has, to date, only been used on an experimental scale but it did show that when calves are given just enough of the sort of solid food necessary to normalize rumen development, enteric diseases can be reduced to the low level considered acceptable in normal calf rearing units. Furthermore, since enteritis triples the risk that calves will subsequently contract pneumonia, respiratory infections were normalized as well. Simply put, the calves were now healthy because their development was normal and because they were healthy they could be run in groups.

Shortly after the publication of this work, the UK government drafted new legislation for the protection of veal calves which requires that:

(1) all calves above the age of two weeks should be provided with a diet containing digestible fibre.
(2) if any calf is confined in an individual crate, the width of the crate should be at least 80% of the height of the calf at the withers.

This legislation effectively destroyed the UK veal calf industry or, to be more precise, completed its destruction since by the time that government delivered their moral *coup de grace* it was a very sick dragon indeed. In the 1950s UK producers went briefly into veal production to exploit the low price of surplus male calves from the dairy industry. By the time of the ban, the price of such calves had already risen to the point where veal production had become uneconomic and nearly all farmers had switched to alternative enterprises like rearing calves for twelve weeks prior to entry into intensive beef units. However, there was and still is (as I write) a substantial export trade in calves from the UK to intensive veal units in, especially Holland and France. Numbers vary greatly from about 200 000 to 400 000 calves per year, a number far in excess of the size of the UK veal industry at the time of the ban. It has to be said, therefore, that the UK ban has had no significant effect either on the European veal industry or on the welfare of calves born to dairy cows in the UK.

The hope was that the principles of the UK legislation would be incorporated into legislation for the entire European Union. Early drafts of this legislation held some promise but the final document for the 'Protection of Calves' (Directive 91/629/EEC) was a grotesque sham. I quote:

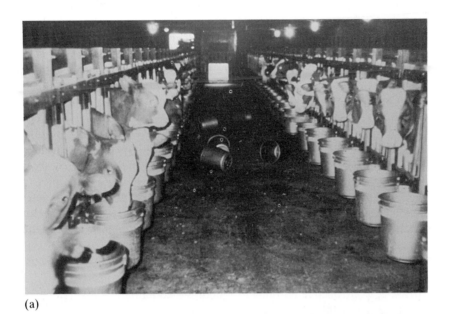

(a)

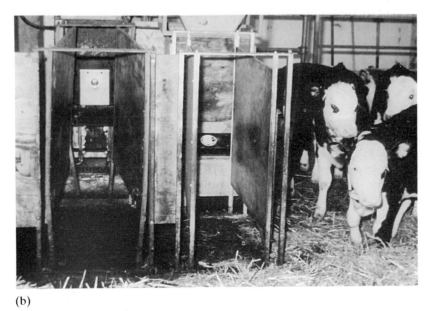

(b)

Fig. 9.3 (a) Veal calves in crates. (b) Veal calves in straw yards fed by the Access system.

'(1)   when calves are housed in individual boxes ... their width must be no less than 90 cm plus or minus 10% or 0.80 times the height at the withers.

(2)   All calves must be provided with a diet adapted to their ... behavioural and physiological needs. However the requirement ... does not apply to the production of veal calves for white meat.'

Many veal calves are now reared to weights over 300 kg when their height at the withers may be over 120 cm. This would require a pen width of 100 cm (in round figures). A 90 cm wide pen less the permissible 10% gives (in round figures) 80 cm, which is the width of the standard pen in present use. After about five years deliberation the Eurocrats elected to do nothing and covered their retreat with a smokescreen of Orwellian doublespeak. The clause dealing with dietary needs is especially bizarre. It is equivalent to stating that 'thou shalt not steal – unless you happen to be a burglar'.

As the advocate for the 'Access' system, I must offer an explanation for why there has been no serious commercial attempt to put it into practice. In the UK the answer is simple. Given existing prices within the UK and competition from conventional units in Holland and France there is no financial incentive to start up any form of veal production. Within continental Europe the veal trade has invested large amounts of capital in expensive, controlled environment buildings containing individual pens. Since the trade is unlikely to expand, producers have neither the incentive nor the money (nor sufficient pressure from society) to invest in alternative husbandry systems.

Gestures are occasionally made, not to improve the welfare of the calves but as sops thrown to the welfare lobby. The most cynical of these is to rear veal calves exactly as before, except that from eight weeks of age they are housed not in individual pens but on concrete slats in groups of four, nominally to give them 'behavioural freedom'. Given the wet and often propulsive nature of veal calf faeces and the sexual precocity of rapidly growing bull calves, animals reared in groups such as these become filthy, sexually harassed and injured through slipping on the slimy slats. When I have challenged producers with the claim that this is even worse than individual crates, the stock answer is 'You know that and I know that, but if that is what the welfarists want that is what we shall give them'.

The production of the whitest of veal for the most 'cultured' of palates may, as explained above, have started innocently enough but it has a squalid history. In the nineteenth century it was common practice to bleed live calves until they collapsed, then let them recover several times before final slaughter. Today, meat colour is regulated by the precise control of dietary iron intake. Very briefly, the red colour of beef is due mainly to myoglobin, an iron-containing compound with a similar structure and function to haemoglobin in blood. It is possible to regulate the iron intake of most calves so that the calves have sufficient haemoglobin to avoid clinical anaemia (manifested, in part, by a failure to thrive) but insufficient myo-globin to redden the meat. However, the variation between calves is such that it is impossible to guarantee meat which is white enough for hypercritical butchers without some calves suffering from clinical anaemia. Butchers who downgrade pink veal are nominally seeking to protect the interests of their customers but also seeking an excuse to pay less for their meat. Although most consumers can easily distinguish between white veal and baby beef, few diners served veal in a restaurant would, I believe, be able to distinquish by sight or taste between white or pink veal. Moreover, in a small taste panel study at the University of Bristol the very few individuals who could make the distinction were equally divided as to which they preferred, pink or white.

I stated at the beginning of this section that I believe that conventional veal production abuses all five freedoms. I do not, however, recommend an absolute ban on the production of veal. This, like so many well-meant ideas could do more harm than good. The veal industry does preserve the cash value of male dairy-type calves, especially Holsteins, which are the wrong shape for beef production. An absolute ban on the veal trade would render such calves valueless and resurrect the practice of shipping 'bobby calves' around between dealers for a few dismal days before being killed for pies and gloves. I would be more satisfied if Europe adopted current UK legislation for veal production, supported perhaps in the short term by incentives to modify buildings and equipment. As we demonstrated with the Access system, it is possible to rear veal calves in a humane way. The system conformed to one of the best of all definitions of good husbandry. I was proud to show it off to anybody.

Sheep production

For most of the last thousand years the British acquired wealth from sheep grown for their wool. The medieval cathedrals and churches of England stand as monuments to the success of the wool trade. In Scotland, the 'Great White Sheep' (actually, medium-sized Cheviots) replaced the crofters during the Highland Clearances because they were deemed to have more value; one of the greater abuses of that much abused word. Today the price of wool (except for the finest fibres) does little more than repay the cost of shearing and the main source of income is from the sale of prime lambs. As with beef production, the economic pressure (when not distorted by subsidy) is to maximize the income from lambs relative to the costs of maintaining the breeding flock. Since ewes are physiologically capable of producing twins or triplets (although they only have two teats) the main route to improved productivity is through improved prolificacy.

Intensification of the sheep industry to date may be said, on balance, to have improved welfare, using the McInerney argument (Fig. 7.1). When sheep or goats are ranched very extensively for the production of wool or cashmere, their individual value is too low to justify much human attention by way of stockmanship or supplementary feeding. Thus, they run a greater risk of suffering hunger and stand a poorer chance of treatment if affected by lameness or blowfly strike (infestation with maggots). Purebred hill sheep are now reared mainly for their lambs, usually one lamb per year. Most of the male lambs are worth relatively little as meat animals, although a few may make very high prices as pedigree breeding sires. More money is made from breeding females, purebred for the hills or 'improved' crossbreds sold to the lowlands to produce twins. On lowland farms most crossbred ewes will be housed over winter in straw yards. Many will be scanned by ultrasound to determine the number of lambs that they are carrying and fed accordingly. The lambs will be born indoors, in the warm and free from exposure to predators such as foxes and crows. There are health and welfare problems for ewes housed indoors over winter then let out again to grass in the spring but on balance their welfare during the winter is almost always better than that of ewes outwintered on the hills.

Income from the sale of lambs and wool is insufficient to sustain hill sheep farming so it is supported, for socio-economic reasons by subsidy. Before 1992 sheep farming subsidies were paid in part directly to hill farmers to support maintenance of the breeding flocks and in part to support the price of finished lambs. Today, there is no subsidy on finished lambs; all subsidy is based on the number of ewes carried on the farm up to an agreed quota. The intention is to reduce total production of lamb meat in Europe while sustaining the hill farmer and thereby the quality of the hill environment. This is an honourable intention but it has the potential to drive sheep welfare back down the McInerney curve to the starting point of poverty and squalor. The previous subsidy payments required the ewes to be productive, i.e. produce lambs. To achieve this they needed to be fed and cared for properly. The present subsidy requires little more than that the ewes are alive and that is a worry.

The worst welfare problems for sheep, such as starvation, lameness and being eaten alive by maggots, arise from the sins of omission and neglect and are too obvious to merit discussion here. It is necessary, however, to consider the question of unnecessary suffering associated with positive acts such as mutilations and other forms of non-therapeutic surgery. The most important procedures are castration, tail docking and laparascopic techniques for insertion of semen or embryos directly through the uterine wall rather than through the cervix. Tail docking undoubtedly reduces the risk of sheep contracting maggots through blowfly strike and is therefore a positive contributor to welfare. Traditionally, lambs were castrated both to prevent uncontrolled and unseasonal breeding and to facilitate fattening off grass. With improvements to nutrition and the demand for leaner meat, it is now preferable to leave male lambs entire to encourage lean tissue growth, provided that they can be finished before the autumn and the start of the next breeding season. However, on many farms, especially hill farms, castration remains an unfortunate necessity.

At present, UK law permits castration by constriction of the testes with a rubber ring, and without anaesthetic under one week of age. Surgical removal of the testes can be performed by the shepherd without anaesthetic up to three months of age. The UK Farm Animal Welfare Council, in their recent *Report on the Welfare of Sheep* (FAWC,1994) has given much attention to the nature and duration of pain associated with the act of castration. Scientific opinion as to the least-worst method of castration is divided but there is now general agreement that it is just as painful on the day of birth as at two or three weeks of age. FAWC's conclusions are as follows:

(1) surgical castration with a knife must be banned at any age, except when carried out under anaesthetic by a veterinary surgeon.
(2) the use of bloodless castrators or rubber rings for castration [without anaesthetic] should be allowed up to six weeks of age.
(3) as soon as a satisfactory and practical way of producing analgesia or administering an anaesthetic without the necessity of injecting it via a syringe and needle becomes available, it must be adopted.

These recommendations have not met with general approval and FAWC indicated that recommendation two, at least, will be reviewed in the light of new knowledge. Briefly, FAWC have recognized that hill farmers are not gathering their lambs for castration by rubber ring under seven days of age partly for the good reason that such a practice would predispose to mismothering. If the process is equally painful in week one and week five then there can be little justification for an unenforceable law that insists upon week one. Recommendation three is a call for research to discover a practical method for reducing the pain and stress associated with castration at any age up to six weeks.

The use of laparoscopy for insertion of semen or embryos direct into the uterus is a classic example of non-therapeutic surgery which carries no benefit at all to the animal and is designed entirely for commercial gain. It is not, in my opinion, sufficient to justify this procedure by legislation to ensure that it is performed under veterinary supervision. Such legislation is directed more towards the welfare of the veterinary profession than that of the sheep. My central argument is that such procedures should be assessed from cost:benefit analysis on a case-by-case basis. I have already indicated that I believe that MOET in cattle, involving implantation through the cervix, is an acceptable procedure. However, I believe, by reference to human experience, that laparoscopy may, in some circumstances give rise to lasting or recurrent pain (see Chapter 5). It follows that I also believe that implantation of semen or embryos into sheep and goats should not be licensed for commercial application until the procedures can be performed safely and humanely without recourse to laparoscopy.

Transport and slaughter

As I write this section, the major animal welfare isssue being addressed by charities like the Royal Society for Prevention of Cruelty to Animals (RSPCA) and Compassion in World Farming (CIWF) is the live export trade in calves and sheep from UK and Eire to the continent of Europe (see Peter Stevenson, 1994, *A Far Cry from Noah*). Export figures from UK for 1992 were 1 373 657 sheep and lambs and 420 620 calves. There can be no doubt than many of these animals will have suffered at some stage of their journey, not least because CIWF and RSPCA have obtained clear evidence that many hauliers are ignoring British law (The Welfare of Animals during Transport Order, 1992) which:

(1) restricts journey lengths for calves and sheep to a maximum of 15 hours, after which animals must be fed, watered and rested (for an, as yet, unspecified period).
(2) requires persons having control of animal transport undertakings to draw up for journeys exceeding 24 hours a journey plan showing

  (i) the arrangements for the animals to be rested, fed and watered and (if necessary) given accommodation appropriate to their species and
  (ii) the arrangements for feeding and watering in the event that the planned journey is disrupted.

I applaud CIWF, RSPCA and others for their outrage because outrage is necessary to get things done. I quote (more or less) Harry Truman's advice to a lobby group whose argument he had just heard in private. 'You seem to have made a very persuasive case. Now go out and put pressure on me!' If I am to help this case, however, I cannot allow outrage to blur my analysis of costs and benefits. The tower of vested interests that sets the rules for the European community is well guarded by a fog of bureaucracy. It will take a lot of people and a lot of courage to topple the tower but we also need a cool eye to guide us through the fog.

In the previous chapter I outlined the acute and chronic stresses that may, or may not, occur when animals are transported. These are:

(1) fear and pain associated with handling and mixing;
(2) thermal or motion stresses during the journey;
(3) hunger, thirst and exhaustion;
(4) risks of infection.

Cattle and sheep face special problems because they are tough. They are far better adapted to withstand thermal stress (especially heat stress) than pigs and poultry (see Fig. 4.1) and they carry greater reserves of food and water in the rumen so can endure longer periods without food and water before they begin to suffer from hunger and thirst. If pigs and poultry were transported without rest, food and water for the times and distances that are common (even when illegal) in the calf and sheep trade, so many animals would die from a combination of heat or cold, dehydration and exhaustion that the trade could not continue unless (i) it reduced maximum journey times or (ii) it radically improved the conditions experienced by the animals in transit.

Although many calves and sheep may suffer during transport, very few actually die. Thus there is no commercial incentive for the industry to change. Improvements to welfare must therefore come from public pressure for new, effective, properly enforced legislation. This will require, as always, rules by which to define 'unnecessary suffering'. When discussing the transport of pigs and poultry in the previous chapter I introduced two general arguments:

(1) Many of the stresses imposed on animals in transit are caused by the design of the vehicle and the handling of the animals and these stresses are not likely to be removed by legislation simply designed to restrict journey length.
(2) If the environmental conditions within a livestock vehicle could be made as good as those experienced by the animals on the farm then they could, in theory, stay on the lorry indefinitely.

It follows from these arguments that legislation to improve the welfare of cattle, sheep (or any other animal) in transit should be based on the 'carrot and stick' approach; proscriptive legislation to restrict journey lengths in conventional vehicles but special provisions for hauliers who can, by improved vehicle design and journey plans, provide an environment that will allow animals to travel for extended periods without unnecessary suffering.

The special problems faced by calves and sheep on prolonged journeys are hunger, thirst, heat, cold and exhaustion. Heat stress can be a particular problem for sheep when lorries are stationary at the roadside or in ferries. Sheep dissipate heat very effectively by panting. Covert videos regularly show lambs on stationary vehicles respiring at over 100 breaths per minute to dissipate excess heat by evaporation. The lambs are able to avoid death from hyperthermia but become progressively dehydrated. We cannot be certain what another animal feels when it is dehydrated, but we do know that some of the most unpleasant symptoms of a hangover in ourselves can be attributed to a degree of dehydration less than that experienced by many calves and sheep after long journeys, especially in hot conditions.

When sheep and calves are densely stocked on lorries and shaken about while the vehicle is in motion, their instinct is to stand up, partly to brace themselves against the motion and partly from fear of being trampled or smothered by the other animals. After some hours, calves and sheep may lie down, if not stocked too densely, presumably because the stress of tiredness is overcoming that of fear. In either event, the assumption must be that these animals do not relax fully while the vehicles are in motion.

On a farm, housed calves and lambs (at two weeks and three months respectively) should have constant access to water and be given food at least twice daily. Realistically, the overnight interval between feeds may often be nearer to 15 than to 12 hours. In practice, sheep may go for longer periods without drinking unless they are lactating or heat-stressed. I can accept current UK legislation which permits cattle and sheep to be transported for up to 15 hours without food and water, provided that the animals are not subjected to heat stress, which increases thirst or cold stress, which increases hunger. I can also accept that lambs can be transported for 15 hours without rest but I believe that any journey that compelled two-week old calves to stand for all, or nearly all, of a period of 15 hours would constitute unnecessary suffering. I suggest that the maximum journey time for calves less than three months of age should be six hours.

This provokes the question, 'How best should the calves or lambs be fed, watered and rested while *en route*?' The ideal rest stop would involve 10 hours in lairage on deep, clean, dry straw with free access to fresh water and rationed access to appropriate feed. In practice, this is not only unrealistic but well-meaning legislation that compelled hauliers to move their animals into and out of overnight lairages may do more harm than good because of the increased stresses involved in loading and unloading. I suggest that any haulier who wished to exceed my proposed maximum journey time of six hours for calves under three months should be able to meet the following conditions:

(1)   The calves should be stocked in such a way as to avoid injury while the vehicle is in motion but, at intervals no greater than six hours, should be able to lie down in comfort while the vehicle is at rest for periods of no less than three hours.

(2)   All calves on the vehicle should be individually fed with milk replacer or an electrolyte solution at intervals no greater than 15 hours and rested then for a period no less than six hours with sufficient space to lie in comfort and with access to fresh water and palatable forage.

For lambs over two months, I would propose that the animals should be stocked on the vehicle in such a way that they will not experience injury while the vehicle is in motion but, at intervals of no more than 15 hours should be able to lie down in comfort while the vehicle is at rest with access to fresh water and palatable forage for a period no less than six hours .

These conditions are by no means impossible to meet, but they would substantially increase the cost of transporting calves and sheep for long distances. This is, of course, one of my main objectives. I would not wish to discourage the export of valuable animals such as breeding stock, so long as they are well cared for *en route*. I do wish, however, to do everything in my power to curtail the cheap and dirty practices involved in the long-distance transport of calves into the veal trade and lambs for immediate slaughter. Legislation by incentive and proscription (carrot and stick) should be designed to encourage animals to be slaughtered as near as possible to their farms of origin.

I have discussed the physical and moral principles that define humane slaughter in Chapter 5. The procedures for stunning of cattle and sheep are demonstrably humane when carried out properly. Most of the stresses experienced by cattle and sheep on the last day of life are those associated with handling, transport and lairage prior to the time of stunning. These problems become more intense for animals that are unadapted to handling procedures, either by virtue of their own experience or of the experience of their species. Thus, newly-farmed red deer are especially prone to fear and injury during handling and transport. Because injury constitutes a commercial problem, this is taken into account by those involved in moving deer to the abattoir. Moreover, it is generally accepted that it is more humane to shoot deer from close range in the field while, for example, at the feeding trough. However, some red deer which are well adapted to the presence of humans can be handled and transported with little stress. Equally, some wild cattle and sheep from the hills are likely to experience extreme fear during handling and transport although they are less likely to injure themselves than deer by virtue of their shape and relative lack of athleticism. The principles for humane handling and transport of animals have been covered well in the recent book by Temple Grandin (1994) and need not be repeated here. I would, however, repeat my proposal that legislation should be amended to read 'at the place of slaughter animals must be handled, rendered unconscious and killed in such a way as to minimize pain and suffering'. The intention of this clause would be to broaden the scope of legislation beyond the simple act of killing. The clause is deliberately flexible so as to encourage the development of integrated systems designed to reduce or eliminate any or all of the stresses that an animal may experience from the time of leaving the farm to the time of death.

There is one more question that I must address in this chapter and that is the casualty or emergency slaughter of sick or injured animals, in particular, the lame, exhausted or collapsed dairy cow. The Welfare of Animals during Transport Order (1992) states:

> '3.2. No person shall cause or permit the transport of an animal that is unfit by reason of it being in the state of being newborn, diseased, infirm, ill, injured or fatigued ...
>
> 3.3. Notwithstanding the provisions of paragraph (2) above, a bovine, ovine, caprine, porcine, or equine animal may be transported to the nearest place of veterinary treatment or to the nearest place of slaughter if the animal is not likely to be subject to unnecessary suffering by reason of its unfitness, but such an animal may not be dragged or pushed by any means, or lifted be a mechanical device, unless this is done in the presence of and under the supervision of a veterinary surgeon who is arranging for it to be transported with all practical speed to a place of veterinary treatment.'

Since an abattoir or knackers' yard is not 'a place of veterinary treatment', this law is explicit. If a large animal like a dairy cow is unable to move, e.g.

from post-calving paralysis, or can only move with extreme pain, e.g. from a broken limb, or is likely to experience pain while in a moving vehicle, then it is illegal to move that animal off the farm to a place of slaughter. There will however, inevitably be borderline cases such as the cow who is being culled for severe mastitis or foot lameness. I have already said that I believe such animals should be culled sooner rather than later but every dairy farmer has, from time to time to weigh in the balance his compassion to one of his old cows against the several hundred pounds' difference in the price he will get from sending her to the abattoir or calling in the knacker to kill her on the farm. The best time for the concerned welfarist to address this particular cost:benefit equation is just after donating 50p to relieve starvation in Africa. The dilemma could be resolved by an insurance policy designed to pay the abattoir price to the farmer for the small proportion of cull cows likely to experience unnecessary suffering *en route* to slaughter. This would require a veterinary certificate, and the costs thereof, but if it paid out on, say, one cull cow in fifty, then I believe the policy and the premium could be made attractive to the dairy farmer. I am uncertain about many things but I do believe that most dairy farmers care for their cows.

10   Horses and Pets

'Moderate the bray and you sow up the donkey'

R.L. Stephenson

The animals that most of us know most about and care most about are the dogs, cats and guinea pigs which we welcome into the home as part of the family or the horse or pony kept nearby in a paddock or local livery stable. We value these animals not for their ability to make money but for the contribution that they, as living individuals, can make to the quality of our lives. At first sight this suggests that these animals are inherently likely to get a better deal. It is necessary, however, to recall from Chapter 1 the parable of the rabbit. A cold, hungry rabbit in a dirty, wet hutch will suffer and the nature of that suffering will be the same whether our motivation to possess that animal was the desire to love a pet, eat rabbit stew, find a cure for cancer or test a new cosmetic. It matters not to the animal how we feel but what we do. Nevertheless, it is usually a help to the welfare of any animal to be valued as an individual,whether for sentimental or economic reasons. It is even more help if caring owners also have the skills and resources to care for their animals properly.

I do not propose to address the welfare of horses and pets on a species-by-species basis. There are plenty of good, practical books dealing with the care of pets and any attempt of mine to condense even the basic principles of pet care into one chapter could only be superficial. Nor shall I consider how pets may improve our welfare since this topic has also been well covered by others (see Fogle, 1981). There is good evidence that pets can help to make us better people by teaching us to care, or help us to live longer by teaching us to relax. My concern, however, is not what animals can do for us but what we can do for them. In this chapter, I shall consider some of the welfare problems of being a pet. I shall assume that the pet is well loved, so exclude sins of cruelty and neglect, and concentrate only on ways in which the actions of man, however well intentioned, may compromise their welfare.

What it is to be a pet

In the natural or wild state, most sentient animals grow up in the company of their own kind. When they separate from their immediate families, they (or their parents) will be motivated almost entirely by self-interest. Most of the time most individuals within most species will treat most other individuals within their own species with indifference or as competitors. Some individuals in some species (which include dogs and horses) will recognize certain other individuals as companions. Individuals of other species will be treated with indifference, as competitors, as predators or as prey. One occasion when an animal will be powerfully motivated to become involved with another of its species is, of course, when it wishes to mate. In the animal kingdom, both male and female are, at the time, motivated to sex by their own self-interest but to serve this self-interest they need a partner even if only for a short while.

The pet that we take into our home or garden has to adapt to a life style that is, by definition, unnatural. To cite an extreme case, the urban lap-dog may be taken from its mother at eight weeks of age and thereafter never again experience any close contact with its own species. It may never mate or rear its own puppies and what social contact it does experience with other dogs may only be when on the end of a lead while being sharply abused by its owner for attempting to behave like a dog. The life of the average pet dog is more unnatural than the life of the pig on the factory farm. This, of itself, is not a problem. It is not essential to the welfare of an animal that its life style is natural; the issue is whether or not the animal can adapt without suffering to the environment and life style to which it is exposed. Some species clearly make better pets than others but no animal classifies itself *a priori* as wild or domestic, working dog or toy dog, vermin or game; it deals with life as it comes.

I shall interpret the welfare of pets, as all animals, in terms of their state of both body and mind. Are the circumstances of a pet animal such that it can act to sustain fitness, seek pleasure and avoid suffering? Are we, who define the life style of our pet, providing it with an environment that will live up to its mental expectations as defined both by its genotype and its experience? To illustrate this point, I ask you to compare the implications of choosing a pet from one of the following pairs:

(1)   a small dog (e.g. a Corgi) or a fox;
(2)   a large dog (e.g. a German Shepherd) or a wolf.

I choose these pairs because a visitor from another planet who studied only their anatomy and physiology but ignored their behaviour might well conclude that the German Shepherd and the wolf were, for practical purposes, almost identical. Most intelligent dog owners would, I believe, consider themselves competent to feed and house a fox but, even if it were legal, probably conclude that it is cruel to 'deny a fox its freedom'. In the case of a wolf they would probably conclude that any attempt to keep it like a German Shepherd would not only be cruel but positively dangerous; if they wished to own a wolf, they could only do so by confining the animal under zoo conditions.

Thoughts of wild animals such as the fox and the wolf generate a further concept of freedom, missing from the famous five, namely the freedom to be free! So far, I have assumed that freedom *per se* is too abstract a concept to affect how an animal feels or is motivated to specific action. What we think of in broad terms as the need of the wild animal to be free may be interpreted by the animal in terms of specific needs for space, sex, and security of food supply in species whose survival has been dependent on the evolution of powerful instincts to hunt and forage. In well designed zoos and game parks it may be possible to meet these needs, or the animal may at least be able to adapt to the conditions to the extent that it does not suffer. At best, it may come to enjoy them. However, a wild animal such as the fox or wolf may, for evolutionary reasons, be more strongly motivated than the domestic dog to make a positive contribution to its own welfare rather than accept absolute dependence on its master. This comes quite close to suggesting that it has a greater desire to be free. I shall develop this theme further in Chapter 11. The central point at issue is that all animals that we take into our lives as individuals must adapt to a way of life that is abnormal for their species. The adaptation required becomes most extreme when we elect to own one puppy or one pony for we immediately deny our solitary pet the company of its kind.

This chapter considers, in general terms, the major welfare problems that may arise when we remove animals from the company of their kind and adapt them to human society. Assuming that the owner does not neglect the animal and has the basic skills to keep it well fed and fit these may include:

(1) boredom;
(2) lack of oral satisfaction;
(3) lack of social contact (with any appropriate species);
(4) sexual frustration;
(5) unnatural breeding;
(6) unnatural extension of life.

I shall illustrate these general themes by reference to horses and the most common pets, the 'companion animals,' an expression which appears to mean exactly the same thing as 'pet', namely an animal which we choose to have as a friend but, in practice, refers to animals which we choose to own, at some personal cost, in order to improve the quality of our own lives. In other words, their value is defined not only in monetary terms. This definition then can include animals such as horses, from the individual pony kept as a pet to the thoroughbred kept in a racing stable holding over 100 animals. Both have been bought for the express intent of giving pleasure to their owners. The child will probably love her pony to distraction. The millionaire may not even recognize his Class 1 thoroughbred in a racing yard, still less think of it as a companion, but will derive enormous pleasure from welcoming it into the winner's enclosure. My working title for this chapter was 'companion animals' but the phrase is both ponderous and imprecise. 'Horses and pets' will do.

Boredom

One of the advantages of being a dairy cow, a sheep on the Scottish hills, or a wildebeest on the African plains is that there is plenty to occupy the mind. Foraging, avoiding and escaping predators, caring for the young or even regular trips to the milking parlour all help to pass the time and increase the motivation to rest and do nothing (i.e. make leisure a pleasure). Young animals raised in the company of their own kind may find that they can do what they need to survive, still have energy to spare, so indulge in play. All these things are conscious actions designed to avoid suffering or seek pleasure. Many pets, much of the time, have no need to hunt or forage, no need to avoid predation, no offspring to care for and no-one to play with. It is no wonder that they get bored.

In Part II, I did not attempt to analyse the psychology of boredom in animals, mainly because I am not convinced by the scientific literature on the topic to date. One does not, however, need science to conclude that the word boredom, as understood in common parlance, offers a very good explanation for the behaviour of a horse isolated all day in a stable or a dog isolated all day in a flat. Moreover, the development of abnormal or antisocial behaviour patterns, such as the horse that becomes a weaver or the dog that tears up cushions, may reasonably be called neurotic and attributed to frustration. The pure psychologist may find these conclusions simplistic but I am not, at this stage, attempting to satisfy the psychologist, I am trying to develop working principles for the care of animals who lack things to do and the company of their kind.

There are two distinct reasons why well-treated pets may suffer more from boredom than farm or wild animals. First, they do not have to work for their living so have more time to kill. Second, they tend to have higher expectations. I have argued that the mind of a sentient animal is determined both by its genetics and its education, itself determined by the impact of experience upon the instinctive nature of the genotype. Thus the pot-bellied pig that is taken into the household as a pet acquires higher expectations than the commercial sow confined in a stall and may display more distress if its expectations are not fulfilled. However, no pig, however petted, ever puts on a display of pure joy comparable to the daily performance of a dog when its owner comes home. Dogs are a uniquely emotional species. This is an unemotional conclusion. I mean much of their emotion is determined by their genes. It can, however, be a source of both suffering and pleasure.

Oral satisfaction in horses and dogs

Animals eat not only to satisfy their hunger but because they enjoy it. In more scientific terms the motivation to eat or forage is not driven simply by the need to ensure an adequate supply of nutrients. For an isolated, bored horse or dog denied social contact or sexual expression, eating may be the only reliable source of pleasure. A typical case in point is that of the stabled horse or pony. The digestive tract of the horse, from the incisor teeth to the large bowel, is designed to process fibrous foods, chopped to a short length and eaten over an extended period of the day. Unlike the cow, it does not have the satisfaction of ruminating on food it consumed earlier. Most horses or ponies in stables but getting regular exercise are given one to three 'hard' concentrate meals per day (depending on their work load) plus a ration of hay which may be consumed at their leisure. Some ponies doing no work can be maintained on hay alone. In most circumstances, such a diet is healthy, nutritionally sound and helps to pass the time. However, feeding hay can cause the following problems:

(1)   if hay is offered to appetite, some horses and most ponies will eat too much and become fat or, at least, pot-bellied and sluggish.
(2)   nearly all hay is dusty and this dust is rich in mites and fungal spores which can provoke allergic, asthmatic reactions in most horses and severe impairment of respiratory function ('heaves' or 'broken wind') in some hypersensitive individuals.

In fact, horses do not actually 'need' to eat hay. They *like* good hay and it can aid digestion by stabilizing fermentation in the large bowel but it contains no essential nutrients that cannot be provided, often as cheaply, from other sources. This means that in some circumstances hay, or substitutes for hay, may be used primarily as a source of oral satisfaction; not so much food as an equine equivalent of chewing gum. Hay substitutes such as chaffed straw, fed plain or molassed, on its own or as a diluent of the hard feed can help a pony to pass the time in an enjoyable way and stabilize its digestion without getting too fat or suffering allergic responses to fungal spores.

Abnormal, stereotypic behaviour patterns in stabled horses, such as weaving, crib-biting and windsucking, may create welfare problems for both the animals and their owners. Traditionally these habits were called 'stable vices,' an unfortunate expression which carries an unjustified implication of immorality. I discussed the possible aetiology of these stereotypies in Chapters 3 and 4 without reaching any firm conclusions. To recapitulate in brief, it is possible that only movement stereotypies such as weaving may be interpreted as a response to barren environments. Oral stereotypies such as crib-biting and windsucking are undoubtedly linked to the sensation of oral satisfaction but are not necessarily a sign of distress. Weaving may be attributed primarily to boredom and isolation, although it is a habit that a horse can acquire from observing others. We do not yet know whether the weaving horse is suffering at the time or has discovered a mechanism to cope with the stress of frustration. In either event, once a movement stereotypy such as weaving has become fixed and emancipated from its initial cause it may reasonably be considered as a visual expression of a disordered (but not necessarily distressed) mind. Compulsive weavers usually lose condition, partly by virtue of their hyperactivity and partly because the more they weave the less they eat. Thus weaving meets the two main criteria for poor welfare, a disordered mental state and a failure to sustain fitness.

Oral stereotypies such as playing with the tongue, crib-biting and wind-sucking may not express distress or even boredom. Horses may do these things initially because it gives them pleasure or possibly (in the case of windsucking) as an aid to digestion. However, they, too, may become compulsive and emancipated from the initial stimulus. A horse has to fix its jaw by crib-biting in order to suck wind into the oesophagus so it is usually possible to prevent these habits from developing by designing the stable in such a way that the horse has nothing to bite on. Radical measures to restrict the compulsive windsucker include the use of collars (Fig. 3.3) or even surgery.

These extreme measures may improve welfare or make it worse. If a horse has acquired a powerful motivation to a particular pattern of stereotypic behaviour then it presumably experiences frustration if it is mechanically prevented from carrying it out. However, the intensity of this frustration may decline with time as it 'loses the habit'. Since 'stable vices' do not constitute immoral behaviour on the part of the horse but coping mechanisms of a gregarious grazing species to abnormal conditions of feeding and housing, then radical measures to restrict these activities can only be justified if the horse is actually doing itself harm. Playing with the tongue is clearly harm-less. Compulsive crib-biters may ruin their incisor teeth. Many owners believe that windsucking can cause colic or otherwise impair digestion. This is unproven. Paul McGreevy at Bristol has studied windsuckers by continous X-ray observations and suggests that they only draw air into the oesophagus and let it out between gulps the way it came in. There does not appear to be a build up of air in the stomach and intestines. If this is so, windsucking may also be relatively harmless. I would not, at this stage, wish to make firm pronouncements on the management of stereotypies in horses beyond the fact that one should, where possible, try to avoid them by attention to feeding, stable design and by trying to make life less boring. When they do occur, they are only a problem if they are positively harmful, i.e if the horse is becoming progressively thin, toothless or stupid.

Since eating is such a satisfying way of passing the time, it is useful to consider whether oral satisfaction can be exploited as a way of reducing the boredom and frustration experienced by the isolated, housebound dog. Unfortunately, the dog, unlike the horse, tends to demolish a meal con-taining its nutrient requirements for the day in two minutes flat. For dogs, the enjoyment of food would seem to be more in the expectation than the consummation, whether it be the promise of the daily meal or a chocolate. One source of sustained oral satisfaction is the marrowbone which can keep dogs entertained for hours. However, this may not be compatible with wall-to-wall carpeting in an urban flat. Roger Mugford, expert on canine neuroses, suggests that owners who have to leave their pet dog alone in the house all day should, before leaving in the morning, feed it a meal that is bulky without being too fattening, based, for example on cooked vegetables such as potatoes or rice. The meal is consumed as quickly as ever but the dog with a belly full of food that is digested relatively slowly is more inclined to sleep through the day. One disadvantage for the urban dog and its owner is that this practice, by the evening, generates a large quantity of faeces and a powerful desire to void them.

Sex and social intercourse

The fourth freedom acknowledges the right of animals to 'the company of their kind'. In Chapter 6 I listed the reasons why an animal may need the company of another, not necessarily of its own species:.

(1)   for sexual intercourse;
(2)   for security;
(3)   for cooperation, e.g. in provision of food or shelter;
(4)   for education;
(5)   for pleasure.

I shall now examine how these needs may be met or circumvented in the life of a typical pet dog, cat and pony. All three species have adapted well to the life of a pet, albeit using different tactics to exploit our affection to serve their needs, but all three, from time to time, have needs that cannot be met by man. The most pressing of these needs is, of course, sex. As always I shall avoid getting into any quasi-philosophical argument as to whether any restriction of the right of animals to reproduce their kind is an affront to their *telos*, and consider only whether they may in any circumstances suffer from the consequences of sexual frustration, sexual excess or enforced asexuality, i.e. castration or ovariectomy.

Sexual continence is something we expect of ourselves but impose on our pets. We restrain our human sexual behaviour on moral grounds, or because we fear the long term consequences of our actions – unhappiness, poverty, sickness or death. (There is a blurred distinction between morality and practical future planning.) If we are able to overcome acute urges to commit unwise sexual acts we may feel better in the longer term. Our actions have led to a more satisfactory resolution of conflicting motivations; we have moved to a more serene spot in MacFarland's egg. Our pets, however, are amoral creatures. They are motivated to seek pleasure and avoid pain, neither fearing future consequences nor rueing the past. I would therefore be guilty of anthropomorphism if I did not consider the possibility that pet animals might actually *suffer* from sexual frustration, since it is but one example of an argument central to the whole welfare debate, namely that animals are motivated by powerful internal and external sensations and may suffer if they are unable to resolve these sensations by conscious action (see Dawkins, 1993; MacFarland, 1989).

The sex urge differs from the sensation of hunger, thirst or exhaustion in that it does not *have* to be satisfied. Male horses, dogs and cats have the potential to be aroused at any time but the motivating stimulus to action is usually external, i.e. the presence of a female on heat. Once out of sight (or smell) they are usually out of mind. Mares, bitches and queens are uninterested in sex until switched on largely by oestrogen from the developing ovarian follicles prior to ovulation. These sensations may, in a general sense, be compared with other motivating forces which do not have to be satisfied such as the motivation to avoid isolation, to explore or seek increased space, to build a nest before laying an egg, or giving birth to piglets. All these denials of 'behavioural needs' are matters of prime concern among advocates of improved welfare standards for animals on farms, in zoos or laboratories. I make this comparison not to espouse the cause of free love for pets but to make the general point that most animals, including man, have to live with many sources of acute frustration and that the case for improved welfare cannot be based on *acute* frustration alone. As I argued in Chapter 6, frustration may only lead to suffering when an animal is chronically unable to resolve problems such as curiosity and fear, pain, hunger and discomfort experienced singly or in combination, and its mood shifts to a chronic state of anxiety or hopelessness.

This argument is slightly unworldly but it leads naturally to one of the most important of all practical questions: 'When, if ever, is it acceptable to neuter a pet animal?' My views on this subject are personal, largely unsupported by scientific evidence, but consistent with the logic of my central argument. I repeat, to achieve a satisfactory state of welfare, an animal must be able to sustain (physical) fitness and avoid (mental) suffering. The effects of neutering (castration or ovariectomy) must therefore be assessed in terms of

(1) pain and suffering associated with the mutilation itself or its immediate consequences;
(2) long-term effects of neutering on the physical or mental state of the animal;
(3) long-term effects of uncontrolled sexual drive or activity on physical or mental state.

Correct anaesthetic procedures can eliminate pain associated with the act itself and reduce (although not eliminate) pain and suffering during the recovery period. If the mutilation can be justified by its long-term consequences then the suffering may be defined as necessary. The question that remains is 'will the quality of life of the neutered animal be impaired, improved or largely unaffected?' I believe that there is no general answer to this question; it must be addressed on a species-specific and sex-specific basis.

The female dog normally comes on heat, i.e. is sexually aroused, for two periods per year, each lasting not more than ten days although she will display vulval bleeding and be attractive to males for rather longer. In most households these occasions come and go with little, if any, apparent disturbance to the bitch or her owner. If there are male dogs in the house or immediate vicinity, management becomes a little more difficult. Male dogs are powerfully aroused by the presence or smell of a bitch on heat but not, I believe, to the point of suffering. For nearly all bitches and most male dogs, I believe that sexual frustration does not constitute a serious welfare problem, although I recognize that some neurotic males (and the occasional female) are a menace to armchairs, neighbours' legs and similarly embraceable objects.

The bitch that is left intact but unmated has an increased risk of abnormal uterine development leading to pyometria and the probability that she will need major surgery for removal of an enlarged, inflamed uterus while she is sick. This risk is much reduced in the bitch that has one or more litters of puppies. Bitches that have reared puppies may also be less likely to develop neurotic behaviour patterns such as furniture abuse or irrational fear or aggression in the presence of strange people or other dogs. In my (unscientific) opinion, the ideal situation for the bitch is to be left intact but allowed to rear two or three litters of puppies. Neutering does affect both the temperament and the physical form of both male and female dogs. Both sexes tend to become more placid and, since both male and female hormones are involved in the growth and maintenance of muscle, both sexes are more inclined to get fat. My personal view is that since the sexual activity of domestic dogs can usually be controlled by their owners, and neutered dogs may show a reduced enthusiasm (or physical capacity) for many of the pleasures of life such as a good walk, neutering should be avoided wherever possible. However, I do not believe that the neutered dog actually suffers in the long term from the psychological consequences of neutering. The hyperactive, sexually obsessed male dog that is regularly punished for his obsessions will, I am sure, enjoy a better quality of life after castration.

The circumstances of the cat are entirely different. The case for neutering cats that are not wanted for breeding purposes is, I believe, overwhelming. Once again, the owner may prefer to delay neutering queens until after they have had at least one litter, possibly because the delay may affect their physique and temperament but mainly because kittens are such good fun. There are, however, powerful reasons why not neutering cats may directly impair their quality of life. Cats are normally left to roam and so are regularly presented with sexual opportunities. Female cats usually have two breeding seasons in early and late spring, lasting, in total five to six months, although when cats are exposed to artificially extended light periods (i.e. live indoors) the season may be longer. During the breeding season they come on heat repeatedly. They ovulate only when they mate. If they do not mate these periods may last up to 10 days. Most entire females therefore spend much of their adult life either 'calling' (on heat), pregnant or lactating. In these circumstances, they usually fail to sustain fitness and I believe they suffer. Male cats do not have to suffer the long-term consequences of past copulation but are compelled to fight for the right to continue. Finally, most neutered cats seem to maintain an active enthusiasm for hunting and other pleasures of the outdoor life, in between long, voluptuous, entirely natural periods of sleep on radiators, in airing cupboards, etc. I am convinced that, on balance, the quality of life of the average pet (or feral) cat is positively enhanced by neutering.

With horses and donkeys, the standard practice is to castrate the males and leave the females entire. This is largely for managemental reasons since geldings are nearly always very biddable, mares biddable most of the time but stallions can be hot-tempered and potentially dangerous. The expensive stallion at a top-class stud not only gets plenty of sexual action but also gets treated like a lord between times. Less valuable stallions are likely to be ridden less and isolated more than geldings (because they are potentially dangerous) which means that their life may be inherently more boring than that of the average gelding before counting in the added burden of sexual frustration. Once again, I think it easier for a gelding to maintain its serenity.

The next issue to address is whether pets may suffer from the lack of other individuals of their species as companions rather than sexual partners. The dog is a truly companionable animal. Wolves and wild dogs operate in packs usually based on extended family groups. Members of the pack not only show deference to the leader but also work together for the good of the family/pack and reinforce their mutual bonds of companionship by conspicuous displays of affection and play. The evolutionary history of the dog has prepared it well for a life style in which it is happy to adopt a subservient role to an adored human leader. The fact that the feelings and behaviour of a pet dog with respect to its owner are fundamentally similar to the instinctive behaviour of a subservient wolf to the pack leader does not detract from the fact that most people and dogs who live together are aware that they love each other's company.

By and large, therefore, man is able to satisfy the desire of the dog for the security and pleasure of a trusted companion. The lap-dog, in constant receipt of human affection but isolated from contact with other dogs may have rather distorted perceptions of what it is to be a dog but, so long as it stays healthy, there is no reason to suppose that it actually suffers. However, dogs, more than any other domestic species, demonstrably revel in each others company and play for hours, simply for pleasure rather than to make a social point (e.g. establish their place in the hierarchy). Kittens also play for hours with their litter-mates and may, at this time, form bonds of friendship which last for life. However, adult cats are more likely to be solitary or (as in the case of feral cats) come together for reasons that carry an obvious advantage to themselves or their genes, such as food, sex or status.

It is argued that the psychological development of the dog is arrested at an infantile stage by the presence of the human 'pack leader' or alpha male, in the same way that the physiological development of sexual maturity is inhibited in wolves while they remain relatively subordinate members of extended families. Once again, the reason for the behaviour may be primitive but if we elect to exert our dominion over a species that can experience joy at any stage of its life then I believe we have a responsibility to allow it to express that joy. I do not want to get sidetracked into a discussion of dog training but this responsibility requires us, at least, to allow dogs to socialize with other animals. This applies especially at the psychologically important age directly after weaning when they must learn by experience to manage the primitive, opposing sensations of curiosity and fear so that they do not lead, on the one hand to foolhardiness or, on the other, to anxiety neuroses. The adult dog should also be sufficiently well trained (i.e. subservient) that its owner can allow it to play freely off the lead with other dogs, secure in the knowledge that it will come when called.

Our need to assume absolute dominion over the dog becomes most extreme when we require it to work for us. Consider two examples: the working sheepdog and the guide dog for the blind or otherwise disabled. The working sheepdog is expected to sublimate its natural instinct to attack sheep in order to move them, with minimal distress, according to the wishes of its owner. I am convinced that well-trained, successful sheepdogs hugely enjoy their work, partly for the satisfaction of pleasing their owners and partly because this redirected expression of the killer instinct may be quite as satisfying as the real thing. On the other hand, the life of a guide dog for the blind or disabled appears to us to be one which involves extreme self-sacrifice and very little fun. I am hugely impressed by the behaviour of guide dogs, not least because I cannot explain their motivation in a way that is consistent with my very limited understanding of the dog mind. In essence these animals have been trained by a dominant human to sublimate almost all their natural instincts to serve a different human whom they may not recognize as dominant. I offer two, profoundly different explanations for this behaviour. Either they have become less sentient, i.e their decisions have become entirely programmed. Alternatively, they have, by training and experience, become aware of the needs of another (in the instinctive life of a dog, one of the family) and made the conscious decision to fulfil those needs; in other words they have discovered true altruism.

Horses and donkeys, being herd animals, may reasonably be expected to seek the company of their kind for reasons of security. However, there is good evidence that both species also form close, non-sexual bonds of companionship with selected individuals who may or may not be related to them. When such bonds are broken horses and especially donkeys may not only display lasting signs of behavioural distress but actually experience a physical decline. I think it fair to conclude that these species can truly be said to form friendships. This implies that it can be cruel to isolate a horse or pony or remove it from a stable relationship (no pun intended). This means that many well loved ponies are being made to suffer by their adoring owners.

In the absence of further and better particulars as to the minds of our most popular pets, I am inclined to suggest that the powerful need for a friend, as distinct from the security of company, may be restricted to dogs and equines. My family have experienced life with most small pets, rabbits, rats, mice, guinea pigs and cage birds. Undoubtedly a small menagerie of guinea pigs, or guinea pigs and rabbits together are more active and more entertaining than an isolated individual in a pen. However, I know of no good scientific or anecdotal evidence to suggest that they form special friendships or suffer from isolation *per se*. However, the pet rat, rabbit or guinea pig kept in a solitary cage or pen needs attention, handling and stroking from its human owner, not only for the pleasure of the moment but also to keep it constantly exposed to novelty and so avoid the increasing fear of the unknown that can accumulate when all exposure to environmental stimuli is denied.

Breeding and welfare

The breeding strategies of wild animals are successful, by definition, because they have been tested by natural selection and led to the survival of the fittest. When man first domesticated animals such as the cow to provide food, the horse to provide power and the dog to aid in the hunt, he discovered that he could improve their utility by arranging matings between superior animals. This selective breeding was unnatural in a strictly Darwinian sense in that the 'superior' offspring may not have been better fitted for survival in the wild, but it was functional in that they were better able to perform the tasks allotted by man. Thus breeds were born. Those humans so fortunate that they did not have to work all day for their survival were able to turn their thoughts to ways of improving the quality of their leisure time. Among this select group a few began to breed domestic animals for their own amusement. This approach to leisure saw its greatest flowering on the estates of the English landowners, individuals whose mission in life was to devise elaborate rituals for passing the time without actually working. These rituals include field 'sports' such as hunting and shooting, which involve the selective breeding of some animals, especially dogs, to make the killing of others, e.g. game birds and foxes, more entertaining. Other dogs were bred to be pretty and pampered and small enough to be carried as fashion accessories.

No other animal species presents such a diversity of physical form as the domesticated dog. The wild hunting dogs of East Africa have acquired by natural selection a reasonably uniform size and shape. The pariah dogs of Asia, a mixture of wild and feral animals derived not entirely by natural selection, present a number of different forms, not dissimilar to the Spitz, greyhound and working collie (Menzel, 1948) but functionally they are very similar, of middle size and athletic (if half-starved) proportions. A combination of natural and artificial selction has produced horses and ponies as different in size as the Shire and the Shetland. However, there is nothing in nature that compares with the differences in both size and form between the St Bernard and the Chihuahua, or the Borzoi and the bulldog.

Dogs can identify others as individuals from several cues including sight and smell but they display no breed prejudice, as is obvious when it comes to the time of mating. The concept of breed has no place in their mind and therefore no direct bearing on their welfare. They are neither troubled by their personal appearance nor concerned with their status as a working dog, sporting dog or toy dog.

The effects of selected breeding on dog welfare may therefore be assessed according to the same rules as those used to assess the breeding of animals for food, for work or for research, whether by natural mating, artificial insertion of semen or fertilized embryos, or by genetic engineering. The Farm Animal Welfare Council (FAWC) defined the following potentially harmful consequences of artifical breeding (and other 'unnatural' procedures). These are 'the manipulation of body size, shape or reproductive capacity by breeding ... or gene insertion in such a way as to reduce mobility, increase the risk of pain, injury, metabolic disease, skeletal or obstetric problems, perinatal mortality or psychological distress'. The importance of this sentence is that it defines the welfare implications of artifical breeding and other forms of tinkering not by the method used to manipulate the animal but by its consequences. I have already stressed that it was conventional selection procedures, not genetic engineering that crippled the heavy breeds of broiler fowl. If the genetic engineers ever wished to produce a pig or a mouse so grotesquely unfit as the bulldog, they would be required by the Animals (Scientific Procedures) Act 1986 to convince the authorities that they could promise a benefit to man sufficient to justify such a cost to the animal, like a cure for cancer. They would also be prime targets for animal activists, many of them dog lovers.

In Table 10.1 I list some examples of abnormalities in dogs that can be attributed wholly or in part to selective breeding. I identify three categories:

(1) *Accidental:* abnormalities associated with recessive genes which emerged by chance within inbred populations.
(2) *Unfortunate:* abnormalities which were not foreseen but which can be attributed, at least in part to deliberate selection, especially for body shape.
(3) *Deliberate:* abnormalities which have been deliberately induced by selective breeding because they are thought to be aesthetic, amusing or simply different.

Some accidental congenital abnormalites, such as progressive retinal atrophy in Red Setters, are clearly associated with single lethal recessive genes. Others, such as epilepsy in Dachshunds and German Shepherds, appear to have a strong familial predisposition but are genetically less clear-cut. These abnormalities are encouraged by inbreeding but, in the first instance, they are nobody's fault. Sins of commission can occur when individuals show and breed dogs who are known to carry recessive genes for these abnormalities. However, most breed societies work hard to eliminate problems such as retinal atrophy for the obvious reason that no owner will derive satisfaction from breeding dogs that will go blind in middle age. For a comprehensive list of genetic abnormalities in companion animals see Foley, Lasley and Osweiler (1979).

Table 10.1 Some abnormalities in dogs associated with selective breeding.

	Abnormality	Susceptible breeds
Accidental	Retinal atrophy	Red Setters, Springer spaniels
	Epilepsy	German Shepherds, Dachshunds
	Gout	Boxers, Great Danes, German Shepherds
Unfortunate	Hip dysplasia	German Shepherds, Old English Sheepdogs
	Osteosarcomas	Giant breeds; Great Danes, St Bernards
	Slipped lumbar discs	Dachshunds
Deliberate	Locomotor disorders	Bassets, Bulldogs
	Ectropion and skin disorders	Bassets, Bulldogs, Bloodhounds
	Breathing difficulties	Bulldogs, Boxers
	Obstetric problems	Chihuahuas

I have called the second category of abnormalities 'unfortunate' because they can be unforeseen consequences of selection for appearance. The 'long sloping rump' favoured by judges of the German Shepherd looks good and is associated with extreme athleticism in most young animals but has predisposed to hip dysplasia (partial or complete dissociation of the head of the femur from its socket in the pelvis), a progressively painful and crippling condition which can develop at an early age. This condition, which appears in many breeds of dog, cannot be attributed entirely to genetics, certainly not to a single gene, so is less easy to control.

Another major welfare problem which falls into the 'unfortunate' category is the high incidence of osteosarcomas, or bone cancers, in giant breeds of dog like the Great Dane and St Bernard. These conditions are not genetic, in the strict sense of the word, because there is, to my knowledge, no direct familial association. The cancers develop at the points of the limb where the bones are subjected to the greatest mechanical stresses. Selection for giantism in the dog imposes abnormal mechanical stresses on the limbs and has significantly increased the risk that these animals will experience pain, disease and premature death.

The third group of abnormalities can only be defined as 'deliberate.' Breeds with loose skin and deep wrinkles in the face and head, like Bulldogs, Bassets and Bloodhounds, are especially prone to chronic inflammation and infection of the skin and mucous membranes of the eyes. Bulldogs and Bassets have reduced mobility. Bulldogs usually have mechanical difficulties in breathing because their nose is too short, distorted and their soft palate too big for their throat. Chihuahuas have an abnormally high incidence of obstetric problems not because they are so small but because fashion has dictated that they should have heads that are too big relative to the dimensions of the birth canal.

It should, of course, be the business of the breed societies to put their own houses in order. Some are better than others. It should be clear that I find some breeds objectionable but I must, as always, try to avoid my own prejudices and think like a dog. I am satisfied that most dogs have the capacity to enjoy life whether they are big or small, herding sheep, retrieving pheasants or being fed chocolates on a perfumed lap. Nor, I suspect, are they much distressed when made to wear clothing that appears ridiculous to me unless it is actually uncomfortable to them. Size, breed and physical appearance *per se* have no intrinsic impact on the welfare of the dog. It is, however, cruel deliberately to distort the shape and form of a dog in such a way as to reduce its ability to run and play, or to predispose it to the chronic discomfort of an itchy skin. This argument must be the same for the dog as for any other sentient animal and the same whether the abnormality and loss of fitness have been perpetrated by traditional breeding or by new biotechnology. No advocate of animal rights can oppose genetic engineering in animals without, at the same time, calling for a ban on the Bulldog.

Euthanasia

When we bring a pet into the family we free it from many of the rigours of natural selection, not least the ruthless elimination of individuals that fail to sustain fitness. Development of the skills necessary to combat the ravages of injury and disease and so preserve not only life itself but also the quality of life for ourselves and for our pets has to be one of the greatest achievements of the human species. Having acquired this power, we are then faced with the responsibility of deciding when to let go; when, in fact, death becomes the kinder option. In most societies, the preservation of human life is given a near-absolute value and euthanasia is illegal. This largely frees the medical profession from the need to make difficult decisions on a case-by-case basis. The veterinary surgeon forced into a value judgement as to whether a sick or injured pet should receive treatment or be put to sleep has to balance conflicting responsibilites to three different parties, the animal, the owner and him(her)self. This generates three unavoidable questions:

(1) how much will the animal suffer if I elect to prolong its life?
(2) how much will the owner suffer from the death of the loved pet or, alternatively, the cost of paying for treatment?
(3) how much money can/should I make from attempts to prolong this animal's life by radical surgery or prolonged medication?

The classic example of this dilemma for the veterinary surgeon is the case of the sick old dog in the home of a sick old man. The vet is operating on the basis of his professional oath that 'my constant endeavour will be to ensure the welfare of animals committed to my care'. If, as I have argued throughout, death (i.e. non-existence) is not a welfare problem for the dog, then there comes a time when it is kinder to the dog to kill it than to sustain its life. Compassion for the dog may, however, be unbearable for the owner. If, in this extreme case, the dog could just survive the man, overall suffering, in a strictly utilitarian sense would be minimized.

Andrew Edney (1989) has prepared a list of questions that a vet should ask before deciding whether to recommend euthanasia to the owner of a seriously ill or injured animal:

First, is the animal

(1) free from pain, distress or serious discomfort which cannot be effectively controlled?
(2) able to walk and balance itself reasonably well?
(3) able to eat and drink enough for maintenance without much difficulty and without vomiting?
(4) free from tumours which cause pain or serious discomfort and are judged inoperable?
(5) able to breathe without difficulty?
(6) able to pass urine and faeces at normal intervals without serious difficulty or incontinence?
(7) Finally, is the owner able to cope physically and emotionally with any nursing and medication which may be required?

This is a very good check list so long as it is not applied too zealously. On these terms, most bulldogs and plenty of middle-aged vets could qualify for euthanasia on grounds of breathing difficulties or chronic back pain respectively. Chronic pain is a severe form of suffering and can be sufficient reason for euthanasia in an animal that has nothing to live for, like an old neglected pony, or a dog with inoperable tumours for whom the prognosis is hopeless. However, the old dog, almost crippled with arthritis may still experience the pleasure of the daily meal and joy at the sight of its master. If the sick old man can still feed and care for the sick old dog, each can, I believe, derive dignity from sharing each other's suffering.

To justify my use of the word dignity to describe the mind and behaviour of a dog, I ask you to consider the condition of the old dog who can no longer control its bowels or bladder. The understanding owner will not punish the dog and may indeed commiserate but the dog will continue to display shame. If a dog can experience the indignity of incontinence it can also experience the dignity of hobbling over to its master's chair.

My argument is beginning to sound emotional but it still conforms strictly to the pleasure/pain principle. The old dog and its old master may both experience a lot of pain but still have the real pleasure of each other's company. Old, lame horses can also enjoy the pleasure of each other's company during their final years at pasture . Consider, however, the case of the solitary old pony. The child, who once devoted half her life to this pony has now outgrown it and left home, except perhaps for weekends. The pony is no longer ridden. It has some chronic arthritic pain and is kept in isolation in a box or small paddock denuded of all but rank weeds and visited for perhaps ten minutes per day. This animal would not qualify for euthanasia according to Andrew Edney's criteria. However, it once knew the pleasures of companionship and exercise but now has nothing left to live for. The owner who decides to end this pony's life should not reproach her(him)self. The alternative – keeping that pony alive (but no more than that) simply because 'I can't bear to let him go' – is unfair.

Finally, before I switch out of preaching mode, I must express my greatest concern in this context, which arises from the increasing capacity of vets to perform heroic, expensive surgery on companion animals, e.g. hip replacements in ageing Alsatians. Such procedures are professionally satisfying and most owners who agree to these procedures are insured or happy to pay to extend the life (or quality of life) of the individual pet in question, i.e. they satisfy the second and third criteria I posed at the outset; they give pleasure to the owner and the vet. The primary responsibility of the vet must, however, always be to 'the welfare of animals committed to his care'. There is no doubt that some of the heroic procedures now being carried over from human into veterinary surgery can restore quality of life for a pet animal. However, the vet has a special obligation not 'to strive officiously to keep alive' and this obligation is most severely tested when set against the opportunity to make a lot of money or enhance his professional reputation. A sour colleague recently accused veterinary schools of training their students 'to prolong the suffering of geriatric pets'. It is an extreme position but he has a point.

11 Wild Animals

'For most of history, mankind has managed to keep a reasonable balance between thinking nature's adorable and thinking it wants to kill us.'

P.J. O'Rourke

Part III of this book, 'What we can do for them', is primarily concerned with the impact of man on animal welfare. When it comes to wild animals I believe that the best thing we can do for them is to leave them well, alone (the comma is essential). By this I mean that wherever possible we should seek to protect their habitat and then simply leave them to it. The conservation of habitat and the need (or not) for culling strategies to preserve the balance of nature are important and complex issues but they fall outside my remit. In this chapter I shall deal only with those circumstances where man impacts directly on the welfare of individual wild animals. This occurs when he confines them in zoos, works them in circuses, but mostly it occurs when he chooses to kill them.

Given the shortage of good experimental studies on the welfare of wild animals I have no option but to work from first principles. The welfare of any sentient animal is, I repeat, defined by how it feels at the time and by its ability to sustain fitness. How it feels is determined by the impact of environmental factors, such as the presence of food and water, heat and cold, friends and foes, on its internal state. Some features of internal state, such as metabolic hunger and oestrus, are primitive and similar in all sentient species. Other drives and moods, such as anxiety and the hunting instinct are more specific to the species and the individual, being determined both by genotype and experience. Thus, while there are clear differences in motivation and behaviour between the wild wolf and the domestic dog, these are essentially differences of degree. Both species operate according to similar basic rules.

It is man who classifies animals first as wild or domestic and then further subdivides wild animals into protected species, game and vermin. The first classification into wild and domestic has some parallel with the way the animals themselves view the world. Wild animals are more strongly motivated than domestic animals to fend for themselves, although this species-specific drive, in both categories, can be profoundly modified by experience. Wolves can become quite tame and dogs can become extremely feral. The second classification of wild animals into game and vermin would be incomprehensible to the species so defined. Game defines animals where man elects to kill individuals (the word game implies for fun) but preserve the

216

habitat and the species; vermin defines a species which we try, if possible, to exterminate by killing the animals directly and/or by destroying their habitat.

Since the expression 'wild' has no absolute meaning when viewed from the point of view of the animal I shall not attempt to define it in biological terms. Instead, I shall use it, arbitrarily, to describe any species of animal that normally seeks to sustain itself and its descendants without assistance from man, whom it views as a competitor or, more likely, a predator – in brief, one who, by circumstances and by choice, leaves *us* well alone. When we elected to domesticate and exploit animals for our own advantage, whether for food, for company or for reasons of science, then we took upon ourselves responsibility for their welfare. This was only fair. However, whenever we do not actually *need* a species of animal I suggest we should try, wherever possible, to stay out of their lives. This, too, is fair.

Unfortunately for us, it is not that simple. The grander the strategic aim (or moral principle), the more difficult it is to reconcile with the necessity to make tactical decisions on the spur of the moment. Albert Schweitzer had the grandest of moral principles. He based his doctrine of reverence for life on the premise that all animals have a 'will-to-life' but only man recognizes the moral problem of killing because only man can recognize the will-to-life in others. In *My Life and Thoughts* he writes:

> 'To the man who is truly ethical all life is sacred, including that which from the human point of view seems lower in the scale. [Man] makes distinctions only as each case comes before him, and under the pressure of necessity; as, for example,when it falls to him to decide which of two lives he must sacrifice in order to preserve the other.
>
> I buy from natives a young fish-eagle which they have caught on a sand bank in order to rescue it from their cruel hands. But now I have to decide whether I will let it starve, or kill every day a number of small fishes, in order to keep it alive. I decide on the latter course, but every day I feel it hard that this life must be sacrificed for the other on my responsibility.'

The tale of the fish-eagle is instructive for several reasons. First, Schweitzer has disrupted the balance of nature in the wild by electing to own a young carnivore. The fish-eagle is, by my definition, no longer truly wild since it is now his responsibility. Having acted to save this fish-eagle in accordance with his 'truly ethical' principle of reverence for life, he now has to make a tactical decision. He has three options:

(1) to set the young bird free;
(2) to hand-rear the bird by catching and killing many fish;
(3) to kill the bird humanely to spare it from further suffering.

He rejects option 1 on strictly pragmatic grounds. He thinks the bird is too young to fend for itself so will die slowly of starvation or more quickly in the jaws of another predator. He elects, with regret, for option 2 which will involve the killing of many fish. He gives no indication that he ever considered option 3, which involves killing one animal humanely to save it from further suffering. He has, apparently without considering all the options, accommodated within his general principle of reverence for all life the conclusion that the life of one sea-eagle is more valuable than the collective lives of an unspecified (but large) number of fish. Was it because he believed the bird to be more sentient or simply more beautiful? The final message which can be drawn from this tale is that if man, in the form of 'the natives' had not captured the fish-eagle in the first place, neither Schweitzer, nor the fish-eagle would have had a problem. The fish, in either event, would have continued to eat and be eaten.

I have, throughout this book, studiously considered moral arguments relating to animal welfare but, equally studiously, tried to avoid getting bogged down by them. I accept, absolutely, Schweitzer's maxim that 'man should extend the circle of his compassion to all living things', but I have no more intention of debating how many dead fish are morally justified by the life of one fish-eagle than I would debate how many angels can fit on the head of a pin. The practical application of compassion for animal life, especially wildlife, must be based on a robust acceptance of the inevitability of suffering and death (which is the end of suffering). Whenever we intervene in the balance of nature in the wild, and it is almost impossible not to intervene, we adjust the pattern of suffering and death, leaving some winners and some losers. The winners are usually those species that are becoming very rare, because they are ill-adapted to the environment we have left for them, dramatically beautiful, or merely cuddly. The Giant Panda, symbol of WWF, the Worldwide Fund for Nature, fulfils all three criteria. It is singularly inept at survival but, fortunately for the Panda, it is our sort of animal.

Although my basic premise is that, wherever possible, we should leave wild animals well, alone, I must consider the welfare implications of man using wild animals for his own devices, whether we elect to kill them by hunting or fishing, or to keep them as living displays in zoos, circuses and game parks. The rules will include, as always, the moral aim to minimize suffering in the live animal, and the pragmatic principle that the welfare of any individual animal or species is likely to increase in direct proportion to its value to man.

Hunting and shooting

Man hunts and kills wild animals in order to eat their meat, wear their hides, make money, remove their competition with himself, regulate their numbers to preserve their habitat, or merely as an enjoyable way of passing the time. Most people who kill wild animals can cite more than one of the above reasons to justify their actions. Thus, the manager of a deer estate in the Scottish Highlands will justify stalking on the grounds that it maintains the health and vigour of the stock by preventing overpopulation, it produces highly prized meat, it gives some people great pleasure and those people pay for their pleasure by bringing wealth and employment to the locality. The Master of Foxhounds, if he feels the need to justify his 'sport' at all, will usually base his argument on the premises that fox numbers need to be controlled and that the hunting fraternity have, in fact, preserved the fox population by ensuring that their farms retained sufficient natural cover.

My brief is not to argue the morality of man's justification for killing wild animals, still less the morality of killing for pleasure, since these conceits are of no direct concern to the animals involved. My brief is to consider the impact of hunting and shooting on the welfare of wild animals, as individuals and as populations. This will be determined by the following:

(1)   the habitat and quality of life when undisturbed by man;
(2)   fear and stress during the hunt;
(3)   pain and distress associated with the intended act of killing.

The huntsman's argument that his fraternity has preserved the fox is valid. If the English country gentleman had not taken such pleasure in hunting during the centuries when his compassion for living things extended no further than his best friends, his horses and hounds, then the fox would have been exterminated from managed farmlands by bullet, poison or destruction of habitat long before it discovered that it could adapt to a new form of co-existence with mankind in the humane suburbs. Whether hunting is still necessary to preserve the fox in these gentler times is a moot point but it is fair to argue that it has conferred some benefits on the fox population of the UK, which has been allowed to live free in a habitat to which it is well adapted. Against this, we must set the cost to the fox of fear and stress during the hunt, whether successful or not and, if successful, the pain and distress associated with the act of killing.

Stalking of stags and deer on the Scottish Highlands appears, at first sight, to present no welfare problems at all, since the intention is to get in position for a killing shot without the animal being more than remotely aware of the presence of the hunter. Assuming the animal is killed cleanly, if not by the hunter-punter then by the ghillie, the whole system would seem to be a most humane way of obtaining meat from sentient animals since each animal is allowed to roam free in a natural habitat until, in an instant, it is rendered non-existent without any of the stresses involved in handling, transport and stunning in the abattoir.

As usual, the welfare argument is not that simple. Highland deer may enjoy a great deal of freedom but, unlike the fox, they are not in their natural habitat. Red deer evolved in Northern woodlands where winter temperatures can be as cold as, or colder than in the Scottish highlands, but there is far better shelter from the chilling effects of wind, rain and snow and usually a better supply of winter food. Death rates from a combination of cold stress and starvation can exceed 50% in deer calves during their first winter on the Scottish hills. A more intensive form of ranching deer that involved some element of shelter and supplementary feeding for the young stock would lead to a net improvement in welfare according to the McInerney principles illustrated in Fig. 7.1, especially if the deer were still shot efficiently while on open range. In the real world, of course, those who pay big money to stalk deer might decide that these better-managed animals had become too tame, were no longer 'good sport' and pay less or go elsewhere, thereby reducing the value of the animals and driving their quality of life back down towards the Malthusian end of the McInerney curve. Nevertheless, I cannot raise a single objection, in principle, to a system of wildlife management that allows the animals to control the quality of their own existence and thereby sustain physical fitness right up to the moment of sudden, unexpected death.

On a rather more mundane level but for the same reasons, I believe there are few welfare objections to the semi-natural rearing of gamebirds such as pheasant to be shot for the table. I do not shoot pheasant myself. However, I will eat shot pheasant with great pleasure whereas I do not eat the heavy strains of broiler chicken. This is because the game pheasant has been permitted by man to enjoy a reasonably natural, free-living but well-fed existence, whereas too many broiler chickens have been condemned by man to spend the last third of their lives in pain. Pheasant rearing is able to achieve the moral aim to minimize suffering in the live animal only because the value of each bird has been greatly elevated by the fact that grown men are prepared to spend good money to shoot them out of the sky. Take away the sport and table pheasants would be reared like broiler chickens.

According to my first criterion of good welfare, habitat and quality of life when undisturbed by man, many wild animals fare better than many farm animals. The distinction is not absolute. It depends how their quality of life rates on the McInerney curve (Fig. 7.1). Sheep housed over winter will fare better than deer left out to starve. Pheasants reared in woodland will fare *much* better than broiler chickens.

The second, most contentious welfare issue is that of fear and stress during the hunt itself, especially the hunting with hounds of foxes and deer. The hunted animal will certainly experience acute fear and may suffer from exhaustion during the chase. Unpleasant memories of previous hunts may also induce a chronic sense of anxiety. On the other hand hunters will argue that it is natural for a wild animal to be hunted. Wild ruminants on the African plains are exposed to predators every day. The red deer will make no distinction between being hunted by hounds (with man in somewhat irrelevant pursuit) or by a pack of wolves. These analogies need to be examined with care. The antelope or gazelle on the African plain almost certainly does not live in constant terror of the lion or leopard. Moving in herds, they observe their predators carefully and try to ensure that they keep at a safe flight distance. They do not appear to be distressed if another, unrelated member of the herd is chased. If they are chased themselves they take off at speed and, on all occasions but the last, escape within a matter of seconds or minutes at the most. They learn that if they take appropriate action they can resolve the problem of acute fear (Fig. 6.1). In the presence of predators, therefore, they may well feel alert but not anxious, rather in the manner of an experienced city dweller setting out to cross a busy road.

If men hunted deer the way that leopards hunt gazelles then the element of enforced suffering, and therefore (in our case) deliberate cruelty, would be small. Unfortunately they don't. The leopard identifies the easiest animal to catch and hunts it down as quickly as possible and with minimum expenditure of energy. If its first choice of prey escapes it will seek another. Hunting deer with hounds is, however, akin to the method used in the wild by African hunting dogs or a wolf pack. The hunt tends to isolate a stag or hind and hunt it 'for up to five hours ... until cramp and exhaustion prevent it from running further' (to quote a motion to ban deer hunting on National Trust property) or (to quote a hunter) 'give it a good run until it is starting to get dark or getting on for opening time' before going in for the kill. The selected stag discovers that its natural talent for evading predators fails so the stress of fear is prolonged and progressively compounded by an increasing state of exhaustion. The prolonged chase of an individual deer is usually unnecessary and will undoubtedly cause the animal to suffer. It is therefore unnecessary cruelty, and if the deer were a domestic animal it would be criminal. As I write, the National Trust are agonizing once again as to whether they should permit deerhunting on their property. This involves setting up a working party to ascertain whether it is cruel. Of course it is cruel! The committee may decide that this degree of cruelty is justified for sociological and ecological reasons, including preservation of the value and therefore the continued existence of red deer on areas such as Exmoor. They may also argue that on balance the life of the deer is far better than that of, say, the veal calf. They cannot, however, wash their hands of the offence of cruelty. The question I would address to any member of a deerhunt who argues that it is not cruel to pursue and kill a large sentient herbivore, is 'Would you do it to a horse?' Somewhat after the fashion of Jonathan Swift's 'modest' (satirical) proposal for preventing the children of Ireland from being a burden to their parents or country, namely 'that a young healthy child well nursed is at a year old, a most delicious, nourishing and wholesome food' may I suggest that the deerhunt on Exmoor might preserve the quality of the moor better if they were to hunt and kill deer and ponies on alternate weeks within (of course) the proper season?

Hunting of the fox with hounds involves elements of cruelty which are identical to hunting of the deer. The Protection of Animals Act (1911) makes it a criminal offence to 'ill-treat, over-ride, torture, infuriate or terrify' a horse or dog. Some may argue (without strong evidence one way or the other) that a horse may be more sentient and have an increased capacity to suffer than a red deer. However, the genetic similarity between the dog and the fox is so close that we must assume that they have a similar capacity to suffer fear, pain and exhaustion. It is thus no more nor less cruel to hunt a fox than it would be to hunt a dog.

The third problem with hunting and shooting concerns pain and distress associated with the intended act of killing. The law requires that when domestic animals are killed 'they should be slaughtered instantaneously or rendered instantaneously insensitive to pain until death supervenes'. I have argued in Chapter 5 that the law might be redrafted to read 'at the place of slaughter animals must be handled, rendered unconscious and killed in such a way as to minimize pain and suffering' since I believe that this would encourage the development of new systems designed to minimize all the stresses experienced by these animals in the last hours, not just the last seconds of life. The same principle should apply to the intended act of killing wild animals whether by hunting, shooting, trapping, gassing or poisoning. The word 'intended' is included because, in the wild, the intention to kill (e.g. by shooting) does not always succeed and injured animals may be left to suffer from the chronic, increasing pain of untreated wounds. One of the valid arguments in favour of hunting with hounds is that the quarry either escapes unharmed or the kill is guaranteed. The same will nearly always be the case when stags are shot on the treeless Highlands of Scotland. When there is plenty of cover, the shooter cannot guarantee a clean kill, although retriever dogs will usually pick up badly injured birds. Sometimes birds are picked up one or two days after they were shot because they have, by this time, become crippled and easy to catch. These birds have undoubtedly suffered, although probably no more, and for a shorter period of time than the crippled broiler fowl.

In the matter of hunting and shooting, like most other complex issues relating to the impact of man's actions on the welfare of other animals, I shall not (to the despair of some) propound any absolutist statements of what is right and what is wrong. My intention, as always, is to advocate the case for the animal and leave it to individuals to weigh that case against their own interests, I hope in a moral sense. My belief (which I cannot expect everyone to share) is that the killing of wild animals should only be done as a matter of necessity, e.g. to preserve their habitat or to prevent the spread of disease. When it is necessary to kill an animal the method should be that which is likely to cause the least suffering, by ensuring that the duration of distress prior to the point of killing is as short as possible and/or by ensuring a clean kill. By these criteria deer-stalking is humane, hunting with hounds is cruel.

Fishing and whaling

Commercial fishing involves harvesting wild animals from the sea, usually with nets, or farming fish such as trout and salmon in fresh water ponds and sealochs respectively. The necessary killing of these animals is, for sound commercial reasons, done by the most efficient possible method. When fish are netted from the sea in large numbers, there is no real alternative but to leave them in air to die from asphyxiation. A variety of more or less humane slaughter techniques has been developed for farmed salmon and trout. Current practices include:

(1)   electrocution;
(2)   mechanical stunning;
(3)   stunning with carbon dioxide gas in water;
(4)   exsanguination without prior stunning;
(5)   asphyxiation in air.

Techniques 1–4 are used for salmon; 1,4 and 5 for trout. Electrocution and mechanical stunning with a club (or 'priest') both achieve 'instantaneous insensibility to pain'. Stunning with carbon dioxide in water causes loss of consciousness after about two to four minutes but there is an initial period of hyperactivity lasting perhaps 30 seconds. The alternative is to cut the blood vessels deep in the gills, return the fish to a tank and allow them to swim around until they lose consciousness. The time taken to lose consciousness is about twice as long as when carbon dioxide is used but there is no period of hyperactivity. It is not possible to conclude, on the basis of current evidence, which of methods 3 and 4 is better. Neither method achieves the aim of inducing instantaneous killing or insensibility to pain. When fish are netted from the sea or farmed trout are removed from ponds and left to asphyxiate, the time to loss of consciousness is much the same as when they are bled out (three to four minutes).

More serious welfare issues arise in relation to 'sport' fishing with hook and line, partly because this practice can seldom be justified on grounds of necessity and partly because we cannot, in all honesty, dismiss the possibility that it might cause both fear and pain. A Committee chaired by Lord Medway (1976–9) and sponsored by RSPCA investigated welfare aspects of shooting and angling. There was, at the time little scientific evidence to work on. Anecdotal evidence was of the following type:

'I do not believe that salmon or any other fish feel very acutely, a reassuring theory for the tender-hearted fisherman. The desperate struggle of the fish to get free confirms the same view. Not all the instinct of self-preservation would induce a man to put a strain of even a pound on a fishing-rod if the hook was attached to some tender part of his flesh.' (Gathorne-Hardy, 1898: *The Salmon*)

This argument has interesting strengths and weaknesses. If the instinct to self-preservation will persuade a salmon to exert all its considerable strength to pull away from the hook in its mouth then one might reasonably conclude that the problem of pain is not paramount. If this action is entirely instinctive then the distress may also be slight. However, if the fish is, in the words of Gathorne-Hardy, 'desperate' then it may be in a conscious state of acute fear.

The Medway Committee concluded, largely on the basis of neuro-anatomical evidence, that fish probably do feel pain. They also expressed concern for fish that may be returned to the water after injury, not so much to their mouths but to their flanks after handling and restraint in keep-nets. Their recommendations include the following:

(1) Every angler should review his appreciation of the sport in the light of evidence presented on the perception of pain.
(2) Hooks and keep-nets should be designed to cause as little injury as possible.
(3) Prolonged 'playing' of fish is deprecated, particularly for those fish destined to be returned to the water.
(4) The use of vertebrates as live bait should be banned.

In more recent years Verheijen and his colleagues at the University of Utrecht have carried out elegant experiments (with the most humane of intentions) to discover whether freshwater fish (mainly carp) experience sensations similar to pain and fear when hooked and captured. The experiments involved either (i) hooking alone, (ii) hooking and 'playing' (applying tension to the line), (iii) electrical stimulation by telemetry of the mouth of free-swimming fish, (iv) triggering alarm responses by release of pheromones from damaged skin. A variety of behavioural and physiological stimuli were used to indicate alarm or stress. Fish responded rather similarly to all stimuli, hooking, electric shocks to the mouth and the presence of alarm pheromones. When the hook was left in the mouth, but there was no tension on the line, the alarm responses diminished. When the line was pulled and the fish sensed that it was captured, the alarm response was greatest. The results of these experiments make it impossible to avoid the conclusion that hooked fish experience sensations for which we have no better words than fear and pain. Any angler who, in the light of this evidence, argues otherwise is guilty of wishful thinking.

Most debates concerning the slaughter of whales concentrate on their high degree of sentience, and therefore capacity to suffer, and on the need to preserve them from extinction. These important arguments are, however, outside the scope of this book. My concern is how well, or badly, killing methods rate against the ideal of achieving instantaneous death or insensitivity to pain until death supervenes. Kestin (1995) has reviewed the efficiency of killing methods used by Norwegian whalers in the period 1992–3. These whales were initially struck with a grenade-headed harpoon. Approximately half (394/811) were killed 'instantaneously' (within 10 seconds). Over 90% were dead within 10 minutes but a few survived as long as 50 minutes. These figures are better than previously recorded during commercial whaling in 1984–6 when 16% were still alive 15 minutes after first strike. Moreover, they do not take into account any element of fear and exhaustion which the whale may (or may not) suffer during the chase which may take up to an hour. The humanitarian and ecological arguments in favour of saving the whale are very strong. All I wish to point out here is that modern, ruthlessly efficient commercial methods for killing whales submit the animals to a far shorter period of fear and stress than that involved in most forms of 'sport killing' whether with hounds or with rod and line.

Wildlife parks, zoos and circuses

The welfare of wild animals confined in zoos or parks, or confined and exploited in circuses may be assessed using the cool logic of the five freedoms, modulated slightly by the rather fuzzier concept that wild species are more highly motivated than domestic species to make an active contribution to the quality of their own existence so may be more inclined to appreciate the 'sixth freedom', the freedom to be free.

I prefaced Chapter 8, on the intensive farming of pigs and poultry, with a quotation from *Animals and Ethics* (Carpenter, 1980). 'Diligent human care for the welfare of such animals as are confined in a few advanced zoological parks can act as a touchstone for the welfare standards of these managed animals.' This comment recognizes that the owners of the best zoos and wildlife parks can demonstrate with pride that they are keeping their animals healthy and in an attractive, enriched environment. There are, of course, still some zoos in Europe where it is possible to isolate a sick lion in a barren cage and (to quote a recent television programme) 'make people pay money to watch it die', but most good zoos can achieve the first three freedoms. Their animals are well-fed, comfortable and healthy.

The main welfare problems for animals in well-kept zoos are likely to be psychological. These include:

(1) boredom and frustration, because they are prevented from acting upon strongly motivated patterns of active behaviour such as hunting and exploration;
(2) anxiety, because they are prevented from carrying out strongly motivated patterns of passive behaviour such as hiding, especially the hiding of offspring.

The aim of any good owner of a zoological garden or wildlife park is, of course, to make the physical and social environment for the species as natural as possible. However, except in the most extensive of wildlife reserves which are, in effect, preserved areas of wilderness, he cannot permit his predators to hunt and his prey species to get killed, nor can he allow his animals so much natural cover that they cannot be seen by the fee-paying customers.

Species as diverse as hunting carnivores, lions and tigers, and fruit-eating monkeys, marmosets and tamarins, may experience frustration of their motivation to gather food even though they are fed a ration that meets their nutrient requirements. Much can be done to encourage primates to pass the time in a pleasantly rewarding fashion by working for food. I can see no way of satisfying the motivation of large carnivores to hunt within the environment of a zoo. However, I am satisfied, in the absence of any scientific evidence to the contrary, that lions – for example, in well-managed wildlife parks within the UK – have, on balance, as good a life style as they could get anywhere.

Of greater concern is the problem of anxiety in higher animals, especially primates confined in small, barren enclosures in constant sight of man. There is good scientific evidence that small, vulnerable monkeys like marmosets and tamarins protect themselves in the wild by operating in family groups where most of the family stay under cover and a few, usually young males, take it in turns to act as lookouts. Experience with these species in research laboratories has shown that if they are kept in small cages without hiding places they display extreme signs of anxiety when humans approach within their flight distance because they have neither a hiding place nor an escape route. There is also good circumstantial evidence that tamarins in these circumstances are highly prone to develop stress-related diseases like ulceration and cancers of the colon. One cannot, in a commercial zoo, create an environment in which the animals stay semi-permanently out of sight of man. It is, however, possible, by use of natural or artificial materials, to create the partial cover that these animals enjoy within the forest canopy. In such an environment, in family groups and with sentinels on watch, these instinctively timid creatures appear to be able to live without anxiety, or, at least, anxiety-related disorders like ulcerative colitis. The compassionate visitor to the zoo is also more likely to be impressed by glimpses of monkeys behaving naturally within a reasonable simulation of their natural habitat than shrieking with fear at the back of a small, barren cage.

I wish, finally, to say something about the impact on wild animals of man's desire to communicate with them in more intimate fashion, whether to exploit them for commercial gain like an elephant in a circus or to express a sense of love for a wild and beautiful creature such as a tiger in a private zoo. The welfare implications of training animals to perform 'unnatural' acts needs to be assessed according to:

(1) the natural affinity of the species with man;
(2) the extent to which the training can be achieved by reward and without inducing a chronic sense of anxiety;
(3) the quality of life for the circus animal when not 'working'.

It is, for example, entirely reasonable to argue that dogs can be trained entirely by reward to perform circus tricks since they can be motivated entirely by the wish to give pleasure to their owners. Species such as horses, elephants and seals can be trained by a fairly benign application of the principle of carrot and stick. With the large cats, training must be based on the principle of absolute dominance and submission. Nevertheless, Marthe Kiley-Worthington, who has a powerful but rational concern for animal welfare, rather surprised her sponsors, the RSPCA, when she was commissioned to consider the welfare of circus animals and concluded that for many species life in a circus was probably better than that in a poor zoo, because the element of fear involved in training and performance was small and the animals had less time to get bored.

It is said that God made pussycats because it is too dangerous to stroke tigers. I can sympathize with the human who wishes to establish an emotional bond with a wild animal but it is not, I believe, a sensible endeavour. Leaving aside the obvious risks that one might get hurt, there is no reason to suppose that any wild animal, other than some higher primates, will actually return this affection. They will derive physical gratification from easy access to food and some sensuous grooming behaviour, but this can be explained entirely in terms of self-interest. (This argument applies to most domesticated animals as well.) Moreover, it is seldom, if ever, in the welfare interests of a truly wild animal to be seduced into an increased sense of dependence on man, even if, as in the case of chimpanzees or gorillas, this may involve a real sense of empathy. In the natural environment where the rule is survival of the fittest, it is, I repeat, best to leave well, alone.

12   Animals and Science

'It must be received as an axiom that a given experiment should be instituted with the least possible infliction of suffering... Pursued in this manner, the science of physiology will be rescued from the charges of cruelty and will be regarded ... as an essential branch of knowledge.'

Marshall Hall (1831)

This chapter, above all others, calls for a cool head. I must now consider the welfare of animals used by man for 'scientific procedures,' a catch-all phrase which includes:

(1) scientific experiments with living animals designed to advance knowledge;
(2) technical laboratory procedures with animals carried out not to increase knowledge but to ensure safety or meet legal requirements;
(3) biotechnological manipulation of animals in order to increase their value to man.

As always, I shall leave most of the moral arguments to others (for a good mix of both sides of the debate try Linzey,1976; Medawar, 1972; Paton, 1993; Ryder, 1975; Singer, 1990; Smith & Boyd, 1991). My remit is to view these procedures from the point of view of the animals, whose perception of their own welfare is uncomplicated by any concept of the purpose or justification of the things that are being done to them. For most laboratory animals, most of the time, life is similar to that of the intensively housed farm animal. Both are likely to be properly fed but stocked densely in thermally comfortable but barren environments and killed by approved methods to yield a commodity for man, be it liver cells for a diagnostic test or meat for a dinner. The quality of life for these animals is determined mainly by their physical and social environment. Anyone who can justify rearing and killing animals for food cannot reject the principle that it is, at the very least, equally acceptable to rear and kill animals in similar ways to improve understanding or reduce the ravages of disease.

By the same logic, pigs that have been genetically engineered to supply hearts and kidneys that will not be rejected after transplantation into human patients are likely to experience a quality of life at least as good as, and probably rather better than that of the commercial pig on the factory farm. Once again, the animal's perception of its welfare is unaffected by its ultimate fate. Spare parts or sausages, it's all the same to the pig.

Some laboratory animals will, however, be exposed to experimental procedures which, without mincing words, can only be described as legalized cruelty or the deliberate imposition of 'necessary suffering'. This may only involve a small proportion of all animals bred for scientific purposes but it poses the most difficult and searching examples of the utilitarian dilemma. 'Does the benefit to society justify the cost to the animal?'

When addressing welfare issues relating to the use of animals in science it is more important than ever to avoid sweeping generalizations leading to blanket condemnation or blanket approval. Many experiments with animals involve no cruelty at all but some do. The animal rights campaigner who condemns as cruel all scientific experiments with animals is self-deluded, dishonest or simply wrong. However, any scientist who attempts to argue that experiments with animals never involve an element of deliberate cruelty would be equally self-deluded or dishonest. A cruel procedure does not have to involve any element of malice. The scientist who performs an experiment that causes pain may be, and probably is, an extremely compassionate individual but the animal does not know that. It is simply aware that it has been made to suffer.

'Scientific procedures' and 'cruelty to animals'

In the UK the use of animals in science is controlled by the Home Office acting under the authority of The Animals (Scientific Procedures) Act 1986. This Act is designed to protect 'any living vertebrate' used in scientific procedures. It achieves this in part by laying down rules and guidelines for breeding, housing and husbandry of laboratory animals and by enforcing provisions for day-to-day animal care and veterinary supervision of health and welfare. In this regard, it confers better protection for animals in laboratories than on the farm. It also regulates (i.e. permits in special circumstances) 'any experimental or other scientific procedure applied to a protected animal which may have the effect of causing that animal pain, suffering, distress or lasting harm'. The Act requires that the pain, suffering, distress or lasting harm that may result from any procedure must be justified by 'the benefit likely to accrue' such as the prevention, diagnosis or treatment of disease in man or animals, protection of the natural environment, or the advancement of knowledge in the biological or behavioural sciences.

So far as the laboratory animal is concerned, the phrase 'scientific procedures' as used in the Animals (Scientific Procedures) Act 1986 (hereafter ASPA) and the word 'vivisection', as used by the British Union for Abolition of Vivisection (BUAV) have the same meaning – i.e. something done to me (the animal) by man for reasons which are inexplicable (to me the animal) but whose effect has been to cause me pain, suffering, distress or lasting harm. Clearly both definitions have been chosen less for their accuracy in describing what happens to the animal than for their emotional impact on man; the former to sedate and the latter to inflame. The word vivisection implies unjustly that all scientific experiments with animals involve cutting them up while alive. On the other hand, the phrase 'scientific procedures' as used in ASPA (1986) discreetly avoids drawing attention to the fact that the prime purpose of the Act is to define the limits of deliberate cruelty in terms of the cost to the animal relative to the potential benefit to society.

The predecessor to ASPA, the Cruelty to Animals Act 1876 was more robustly phrased. The title acknowledged that the act licensed certain individuals to be cruel to animals. Mincing its words only a little, it 'did not disallow' specified acts 'calculated to cause pain' when performed by licensed persons for approved scientific purposes. In practice, the Cruelty to Animals Act 1876 did afford a reasonable degree of protection to laboratory animals in keeping with the early expression of honourable intent by Marshall Hall (1831) from whom I quote for the heading to this chapter. However, ASPA (1986), despite its somewhat misleading title, is superior to its predecessor in four main ways:

(1) It assumes that there is more to cruelty than pain alone and expands the definition to include 'pain, suffering, distress or lasting harm'.
(2) It submits every application to carry out a scientific procedure with laboratory animals to a cost:benefit analysis to determine whether the cost to the animal, however slight, can be justified in terms of the potential benefit to mankind or, of course, other animals.
(3) It recognizes that the welfare of animals used in science is not simply determined by the experimental procedures to which it is subjected but also by the quality of its environment, and so pays particular attention to day-to-day care.
(4) It gives final authority for animal welfare to a named veterinary surgeon who is *not* the holder of the Project Licence to carry out the experiments. Thus the named veterinary surgeon who feels that an animal has suffered enough can override the wishes of a research worker who feels that his scientific objectives have not yet been met.

Implementation of the detailed rules and recommendations in ASPA (1986) has done a lot to improve the quality of life for laboratory animals and to reduce the number and severity of procedures likely to cause pain, suffering, distress or lasting harm. I am, however, still troubled by the implications of the title 'scientific procedures'. It has not achieved its political obective since it has done little to improve the image of the scientist in the eyes of the animal rights lobby. More seriously, it may be compromising the welfare of some laboratory animals by failing to hammer home the message that the act is still, like its predecessor, primarily concerned with controlling the deliberate infliction of suffering. Any scientist contemplating experiments with animals that involve pain, suffering, distress or lasting harm, must, like the hunter or the fisherman, face the fact that what he is doing is cruel. He may be able to justify the cruelty of his planned actions on utilitarian grounds but he cannot, on the basis of overwhelming evidence, pretend that the consequences of his cruelty, as perceived by the animals, do not exist. There is a cost to the animals and he has a moral obligation to reduce that cost. The axiom must be that prescribed by Marshall Hall, '*to ensure the least possible infliction of suffering*'. The routes to right action are the three Rs, *refinement, reduction and replacement* (a phrase originally coined by Russell & Burch, 1959).

Table 12.1 lists the numbers of animals used in 1992 for 'scientific procedures' within the meaning of ASPA (1986), i.e. procedures which *may* have the effect of causing pain, suffering, distress or lasting harm. Such procedures are ranked *a priori* as of mild, moderate or substantial severity. Most mild procedures can be very mild indeed, such as the collection of a single sample of blood from a superficial vein and many animals included in this list did not, in the event, suffer at all from the direct effects of the experiment. They may, for example, have been individuals serving as controls in a drug trial and injected only with physiological saline. Table 12.1 therefore exaggerates the number of animals that were actually made to suffer. However, it does not include animals used for scientific purposes that involved no risk of deliberate cruelty. Animals are classified according to the primary purpose of each 'scientific procedure'. Category 1 consists of true scientific procedures subdivided into fundamental and applied studies. Fundamental studies include physiological and psychological experiments intended to discover the workings of the animal body and mind, and medical experiments designed to improve our ability to diagnose, prevent and cure disease. These constitute nearly half of all procedures (47.1%). Applied scientific procedures include

Table 12.1 Numbers of animals used for scientific and technical procedures in 1992. (Source: Universities Federation for Animal Welfare.)

Primary purpose of procedure	Number	0%
Scientific		
Fundamental science: body function and disease studies	1 378 820	47.1
Applied science: e.g. development of drugs and other treatments	627 383	21.4
TOTAL: scientific studies	2 006 203	68.5
Technical		
Production: antibodies and other biologicals	416 127	14.2
Safety testing: toxicology, pollutants, food additives, cosmetics	258 602	8.8
Diagnostic tests	21 942	0.75
Development of surgical methods	15 028	0.5
Education	9 173	0.3
Other: e.g. forensic enquiries, ecological studies	23 187	0.8
TOTAL: technical studies	744 059	25.4
Breeding: harmful genetic defects, transgenics	177 996	6.1
TOTAL: all procedures	2 928 258	100

research, development and testing of potential new drugs for man and animals. These procedures are justified by the attempt to improve knowledge and understanding. Inevitably some will succeed better than others. A very small proportion of all experiments will lead to massive improvements in our ability to control and ultimately cure a disease like diabetes. The gains from most experiments will be very modest and some, for a variety of reasons, will be useless. One cannot guarantee the success of an experiment in advance. If that were the case it would not be worth doing.

Category 2, 'Technical', includes toxicity tests including the infamous LD_{50} and Draize tests, the former measuring the toxicity of a test substance according to the dose that kills 50% of treated animals, the latter being, for many years, the standard test for ophthalmic irritancy of, for example, a new shampoo. These are not scientific procedures (except in a legal sense) but technical procedures deemed necessary in law to protect the public from exposure to untested and potentially dangerous new products. Category 3 includes biotechnological manipulations such as hormone injections to increase the productivity of farm animals and genetic engineering of animals to produce high value products such as pharmaceuticals or organs for transplantation.

Table 12.2 lists the number of animals used in scientific procedures in Britain during 1992 according to species. Total numbers at first sight appear very large, just under 3 million. This number compares with totals in excess of 5 million throughout the 1970s. We are witnessing success in the application of two of the three Rs, namely *reduction* and *replacement*. The reduction reflects in part a reduction in expenditure on scientific research but can be attributed mainly to positive steps taken by the scientific community

Table 12.2 Species of animals used in scientific procedures in 1992. (Source: Universities Federation for Animal Welfare.)

Species	Number used	%
Mice	1 448 960	49.5
Rats	833 004	28.4
Rabbits	79 450	2.7
Cats	3 692	0.1
Dogs	9 085	0.3
Ruminants	34 431	1.2
Primates	5 018	0.2
Other mammals	137 100	4.7
Birds	220 312	7.6
Reptiles/amphibians	18 955	0.6
Fish	138 251	4.7
Total	2 928 258	100

to reduce numbers and seek alternatives to the use of animals in biological experiments. Introduction of ASPA (1986) actually increased by approximately half a million the number of procedures that required a licence from the Home Office, simply by expanding the definition of a scientific procedure. The most direct comparison with reports completed under the 1876 Act reveals that the number of animals used for such procedures has been halved in the period 1972–1992.

Although we have an obligation to inflict the minimum amount of necessary suffering and one case of *unnecessary* suffering is too many, it is necessary to put these large numbers into some sort of perspective. In Chapter 7 I pointed out that the average human omnivore who maintains good appetite to the age of 70, manages to consume 550 poultry, 36 pigs, 36 sheep and 8 oxen. At present we use approximately 3 million animals per year for scientific procedures, of which about half are mice. Given a UK population of 56 million with a life expectancy of 70 years, this corresponds to less than four laboratory animals per human lifetime. For every three human lives, one animal is sacrificed to test the safety of food additives, cosmetics etc. Finally, the number of mice sacrificed to advance knowledge and so improve health and safety for every man and woman in the UK is two! This is not, perhaps, so much to ask of Brother Mouse.

Costs and benefits

The benefits of scientific procedures accrue to society (or animals) in general. The costs (in this context) are paid by individual animals who derive no personal benefit from the exercise, hence our responsibility to minimize these costs.

A Working Party set up by the Institute of Medical Ethics has defined the issues which need to be resolved by any research worker prior to undertaking a series of scientific procedures with animals (Smith and Boyd, *Lives in the Balance*, 1991). These are:

(1)   What are the likely (or possible) costs to the animal?
(2)   Is the goal worthwhile?
(3)   What is the absolute minimum number of animals necessary to achieve the goal?
(4)   Is there a less drastic approach to the same goal?
(5)   Is there a reasonable probability that the experiment will achieve its goal?

Questions 1, 3 and 4 address the nature of the cost. How much will each animal suffer? Can the number of animals who are made to suffer be reduced? Can I refine my approach to reduce or eliminate suffering, either by using a less drastic method or a less sentient animal? The latter question is not necessarily as difficult as it sounds. Paton (1993) suggests that while it would be difficult to discriminate between the sentience of a rat and a rabbit, few people would deny that a tadpole was less sentient than a chimpanzee. Questions 2 and 5 address the nature of benefit. First, is the goal (the benefit to knowledge or society) worthwhile? Second, and highly important, are the objectives and design of the experiment sufficiently well focused that it stands a reasonable possibility of achieving its goal?

Question 5 can be rephrased in rather more abrupt terms: 'Is the experiment worth doing at all?'

I believe in the power of science to improve our understanding of the world, free us from the burdens of ignorance and superstition, and improve the quality of our lives. However, nobody can go through a career in science without coming across some experiments (including some of their own) which were worthless because they were badly designed, because they did not ask the proper questions, because the solution sought was beyond the limits of resolution of the method, or because the answer to the question they put was known already. Any honest scientist would do well to begin each day with the question 'Is my experiment really necessary?' Any honourable scientist doing experiments involving the risk of pain, suffering, distress or lasting harm to his animals, would do well to ask also 'Have I the right to impose this cost?'

The five questions from *Lives in the Balance* provide an excellent structure for the formal evaluation of any application to conduct experiments with animals. In the UK the formal procedure for consideration, modification and final approval of Scientific Procedures is undertaken by the scientific project leaders in association with Home Office Inspectors responsible for the implementation of ASPA 1986. However, many scientific establishments these days also have their own procedures, such as Ethical Committees, for assessing the ethical and technical issues involved in each application before it is submitted to the Home Office. I believe that Ethical Committees can make a significant contribution to the improved welfare of animals used in science, provided that it is understood by all parties that the ethical and technical issues are inextricably linked and cannot be addressed as absolute values and in isolation. Thus the cost to the animal cannot be assessed without some non-anthropomorphic understanding of the nature of animal mind and animal suffering. The questions 'Is the experiment worthwhile?' and 'Is there a less drastic approach to the same goal?' can really only be addressed by someone with knowledge of the area of science under review. Ethical Committees therefore need

(1) scientists, mainly to consider the goals and the most cost-efficient ways of achieving them (in all senses of the word cost);

(2) the named veterinary surgeon to ensure professional care and concern for the welfare of the animals to be used in the experiment;

(3) a layperson (A.P. Herbert's 'reasonable man') who needs to be convinced that the experiments are likely to be worthwhile.

Decisions as to the proper use of animals in science must necessarily involve questions of science but that does not mean that decisions should be left to the scientists alone. The named veterinary surgeon offers laboratory animals the added protection of a competent individual who has no direct conflict of interest between his concern for animal welfare and experimental success. The scientist should also be able to justify his experiments with animals to a reasonable layperson, in exactly the same way as a farmer should be able to justify his animal husbandry. If either has difficulty in justifying his methods to a 'reasonable man' he should seriously question whether he can justify them to himself.

Assessment of costs

Table 12.3 presents examples of the ways by which animals may be made to suffer by scientific procedures. As always, it is essential to dissociate our perception of the image invoked by a particular scientific procedure from the way it is likely to be perceived by the animal that is directly involved. Consider, for example, one of the most evocative of images used by the anti-vivisection movement, the cat with its skull exposed and electrodes inserted into its brain. The image is instantly shocking to us and even if we start to think about it, it is likely to remain shocking because we identify with the cat and experience fear both at the visual image of the top of our head being removed and replaced by scientific apparatus and at the thought of a scientist controlling our minds by electricity.

The cat *may* suffer from the presence of this implant to its skull but for different reasons. Tie a handkerchief around a cat's tail and it will almost certainly try to remove it. The handerchief is clearly seen as 'not-self' and an irritant. Tie a collar round its neck and the cat may, at first, scratch at the collar, because it feels its physical presence as uncomfortable or merely

Table 12.3 Examples of the costs to animals incurred by scientific procedures.

	Severity		
	Mild	Moderate	Substantial
Hunger	Unbalanced diets		Starvation
Metabolic stress	Acute heat or cold		Swimming to exhaustion
Pain	Single injections	Recovery from surgery	Burns, fractures
Malaise	Mild infections, tumours		Fulminating infections, tumours
Acute fear		Isolation restraint	
Chronic anxiety	Prolonged isolation		Anticipated pain, exhaustion

unusual. In time, however, it will become unaware of (or unconcerned by) its existence. Implant an arrangement of plastic and stainless steel to the skull of a cat and it will, at first, certainly be aware that something is different. Like the new collar, it may try to scratch, rub or remove it, especially if it is physically uncomfortable but it is unlikely to be concerned by either the appearance of the implant or its implications. The ability to recognize oneself in the mirror as an individual appears to be restricted to man and (possibly) some of the higher primates and there is no way that a naive cat could know either that the attachment to his head made it look different or presaged experiments with its brain. The implant *could* cause the cat to suffer if

(1) it induced chronic itching, pain or infection;
(2) the cat learnt to associate subsequent manipulation of the implant with unpleasant procedures such as severe restraint, pain at the skin surface (there is no local sensation of pain or touch within the brain), or mental sensations like fear or anxiety.
(3) if, to protect the implant, the natural behaviour of the cat was severely restricted.

It is inevitable that cats with such implants will suffer to some degree from restriction of normal behaviour. However, if the implant were neither uncomfortable nor associated with unpleasant experiences, we may assume that in time it would become no more troublesome than a collar. Indeed it might reasonably be compared with a collar with a bell on it, since both, indirectly, frustrate normal behaviour (e.g. hunting).

The logic used in Table 12.3 to identify possible sources of suffering associated with scientific procedures is, of course, that of the five freedoms. An animal made to eat unbalanced diets is likely to experience a metabolic hunger for specific nutrients. The severity of this is likely, in most circumstances, to be mild. The cost to an animal of an experiment that deprived it of food altogether to study the metabolic consequences of starvation would be substantial. Many experiments involve some degree of metabolic stress. Mild examples include acute exposure of animals to tolerable intensities of heat or cold. Forcing rats to swim to exhaustion imposes a very severe cost which, in my opinion, can hardly ever be justified. When the costs are this severe, the experiment cries out for refinement. There must be a less drastic approach to the same goal.

The most obvious welfare abuse associated with scientific procedures is that of pain. This may be mild, such as that associated with a single injection of a non-toxic substance or the withdrawal of blood from a superficial vein. Experimental surgery must, of course, be performed under anaesthesia but, as I indicated in Chapter 5, moderate to severe pain can occur during recovery from surgery and maybe for some considerable time thereafter. It cannot be assumed that anaesthesia during experimental surgery eliminates the problem of pain. However, the more competent the operator in the skills of premedication, anaesthesia and analgesia, the lower the cost to the animal in terms of suffering. Anyone seeking to perform experimental surgery on animals must be educated in or exposed to the most modern approaches to humane anaesthesia.

A very few experiments, such as the deliberate induction of bone fractures or burns, involve the deliberate imposition of chronic, severe pain. It must be honourable to steel oneself to carry out a minimal number of these distressing experiments if they offer a realistic prospect of reducing the risk that a severely burned child will be disfigured for life, or die of shock because he or she cannot maintain electrolyte balance. It is not, in my opinion, acceptable to burn rats because this has, for example, interesting effects on protein turnover in muscle and skin, which might have some bearing on post-trauma oral or parenteral nutrition, since these are conclusions which could have reached by application of first principles and the design of a less drastic experiment.

In general, great care is taken to minimize suffering in experimental animals, especially in Britain since ASPA (1986). However, I continue to be angered by publications describing experiments with animals where I cannot personally accept that the end justifies the means, sometimes because the cost appears to be so high but more often because the benefit appears to be so trivial.

Deliberate induction of disease by infection or neoplasia will obviously impair welfare by creating a 'disturbance to normal health'. In most cases the animal will also suffer malaise; in simple words, it will *feel* ill. If the infection is brief and the symptoms are slight, then the degree of suffering invoked may be described as mild. If the infection or induced neoplasm is chronic or leads to a slow death associated, for example, with gastric ulceration, liver or kidney failure, then the severity is very substantial and the experimenter must, once again, seriously consider whether it is possible to achieve his objective at less cost to the animal. I discuss this issue in more detail below in relation to toxicology testing.

Perhaps the most striking of all images used in the campaign against vivisection is that of the animal in terror of the shadow of the knife. This image of the professional scientist is, of course, quite unfair since it portrays a criminal act. It does, however, personify one of the greatest real concerns relating to the welfare of animals used in scientific procedures, namely the extent to which the procedures themselves may induce acute fear or chronic anxiety. Recapitulating Fig. 6.1, I argue that acute fear is a normal (albeit unpleasant) protective mechanism that may be induced by novelty, innate threats (like a natural predator) or learned responses to an experience that has, in the past, been associated with pain, malaise or some other source of suffering. Almost any novel form of restraint and manipulation by man will arouse fear in an adult animal when first it occurs. If the animal learns that the restraint leads to no further unpleasantness or a very mild sensation such as collection of a blood sample, then the degree of fear will decline with time. Many experimental animals subjected repeatedly to mild procedures become very tame. It is important to be sure that what we interpret as increasing tameness is not, in fact, learned helplessness in an animal that has been stressed into submission. Sometimes this is not too difficult. I have, for example, worked for many years with goats, which I have used repeatedly for nutritional studies or briefly exposed to tolerable degrees of thermal stress. These animals have, over time, shown no signs whatever of increasing fear or apathy. On the contrary they have completely lost whatever sense of caution they might have had at the outset and become more outrageously (or endearingly, depending on my mood) goat-like than ever.

If, on the other hand, an experimental animal associates a repeated procedure with sensations that are painful, such as electric shocks, it is likely to become increasingly anxious with time. If an animal suffers anxiety in anticipation of a scientific procedure then the severity of that procedure will increase with time. This implies that, all other things being equal, it is crueller to repeat the same unpleasant procedure ten times on the same animal than perform it once on ten different animals. Licences to perform experiments with animals are drafted with this principle in mind.

Refinement and replacement

Viewed with the coolest of eyes and from no moral position whatever it is impossible to deny that the antivivisection movement has had a major impact on the welfare of animals used in science, far greater than anything achieved as yet by advocates of improved rights for farm animals. The prime intention may have been to frighten scientists off working with animals. The prime effect has been to force scientists to think more about what they are doing. We have two ways to deal with the problem of suffering in animals under our direct dominion. One is to shut our minds to it altogether, the second is to strive constantly to ensure that suffering is reduced to a minimum and imposed only for the most honourable of reasons. The scientist who deliberately exposes sentient animals to the risk of pain, suffering, distress or lasting harm should feel a special sense of debt to the animals that are helping him to add to knowledge, improve health and safety and, not least, advance his own career.

Science has, during the last 20 years, made great progress towards refinement and replacement of animals used for 'scientific procedures', especially those procedures used for toxicology testing. This can be attributed in part to scientific progress in the development of methods based on, for example, cell cultures rather than the use of live animals, but no scientist could stand, hand on heart and deny that the main impetus for refinement and replacement has been the pressure of public opinion. I shall offer two, very different examples of the way in which pressure of public opinion has forced scientists to adopt less drastic (and crude) approaches to a problem, and in so doing actually improve not only the welfare of the animals but also the quality of the science.

The first example is the classical, infamous LD_{50} test. In its original form this was designed to measure the acute systemic toxicity of a test substance by determining the dose required to kill 50% of a population of animals. The number of animals used per test (and per species) was 60–80 and there was no upper dose limit (see Smith and Boyd, 1991). Diligent application of this crude and cruel procedure led to some animals being forcibly dosed with ludicrously high quantities of test substance so creating conditions of distress quite unrelated to toxicology and others being left to die slowly and in increasing distress. The LD_{50} test has been progressively refined over the years. The acute systemic toxicity test currently favoured by the British Toxicology Society (1987) is a non-lethal test which only uses 10–20 animals per species and permits the animals to be humanely killed as soon clear signs of toxicity are detectable. This not only ends the suffering of the test animals as quickly as possible, it often means that the nature of the toxicity can be interpreted better from, for example, liver and kidneys showing early, toxin-specific signs of cell damage than those at an advanced stage of disintegration in an animal that has been left to die.

My second example of refinement that has led both to better welfare and better science is drawn from an area of research in which I have been directly involved, namely the study of digestive physiology in ruminant animals with a view to improving the productivity of cattle and sheep. When I first entered this field in the 1960s the standard approach to this problem was much the same as in the days when Pavlov was active (1890-1920). In order to discover what was happening to food at various stages of the digestive tract one or more permanent fistulae were made in the gut wall and cannulae inserted to sample (T-piece cannulae) or make total collections (re-entrant cannulae) of the flow of digesta. I accept that the best of the early studies could be justified by the need to discover the basic principles of digestive function. Moreover, I concede that well-managed, phlegmatic animals like sheep, with permanent cannulae seldom show signs of distress or lasting harm. Their welfare can, however, be impaired. They are usually very closely confined to protect the cannulae. Moreover continuous X-radiography of animals with re-entrant cannulae reveals that the passage of digesta is grossly abnormal because of the disruption of normal peristaltic movements. This functional indigestion may cause some degree of malaise.

These procedures are still being used today, although to a lesser extent, because they often fail to pass the cost:benefit analysis. This is not only because they involve some degree of distress, e.g. during recovery from surgery, but also because research methods based on radical, invasive surgery (real vivisection) can be counterproductive to good science. In this case

(1)   radical surgery has distorted the physical processes of digestion.
(2)   the cost of preparation and maintenance of surgically prepared animals severely restricts the rate of scientific progress (e.g. assessing the efficiency of digestion of novel or pretreated feeds).

(3)   the need to confine surgically prepared animals precludes investigation of some of the most important questions, like what happens to grazing animals when they are actually out grazing.

There was a time when physiologists could claim that they were compelled to work with experimental animals because the methods essential to advance knowledge were not acceptable for use in man. In a decreasing number of cases this argument remains true. However, in recent years a new array of non-invasive methods has been developed for the study of human function and human disease. These include high-tech., expensive methods of external scanning based on X-ray tomography, ultrasound, nuclear magnetic resonance, etc. but also cheaper methods based on good ideas and good chemistry such as the use of natural markers in foods and excreta. It is easier now, because of new technology, to avoid the use of procedures that are cruel to animals in the study of the function of man in health and disease. It is also easier to devise more refined, less drastic ways of studying the health and efficiency of animals in their own right. As refinement becomes ever easier, so our responsibility to seek refinement becomes ever greater.

It is a basic axiom of all science that all experimental procedures distort the phenomenon that one wishes to study by experiment. The moral imperative to obtain the maximum benefit to society at the least cost to the animals is therefore usually consistent with the scientific imperative to devise clear questions to resolve the ways that animals deal with important challenges to body and mind, unconfounded by experimental artefacts. The best science is usually done by those who mess their animals around the least.

Animal welfare research

Pressure of public opinion has forced governments to accept that animal welfare is itself now a proper subject for research. Moreover, the major animal welfare charities also accept that scientific research can help to achieve their aims. All this is admirable but unspecific. Problems arise when we have to decide how best to use the techniques of good science (and limited funds) to achieve the moral objective of improving animal welfare. Part II, 'An enquiry into the nature of animal mind and animal suffering', was essentially an investigation of the way that science has been used for the study and improvement of animal welfare and I shall not recapitulate the major themes (pain, fear, frustration, metabolic stress, etc.) here. The Farm Animal Welfare Council (FAWC, 1993) has produced a detailed list of priorities for research relating to the welfare of farm animals and many of these priorities can be carried over to other species.

It is difficult, however, to escape the conclusion that a lot of well-intended welfare research is neither very good science nor very helpful to the animals. Too much welfare research is flawed (in my opinion) either because it is oversimplistic or because it is not so much designed to test preconceptions as to reinforce prejudice. My particular *bête noire* is the experiment which seeks only to obtain a so-called 'objective' measure of something which the researcher preconceives to be a stress, be it a psychological stress such as confinement or a physical stress such as pain. This 'objective' measure usually is cortisol concentration in blood, but if the scientist is more ambitious or better equipped it may be a neurotransmitter in the brain or even a brain gene (e.g. c-fos) 'turned-on' by the stimulus.

Some of the most exciting new ideas in science are emerging from fundamental studies of the physics, chemistry and biology of information transfer within the brain. These studies may also lead to improved treatment of mental disorders in man. However, I am unconvinced that they will make a significant contribution to the strategic objective of improving animal welfare through application of new research.

Animal welfare research also contains too much mediocre science; e.g. derivative experiments which use measurements of cortisol, endorphins or the neurotransmitter of the month as a so-called objective index of stress (e.g. during transport). Such experiments are often guilty of two academic sins, oversimplicity and prejudice. Prejudice is evident both when the scientist uses his so-called 'objective' marker (e.g. endorphins) as evidence that his preconception was correct and when he concludes that because this particular chemical was *not* elevated by a particular stress it must have been the wrong marker. The sin of oversimplification is committed by anyone who believes that he can interpret how a conscious, sentient animal feels about the impact of a particular environmental challenge upon its current state of mind in terms of one, or even a cocktail of biologically active chemicals in blood and other bodily fluids.

This is a classic case of the 'Missing Giraffe Syndrome'. A scientist from the US space programme that landed a probe on Mars was describing on television the elaborate equipment available to test for the presence of life by collecting a soil sample and testing for any evidence of uptake or release of oxygen or carbon dioxide. Having finished his explanation, he added, with great wisdom, 'Of course, if a giraffe passes the window we shall fail to spot it'.

My approach to a question as complex as the state of mind of a conscious, sentient animal is based on the navigator's art of triangulation, i.e. one attempts to get an approximate fix on the problem or position from at least three completely different directions, thereby creating the smallest possible triangle of uncertainty. If, for example, I wished to test the hypothesis that a particular animal was distressed by acute isolation but thereafter did or did not habituate to the stimulus, I might observe the problem from the following, different, directions.

(1) behavioural responses of the animal to short and long term isolation;
(2) motivation analysis to test the extent of aversion to short and long term isolation;

(3)   physiological measurements potentially indicative of stress (e.g. corti-
        sol: I have no objection to this approach so long as it is only part of the
        story);
(4)   effects of mood-altering drugs on 1–3 above.

Such an experiment, with proper attention to controls, should, with luck,
provide a reasonable answer to the specific question, and could be used to
generate recommendations for legislation or codes of practice for the care and
protection of a particular species of farm or laboratory animal. There is
nothing inherently wrong with testing a preconception in science so long as the
problem is real, well-defined and the questions posed are both appropriate and
sufficient. In effect, this means that the good scientist should be designing
experiments not to reinforce his hypotheses but to test them to destruction.

Tinkering: biotechnology and genetic engineering

I wish to deal briefly now with the third important area of conflict between
science and animal welfare, namely the manipulation of animals by biotechnology or genetic engineering, not to advance knowledge or ensure safety
but to increase their value to man. I have discussed some aspects of this
problem in relation to conventional breeding of farm animals and pets.
Before broadening the discussion to consider all current possibilities of using
science to tinker with animals for profit I must restate (again!) one of my
constant themes, namely that the cost to an animal of a particular action of
man must be assessed in terms of its impact on the animal, not the motivation
for that action, nor the method by which it is achieved. Thus the welfare cost
to the broiler fowl of conventional breeding for rapid growth is far greater
than the cost to the dairy cow of regular treatment with the genetically
engineered growth hormone BST, although it is the latter process that has
given rise to much more public concern. The welfare of a mouse that is
genetically engineered to model a congenital disease of man or to test new
forms of cancer therapy will be defined by whether the engineered alteration
causes it any physical or mental distress on a day-to-day basis and by what
happens to it when it becomes involved in an experiment. If it is of no
concern to the mouse whether it is being used to test a new cure for cancer or
a new cosmetic it is equally of no concern to the mouse whether or not it and
its family are the subject of a patent application. The question of patenting
life forms may present us with a moral dilemma but this dilemma has nothing
to do with animal welfare.

I list below the general areas of biotechnology and genetic engineering that
may attract a commercial sponsor as offering a reasonable prospect of
adding value to an animal or its products. I use added value in the broad
sense to mean anything that improves the quality of life for us. It could be a
cheaper piece of meat from a chicken; it could be a new heart from a pig.

(1) Manipulation of animal feedstuffs to increase nutrient yield and composition.
(2) Manipulation of digestion to increase nutrient availability.
(3) Manipulation of metabolism to increase the production or alter the composition of meat, milk or fibre.
(4) Increasing the rate of reproduction in the breeding female.
(5) Artificial manipulation of breeding (genetic progress) by embryo transfer or cloning.
(6) Conferring genetic resistance to infectious disease.
(7) Manipulation of cognition by gene deletion within the central nervous system.
(8) Insertion of human genes into animals for the manufacture of pharmaceuticals.
(9) Genetic manipulation of animals to become universal donors of organs such as hearts and kidneys.

This list has been deliberately drafted not in scientific terms but in words that will appeal to the entrepeneur who has a profound disconcern for how the effects may be achieved; he is only interested in the results. In this sense the animal and the entrepreneur think the same way. The first procedure on this list, manipulation of animal feedstuffs; is unlikely (except in the most unusual circumstances) to have any direct effect on animal welfare. Procedure 2, manipulation of the digestive system, implies an alteration in the animal's physiological state and this should, at the least arouse caution. An idea that has been fashionable for some time involves engineering a cellulase enzyme into the gut of a simple-stomached animal such as the pig or chicken to enable it to digest dietary fibre in a manner similar to that of a cow or sheep. This appears at first sight to be an ecologically attractive idea since it would make these animals less competitive with man for nutrients based on cereals. The image of grazing chickens also presents no obvious abuse to animal welfare. However, this idea is fundamentally flawed since the capacity of animals to digest cellulose is not primarily constrained by the absence of cellulases (all mammals and birds normally have cellulases somewhere in their guts) but by the length of time available for cellulose digestion and this is primarily determined by the anatomy of the gut, i.e. the size of the fermentation vat in the rumen, caecum and colon. I cite this example not because it has anything directly to do with animal welfare but to make the general point that whenever new technology provokes the expression 'Gee whiz!' this should always be followed by a stern 'So what?' In most cases, 'So what?' should include the questions 'Is it sensible? Is it cruel?' and from these, 'Is it fair?'

Manipulation of the metabolism of animals in order to increase the production or alter the composition of meat, milk or fibre has the potential to cause problems. These, as defined by FAWC (1993) include 'the manipulation of body size, shape or reproductive capacity by breeding, nutrition, hormone therapy or gene insertion in such a way as to reduce mobility, increase the risk of injury, metabolic disease, skeletal or obstetric problems, perinatal mortality or psychological distress'. Once again, this statement makes it clear that the welfare implications of new technology need to be defined by their effects on the animal, not the methods used to achieve those effects. This argument does not embrace all moral considerations relating to the manipulation by science of sentient life forms but it deals with a good proportion of them.

I discussed the costs and benefits of tinkering with animal performance by BST, natural breeding, 'unnatural breeding' (e.g. multiple ovulation and embryo transfer, MOET) in Chapter 9. The principles, 'Will the animal suffer; if so, how much?' and 'Who, if anyone, will benefit; if so, how much?' can be extended to all applications of biotechnology and genetic engineering. I also repeat and extend here my suggestion that advances in animal technology, first developed under the protection of ASPA (which, of course, protects not only the animals but also the scientists) should only be licensed for commercial use subject to a cost:benefit analysis to decide whether the cost to the animal (however slight) can be justified by the likely benefit to society. I listed four main cause for concern.

(1) Pain and/or fear associated with the procedure itself or its immediate consequences.
(2) Periparturient problems associated with unconventional breeding.
(3) Physical or psychological problems demonstrable in all (or most) of the genetically modified offspring.
(4) Increased incidence of disease or disability only demonstrable by observation of relatively large populations over several generations.

A valid objection to the imposition of controls on the application of new science is that it holds up progress. This argument is only valid, of course, if the progress can be shown to be humane. The first three of the welfare problems listed above, e.g. the crippling abnormalities of bone development in the 'Beltsville' pig genetically engineered to secrete very large quantities of human growth hormone can, I believe, be resolved (one way or the other) within two generations, or the length of time required for experimentation by ASPA. The genetically engineered strain of Beltsville pigs would never have been licensed for commercial use, which implies that animals subject to tinkering by new procedures such as genetic engineering will be better protected from exploitation than the commercial broiler or pet bulldog. There remains, however, the fourth problem, namely the possible effects of tinkering on complex, low incidence conditions like mastitis and lameness in dairy cattle, which cannot be resolved without allowing the procedure to expand onto a commercial scale. I suggest, therefore, that all new technologies carried out initially under protection from ASPA should be subject to a two-stage review process. If the procedure passed according to the first three criteria, it should be given, in essence, a provisional licence for commercial exploitation, subject to a properly designed monitoring procedure for category 4 effects in practice (such as an increase in the incidence of mastitis) and reviewed after, say, five years, the costs to be met by those promoting the procedure.

The use of biotechnology to impart genetic resistance to diseases in farm animals, whether of infectious or metabolic origin, rates as a very good idea indeed on the basis of a moral cost:benefit analysis since the costs to individual animals are likely to be small and the true added value to farm animals in general (and thereby man) would be high. I would like to think that this was the way forward for farm animal biotechnology but I doubt it. We have here a classic example of the difference between lasting added value for society and short-term financial advantage for the entrepeneur. There is little, if any direct profit to be made from a single action which creates a strain of animals resistant to a particular disease for all time but much potential profit to be made from developing a drug like BST designed to be injected on a regular basis into as many animals as possible. Of course, if the genetic engineer could patent his disease-resistant strain of animal he might consider his investment to be worthwhile. I am quite sure that the healthier animal would not object; in which case neither would I.

In recent years scientists studying the genetic basis of information storage and transfer within the brain of rats have discovered that the deletion of single genes can dramatically impair their capacity to learn from experience. They will, for example, take 'sensible' evasive action if exposed to an aversive stimulus but the experience will initiate no cognitive (or even conditioned reflex) processes designed to modify their subsequent actions. According to most definitions, these rats have become less sentient. Now it is possible to develop the argument that if we elect to exploit animals for food or cause them to suffer in the interests of science then we should be morally justified if we decreased the sentience of the species that we wished to exploit on the same grounds that we should be congratulated for electing to experiment on the tadpole rather than the chimpanzee. This argument leads us into a moral minefield. If we are concerned about the quality of life experienced by farm or laboratory animals then can we overcome that problem by destroying their conception of quality? My instinct is to resist this argument but perhaps I am failing to live up to my own rational standards. I have one immediate practical concern that arises from this specific approach to reducing sentience. While it is possible that an animal that never learns from experience of pain or other aversive stimuli may fail to develop a sense of anxiety, it is equally possible that an animal which grows up in an environment in which everything is always novel would become increasingly anxious with the passage of time. Some psychological studies of humans with brain lesions that impair long-term memory suggest the latter explanation may be more likely, but it is something that could be determined by experiment.

I can think of one justification for the creation of a strain of animals that were less sentient in such a way that they clearly had less capacity to suffer. This would be for use in unavoidable scientific experiments deliberately designed to cause pain or distress, such as the Draize test for skin and eye irritancy. In all other examples I believe it would be an insult both to animal welfare and to human morality to engineer less sentient strains of animals. This is partly for the practical reason that welfare is a matter of both mind and body and sustained fitness depends on the capacity to avoid lasting physical harm by taking conscious action. I also believe that we have a moral responsibility to rear animals for food under humane conditions and lowering our standards of husbandry would therefore be a severe abuse of the concept of reverence for life. I am aware of the inconsistencies in this argument, but then, it is a moral minefield.

The final and most dramatic application of biotechnology, both in a scientific and a moral sense, has been the genetic manipulation of animals to make them more like humans. The genetic engineering of sheep and cattle to secrete human versions of the clotting Factor IX, α-1-antitrypsin or lactoferrin have tended, in my experience, to meet with general approval. These procedures might present special problems for the moral philosopher, because they involve engineering an element of 'humaness' into another species. However, if it is explained to the average reasonable, pragmatic man or woman that milk containing α-1-antitrypsin from a single, genetically engineered sheep could keep 20 sick children alive at a cost of £50 per year, whereas with existing technology it would cost £10 000 to support a single child, then genetic engineering suddenly looks like a thoroughly good idea.

The effects of such genetic engineering on animal welfare are, on balance, likely to be beneficial. There is some cost, probably to large numbers of animals, as a result of the surgical procedures necessary to install the desired gene. Thereafter subsequent generations of sheep secreting α-1-antitrypsin in their milk or pigs carrying hearts and kidneys that would not be rejected if transplanted into a human are most unlikely to *feel* any different. Moreover, they benefit from one of the crudest of all economic laws, namely the fact that the amount of care we are prepared to lavish on an animal increases in direct proportion to its value to us, whether economic or sentimental. Tracey and other ewes secreting α-1-antitrypsin in their milk are being treated as well as racehorses.

I close this chapter with the suggestion that Schweitzer's absolutist argument that the practice of reverence for all life should only be breached under the pressure of necessity has a great deal in common with the pragmatic common sense of the reasonable man. In this debate I have more faith in public opinion than in that of the entrepeneur or the scientist in his thrall. The reasonable man can see the case for genetically engineering a strain of sheep to keep sick children alive. The necessity is great and the cost is small. Public opinion is, however, opposed to the use of the injection of growth hormone (BST) into cattle to increase milk yield or the insertion of growth hormone into the genome of pigs to make them grow faster, not primarily because they are new science but because we do not really need these things. In which case they are not fair.

13 Right Thought and Right Action

'The end of a man is an action and not a thought, though it were the noblest'

Thomas Carlyle, *Sartor Resartus*

The title for this final chapter is taken from the 'Middle Path' or 'Noble Eightfold Path' of Theravada Buddhism. It is, in full, 'right views, right attitude of mind (or motive), right speech, right action (or conduct), right means of livelihood, right effort, right mind control and right serenity (or meditation)'. The path does not necessarily require any element of dogma, it is simply a means to an end, a code of conduct based on the moral principle of reverence for all life and the pragmatic principle that the most effective route to right action is the 'Middle Way'.

The middle way

The 'Noble Eightfold Path' is a very practical philosophy which can be applied to the principles of animal welfare without piety or sentimentality. For example:

(1) The concept of reverence for all life is a powerful deterrent to self-interest.
(2) The concept of the middle way is a powerful deterrent to extremism.
(3) The recognition that within the overall scheme of things, animal welfare is important, but not *that* important, is a powerful stabilizer.
(4) The concept that emotion should be cerebral rather than visceral is a powerful way to stay cool.

My approach to the problem of animal welfare has been to ask four basic questions:

'Where do we stand with regard to the animals?'
'What do we know of their minds and their capacity to suffer?'
'What can and should we do about it?'
'Is what we propose to do likely to work?'

Because the mind of any sentient animal is determined both by its genes and its personal experience, it follows that no two animals will ever feel in quite the same way. Ideally, every animal should be considered as a unique individual. This approach may be impractical, for example, when dealing with a flock of sheep, but it is a useful principle to assume that the welfare requirements of animals should be considered not only in terms of the species and the environment to which they are exposed but also, wherever possible, in terms of their individual needs and expectations. I have argued throughout that problems of animal welfare are complex and need to be analysed in detail on a case-by-case basis. It helps neither man nor animal to reduce the debate to slogans like 'Animal Liberation'. It helps even less to set animals 'free' without any clear idea as to where they would prefer to be.

In attempting to draw together the multiple strings of my argument, I am faced by the trite but true cliché that all generalizations are dangerous, even this one. My first general conclusion actually escapes this criticism because most problems of animal welfare need to be made on a case-by-case basis. There are, however, some basic principles and common rules which can be applied to the analysis and resolution of specific problems in animal welfare, in the same way as there are basic rules for the diagnosis and treatment of disease.

Where do we stand?

The question 'Where do we stand with regard to the animals?' can be built up from four basic premises, indeed, facts of life. The first is that man has dominion over most animals, whether we like it or not. The extent of this dominion varies. At one extreme stands the tiger. We define the nature and extent of the habitat we are prepared to grant to the tiger but thereafter leave it alone to fend for itself. At the other extreme we find the battery hen or lap dog, where, for rather different reasons, we take it upon ourselves to provide all the things we deem necessary for existence and in so doing, almost entirely deny these animals the opportunity to make a constructive contribution to the quality of their own life.

The next fact of life is that we care for animals in direct proportion to their value to us (whether we admit to it or not). Value here implies both wealth and the quality of our own life. We measure the value of the battery hen in terms of its ability to make money by laying eggs. When egg-laying stops this value disappears. The racehorse breeder values his animals because they give him pleasure and *might* create real wealth. When dog owners say that their pets have mere sentimental value they are understating their case. Pet dogs directly influence the quality of their owners' lives; they satisfy a human need quite as directly as the hen that lays a daily egg. The supreme example of a sense of value that is entirely sentimental is our desire to save the tiger. We don't actually 'need' tigers any more than we need wild rats and both are potentially dangerous to man. Taking either species out of its ecosystem would disturb the balance of nature but nature would adjust.

Because we care for animals in proportion to their value to us, it follows that the welfare of an individual or population of animals will increase only in proportion to the extent that we are prepared to increase their value. To achieve this, they must work harder (or produce more) for us or we must work harder (or pay more) for them, or both. Thus matters of animal welfare cannot be considered as absolutes but on the basis of cost:benefit analyses to determine:

(1) the cost to them of the things we do to animals for our benefit (e.g. for food or for science);
(2) the cost to us of acting for their benefit (e.g. by improving husbandry or habitat);
(3) the cost to us of breaking our current association with an animal species (e.g. exterminating the tiger or giving up veal).

The third fact of life is that it matters not to the animal how we feel but what we do. Its capacity to suffer will be related to its sentience and its welfare determined by how well it can avoid suffering and achieve reward. These things are defined by the animal's genotype, habitat and experience, irrespective of whether we classify it as food, pet or vermin and irrespective of our present and future intentions.

The fourth fact of life is that being dead is not a welfare problem for the animal that is dead.

Animal mind, animal welfare and suffering

The welfare of a sentient animal depends on how it feels (in its mind) and on its ability to sustain fitness (in its body and mind). Most of the animal species closest to man – including pets like dogs, cats and horses, farm animals like cows, pigs and chickens, laboratory animals like rodents and primates, 'game' like deer and foxes – are sentient creatures. Though their minds may differ greatly from one another and even more from that of man, they are not 'hard-wired' automata which can only react instinctively to stimuli, in the sense that a moth is instinctively attracted towards a light. Many of their actions are instinctive, as are ours. However, they are also *aware* of sensations from the external and internal environment and use this awareness as a basis for cognitive decisions governing actions designed to avoid suffering or seek reward. The most simple and satisfactory way to interpret the motivation and conscious behaviour of such sentient animals is to accept that:

They are aware of how they feel; *and it matters to them.*

Sentient animals are not only aware that they can feel bad and feel good, they know it *matters* to their welfare to feel good and to avoid feeling bad, not only to sustain fitness but also to maintain a satisfactory state of mind. In an environment where they have to work for themselves they are faced by a number of simultaneous, conflicting, potentially stressful stimuli like hunger, cold, fear and exhaustion. They rank the importance of these stimuli according to how they feel (Chapter 2), and establish a set of priorities for action designed to adjust how they feel away from a state for which there is no better word than suffering and, if circumstances are favourable, towards a state for which the best word is pleasure.

Many of these potential sources of suffering and pleasure, like hunger and appetite, cold and comfort, fear and security, are very primitive and therefore occur in a wide range of species. Other feelings and moods, like boredom and frustration, friendship and loss may be restricted to a very small range of species, or less important to a chicken or a horse than they are to us. However, there is no need to assume that animals suffer in the same way, or for the same reasons as we do, in order to conclude that they have the capacity to suffer. The source of their suffering may be primitive, like hunger or pain, but it still makes them feel bad.

Among the many animals about our house when my daughter was young were stick-insects. Now to deny these animals food, water or an adequate thermal environment would be detrimental to their welfare because they would, eventually, be unable to sustain fitness. It would, however only be cruel if stick-insects have the mental capacity to be aware that they are suffering from hunger, dehydration or cold. I do not wish to speculate as to the extent of sentience in the stick insect. I am, however, convinced by the evidence that mammals and birds have the capacity to experience both suffering and pleasure, which implies that it is cruel to abuse their welfare by 'doing or omitting to do any act'. We may be able to justify our action, or inaction, on the basis of our need relative to the amount of cruelty likely to be involved but we can no longer escape the conclusion that cruelty *is* involved so justification is necessary.

When man either assumed, in Cartesian fashion, that animals had no feelings, or more commonly, simply did not think about the matter at all, we could claim that we were not being cruel because we were not aware of the suffering of other species, in the way that we assume the tiger is not aware of the suffering of the kid. However, man started very early to eat of the fruit of the tree of knowledge of good and evil (and was banished, in consequence, from the Garden of Eden). What is more, we continue to eat avidly and ever-increasing knowledge brings ever-increasing responsibility. The more we learn of the minds of other animals the more difficult it is to escape the fact that we can and do cause them to suffer. The extent to which they will suffer is determined by the nature of their own sentience, not by the way we may classify them as friends or foes of man; pets, farm animals or vermin.

One of the main aims of this book is to help us live with this knowledge and act upon it with a proper mixture of compassion and realism. The rules that help me in this regard are:

(1) It is impossible to eliminate suffering in animals or in man. The aim must be to *minimize* suffering. The utilitarian principle of Jeremy Bentham and Peter Singer requires that this aim should extend beyond man alone to include all animals. Since, by definition, only sentient animals can suffer, this restricts somewhat the extent of our obligation.

(2) It is not necessary to the welfare of an animal that it is given an environment that is without stress, but one in which it can cope with these stresses by taking effective action before they reach an intensity sufficient to induce suffering.

(3) If we are to minimize suffering we need to understand the specific causes of suffering in animals and the specific actions they need to take to prevent these from occurring.

(4) Our responsibilities to animals must always be set against our responsibilities, not only to ourselves as individuals but also to human society. My argument throughout is that we should try to be fair; i.e. strike a reasonable balance between costs and benefits to both parties. I recognize, however, that my definition of fairness is one-sided. One can ask animals how they feel at the time but not in what circumstances it is fair to be eaten.

Sources of suffering and pleasure

Throughout this book I have used the five freedoms as a framework upon which to build a comprehensive series of questions to address what, if any, factors might constitute a source of suffering to animals whether on the farm, in the home or laboratory, in the wild, in transit or at the point of slaughter. To recapitulate, the five freedoms are:

(1) *Freedom from thirst, hunger and malnutrition* – by providing ready access to fresh water and a diet to maintain full health and vigour.

(2) *Freedom from discomfort* – by providing a suitable environment including shelter and a comfortable resting area.

(3) *Freedom from pain, injury and disease* – by prevention or rapid diagnosis and treatment.

(4) *Freedom to express normal behaviour* – by providing sufficient space, proper facilities and company of the animal's own kind.

(5) *Freedom from fear and distress* – by ensuring conditions which avoid mental suffering.

The five freedoms can be said to constitute 'right thought' in a strictly practical sense. They are easily memorized and comprehensive. This means that when they are used as the framework for an evaluation of the welfare of a particular group of animals in a particular environment there is a fair chance that nothing of importance will be forgotten. Many practical husbandry systems and most moral debates on animal welfare can be criticized on the grounds that they tend to be based on incomplete pictures of what constitutes quality of life for an animal. Use of the five freedoms reveals the complexity of most animal welfare problems, so guards against simplistic propositions like 'Ban all forms of cage for the laying hen!' on the grounds that they may do more harm than good. It also acts as a deterrent to impossibilism – seeking too much and ending up with nothing.

The biggest flaw in the concept of the five freedoms is that it is not, in fact, necessary to the welfare of an animal (or man) to have absolute freedom from hunger, cold, pain, fear, etc., only that the animal should be able to cope with these problems by taking effective action to avoid suffering. I have suggested that there should perhaps be a sixth freedom, the freedom to be free or, more specifically, the freedom to exert personal control over the quality of life and so escape not only suffering but also the possibility of limbo (Fig. 2.2). It helps to bear in mind this important, if rather fuzzy, general principle when addressing a welfare problem but it does not fit alongside the first five freedoms which are specific, pragmatic and lend themselves to practical solutions.

Having emphasized that no welfare problem can be considered in isolation, I shall now review, with caution, some of the specific issues raised in Part II and identify those which, in my opinion are currently causing the biggest welfare problems for those animals within our dominion.

Pain

Whatever criteria one uses to rank problems of animal welfare – intensity, duration or numbers of animals affected – pain must rank as the most serious. Our understanding of pain in animals and man is far from complete but the available evidence suggests that animals such as cattle, sheep and horses are as sensitive to pain as man. Animals not only find pain aversive and try to avoid future exposure but also display anxiety if they anticipate that they will be unable to avoid pain or control the intensity of the stimulus. When pain becomes chronic, the intensity tends to increase rather than diminish with the passage of time. All these factors imply that sentient animals do not merely experience pain, they suffer from it.

Complete freedom from pain, like all the five freedoms, is not only unattainable but unnecessary. Some animals, like old dogs and old people, can sustain a reasonable quality of life while in chronic pain provided that they can enjoy good food, good companions and rest in a comfortable bed. However, farm animals crippled with lameness not only have few, if any compensating pleasures but are also unlikely to find a place to rest in comfort. Indeed, their accommodation is likely to have contributed to their lameness in the first place. Approximately 25% of broiler chickens suffer from painful leg disorders for one-third of their lives. Thus at any one time within the UK the average number of broiler chickens in pain is 600 000. This gross departure from the principle of good husbandry which is that animals should be bred and reared for sustained fitness only works in economic terms because the birds are killed at six weeks of age. If, for any reason the slaughter date is postponed by as little as two weeks, the birds begin to die spontaneously at a rate that would alarm even the coldest of accountants.

The other group of farm animals that suffer pain from chronic lameness are the breeding females, dairy cows, ewes, sows and laying hens. In each case chronic pain can cause individual animals to suffer without seriously compromising the reproductive performance of the flock or herd. The problem of lameness, whether in broilers or breeding females, is the most striking and serious rebuttal to the producer who argues that optimal productivity is synonymous with optimal welfare: 'If they weren't happy, their performance would suffer.'

Hunger

Any sentient animal will suffer if exposed to starvation or severe malnutrition. Problems of this severity are most likely to occur to animals in the wild, or ranched in the most extensive conditions such as the Australian outback. Farmers will not normally malnourish their animals because it would be economically inept. Individual cases where farm animals or 'pets' have been neglected and left to starve can usually be attributed to poverty and ignorance – problems which, I regret, will not be influenced in any way by the publication of this book.

In the wild, animals may be chronically hungry but they are usually able to address the problem by taking constructive action, by hunting or foraging. Adult domestic animals fed a ration sufficient only to sustain maintenance (to save money and prevent them getting fat) will not suffer hunger but would experience pleasure, in the short term, from access to more food, and are powerfully motivated to search the environment with food in mind. If we simply wish to avoid cruelty, i.e. we consider the extent of our obligation to a particular species of animal is to minimize suffering, then it may be sufficient simply to meet its nutrient requirements. If we wish to encourage positive welfare, i.e. be kind to an animal, we must recognize that food and working for food are both sources of pleasure and help it to manage its life accordingly.

Fear and anxiety

Fear is one of the most useful properties of the conscious mind because it is conducive to survival. Sentient animals are born curious because they need education to survive and acquire this education usually while under the protection of a parent or parents. They learn to discriminate between real and apparent dangers and, as they mature, become progressively cautious. Having lost the protection of a parent, they rely on their own sense of fear to direct their actions towards survival. When the gazelle learns that the charge of the leopard is truly frightening but once again, manages to escape, it may come to recognize fear as a constructive motivating force that produces its own reward, not as a source of suffering.

Again I appear to have made a nonsense of one of the five freedoms. We are under no obligation to give animals freedom from fear. Our responsibilities are twofold:

(1) to allow the mind of a young animal to develop normally in an enriched environment so that it can learn to distinguish between real and apparent threats before the innate maturation of mood proceeds from curiosity to anxiety;

(2) to minimize the exposure, and repeated exposure, of animals to unpleasant stimuli which they cannot, or anticipate they cannot, escape.

We fail equally in our first responsibility if we keep a veal calf tethered in an individual crate or a puppy chained in a kennel. We fail in our second responsibility when we regularly expose an animal to unpleasant experiences, be they repeated 'scientific procedures' or repeated visits (for some dogs) to the boarding kennels. In each case, they anticipate that an unpleasant experience is forthcoming *and there is nothing that they can do about it*. This can induce a mood of anxiety. 'Freedom from fear' might read better as 'Freedom from anxiety' but it does not sound so good and still needs explanation. The five freedoms were devised to carry the impact of the Ten Commandments (writes Webster with consistent lack of modesty). I have spent the last ten years trying to prevent committees from turning them into the Book of Leviticus.

Stress, malaise and exhaustion
The word stress lacks specificity. There is little point in alleging that an animal is suffering stress (still less in wasting money trying to measure it 'objectively' or 'scientifically') without defining, first, whether the alleged stress is to body or mind, and then to what mechanism(s) of body or mind. Only then can one look to a specific remedy. The least unsatisfactory single-sentence definition of stress is 'the state experienced by an animal when it is having difficulty coping with potential sources of suffering or physical harm, presented singly or in combination'. Implicit in this definition, and in Selye's original concept of the general adaptation syndrome (Chapter 6), is the premise that most animals can cope with most acute physical or mental stresses but chronic stress ultimately becomes exhausting and this abuses welfare because the animal not only fails to sustain fitness but suffers from a progressively greater sense of malaise.

The greatest cause for concern relates to farm animals, 'the workers', especially those in the most intensive production systems (Chapter 7). I have already criticized the commercial production of broiler chickens as a grotesque distortion of the principles of good husbandry. Other systems, such as dairy farming, pig breeding and egg production, rear the breeding females to be physically fit at the start of their adult working lives. However, many cows and pigs, and all hens will be 'spent' – worn out – long before the normal, genetically programmed end of their reproductive life-span. Longevity, *per se*, is not an essential for the welfare of non-human animals but quality of life is. The Protection of Animals Act (1911) makes it an offence 'cruelly to ... override, overdrive, overload ... any animal'. It must be equally cruel to make an animal continue to work to provide, for example, milk or eggs when it is finding it increasingly difficult to cope because of chronic pain or the malaise of exhaustion. A few (very few) spent hens may recover in good homes. It will help the majority of all farm animals far more when production systems and culling policies are both designed to protect them from suffering throughout their working lives and then ensure a gentle death.

'Higher feelings'

It is finally necessary to reconsider what animals, if any, may experience suffering or pleasure from 'higher' feelings such as friendship and loneliness, happiness and grief. These words almost invariably crop up when we humans discuss the welfare of other animals and, like 'stress', they usually reflect sloppy reasoning, in this case, anthropomorphism. The evidence of evolution and psychology indicates that the mind of man differs greatly in degree from that of other animals and that the development of mind only began to acquire greater significance than the development of body within the primates (Fig. 2.1). Many aspects of higher feelings, such as empathy and grief are probably restricted to a small range of species, perhaps only a few species of higher primate. The capacity for friendship, as distinct from the exploitation of another individual for reasons of sex or security, may be more widespread and include two of our favourite pets, the dog and the horse. The bonding of parent to offspring is more primitive and widely distributed, which implies that a wide range of parents can suffer grief when untimely parted from their young. The extent of grief will be determined by the extent to which the instinctive bond has been reinforced by experience. Thus the cow whose calf is removed at birth will grieve but she will grieve longer if she loses her calf at two weeks of age. The calf removed from its mother at birth may experience hunger and will call, instinctively, for attention but it will no more experience higher feelings like 'missing its mother' than would a newborn baby.

The final question, to which there is, as yet, no clear answer, is 'Do animals suffer, when in limbo, from boredom or frustration?' We know that they are motivated to actions designed to avoid suffering. When in limbo, and with nothing constructive to do, many animals do nothing at all. This may be a sign of serenity or learned hopelessness. Others develop apparently pointless patterns of behaviour which we call stereotypies. Such behaviour can be taken as evidence that the environment is lacking in interest or reward but we do not yet know whether they indicate that the animal is suffering from frustration, or attempting to cope with a problem of frustration before it reaches the point of suffering, or has simply discovered a pointless but satisfactory way of passing the time. The British pride themselves on having given so many games to the world. We should perhaps admire the pig for its capacity to devise ways of amusing itself.

The capacity of animals to have higher thoughts and feelings like boredom, empathy and grief are proper subjects for research, partly because they may have an important bearing on their welfare, partly because we have a responsibility to learn more about the minds of the animals which we choose to exploit, and partly because the subject is absolutely fascinating. However, if we are to fulfil our practical responsibility for the welfare of the animals in our dominion, we must not give too much emphasis to these higher feelings which may or may not be important. Attention to welfare requires attention to all five freedoms. Most sources of animal suffering are primitive – pain, hunger, heat, cold, anxiety, etc. – but they are sources of suffering nevertheless. Jeremy Bentham's maxim must apply. 'The question is not, Can they reason? Can they talk? but Can they suffer?'

Right action

So far as the animals are concerned it matters not what we think or feel but what we do. So far as we are concerned, '*The end of a man is an action and not a thought, though it were the noblest*'. However, right action depends on right thought. This is not necessarily a moral argument. It simply helps to know what you are doing and why. The main aim of this book has been to help man to improve the welfare of animals:

(1) by raising our consciousness of the nature and specific sources of animal suffering and pleasure;
(2) by exploring how, in our contacts with animals, in the wild, in the home, on the farm, or in the laboratory we may strive to minimize suffering;
(3) by suggesting action for change where change is necessary.

The approach throughout has been deliberately cool, i.e. rational and unemotional. My final approach to right action will be the same, and based on academic principles of research, education and legislation – research to improve our understanding of what is right, education to bring human perceptions of what is right closer to the way that animals feel about it themselves, and legislation to enforce the right when it conflicts with self-interest, market forces or 'short-termism'. I would, however, be less than rational, indeed, a complete idiot, if I thought that this approach would work on its own. There can be no doubt that the welfare of animals depends, too, on the strength of our emotions, particularly the emotions of compassion and anger.

Compassion and anger

Humans have the mental capacity to be cruel but we have also the capacity to be kind. Animal behaviourists have a tendency to dismiss expressions of kindness and altruism in all species, including man, as motivated by self-interest. 'Mother Teresa only acts the way she does because she wants to get into heaven/onto television.' Such arguments are rubbish. The motivation to many human actions can only be interpreted in terms of kindness and compassion, with only the most tenuous element of self-interest. It is, for example, very difficult to attribute to self-interest the desire of some people to improve the life of the battery hen. They might feel better if they achieved their goal, but there are simpler ways of feeling good.

It is also an inescapable fact of life that the welfare of animals has been improved by those who have expressed outrage, even if the outrage has been misguided, offensive or even criminal. I am not advocating violence in the cause of animal liberation. Indeed, I abhor it, but I cannot pretend that has no effect. Expressions of public outrage against, for example, the use of animals in science, or the rearing of veal calves in crates, have brought about change which has, on the whole, been for the good. Whenever there is widespread public outrage, whether about animal welfare, or the politics of Northern Ireland, it will always attract an extremist fringe who are both dangerous and evil, but whenever there is widespread public outrage it is a sign that there is something wrong.

Outrage will, however, only draw attention to a problem, it will not solve it. Solutions call for a cooler head. The Noble Eightfold Path does not reject emotion (although it is not too keen on self-indulgence). It suggests that emotion should be cerebral rather than visceral. I interpret this to mean that it is more compassionate to preserve the natural habitat of a woodland than to put a bandage on a hedgehog. I (though not the Buddha) also interpret it to mean that anger works best when it is served cold.

Research

Research is the pursuit of knowledge and understanding. Once it was simply called philosophy. However, the approach to biological knowledge has come to depend increasingly on the application of scientific method which is, or should be, the creation of hypotheses and then the attempt to test them to destruction. It is difficult to fault the disinterested pursuit of knowledge on grounds of principle but, on the whole, scientists are not greatly loved by the advocates of animal welfare. There are faults on both sides. Many anti-vivisectionists make up their minds in advance and resist all attempts to allow facts to influence their preconceptions. Many 'pure' scientists have been motivated entirely by scientific interest or self-interest without a proper leavening of compassion. Most applied scientists have, until very recently, been directed by the need to produce more food, or to control disease in man, or to create wealth. This motivation to serve human self-interest is highly understandable and highly proper in the face of human hunger, poverty and disease.

When society achieves stability and affluence, it is then equally proper to redirect scientists to other human aspirations like animal welfare and the quality of the environment. Agricultural scientists, in particular, have taken a lot of stick in recent years for working to increase the productivity of the land and the food animals. However, this is what society wanted at the time. We did what people asked for and we succeeded. If it is now the wish of society that we should, by improvements to knowledge, improve the quality of the environment and the welfare of the sentient animals then we can do that too.

I must, however, add a note of extreme caution with regard to the application of science to animal welfare. Much so-called welfare science is really not very good for reasons I have already discussed in some detail. It is either trivial, or fundamentally flawed because, while it purports to achieve objectivity, it merely seeks quasi-scientific measurements to reinforce subjective preconceptions. The top priority for welfare science is, I suggest, not to publish ever more papers on things which we already know to be cruel, or at least unpleasant, but to seek to understand the minds of the animals whose lives we control; their powers of perception, decision making, self awareness, capacity to learn from others. The new generation of cognitive psychologists have developed methods for the study of animal mind that are infinitely more subtle than those based on simplistic stimulus-response theory (see Toates, 1986; Dawkins, 1993). This approach poses subtle questions to animals set in a form which they can understand. As the questions become more interesting so, too, do the answers. Fundamental research into the animal mind is, of course, completely open-ended but it does offer the most constructive approach to welfare questions which we cannot possibly judge *a priori*, such as the extent to which the genotype and experience, or education, of an animal can affect its strength of motivation to and from specific sources of pleasure and suffering, its motivation to make an active, constructive contribution to the quality of its own life and the frustration it may feel if it is thwarted in these devices and desires.

The danger here is that scientists can stand in the way of progress by constant calls for 'further research in this area', possibly through self-interest but more probably due to ingrained liberal indecision. Although we have hardly begun to understand how animals perceive the world there are some things that are simply not acceptable in a society that recognizes animals as sentient creatures. Classic examples include the problem of chronic pain and the deficiencies of the battery cage for laying hens. These things require action now. If legislators had allowed themselves to be influenced by scientists at the time of the drafting of the Protection of Animals Act (1911) they would have had extreme difficulty in drafting the phrase 'unnecessary suffering'. Scientists and others more interested in thought than action would have wrangled endlessly (indeed, still do) over 'What do you mean by suffering?' and 'What do you mean by unnecessary?'

Although scientists and scientific research can contribute to the animal welfare debate and suggest courses of action to be taken or avoided, the topic of animal welfare and what we should do about it goes way beyond science. It involves economics, morality and politics as (we hope) the public expression of morality. I have only skirted around the edges of these themes, preferring to concentrate on an analysis of how animals feel about what we do to them. My role is to act as advocate for the animals in the debate but to accept the judgement deemed to be most fair when all parties have been heard.

Legislation

A.P. Herbert wrote 'The common law of England has been laboriously built about a mythical figure – the figure of the Reasonable Man'. This wise comment illustrates two themes central to any discussion of the law as it relates to animal welfare. First, most law is no more than an attempt to strike a fair balance between the differing objectives of reasonable people. This is why it tends to be unpopular with extremists. Second, the law relating to animal welfare is decided by reasonable *men* (usually: it is difficult to avoid sexism here); animals have made no contribution to the discussion. From the animals' point of view, the law is, at worst, despotic and, at best, paternalistic. This comment is not frivolous. Most animal welfare law is drawn up by legislators under pressure from industry (agriculture and pharmaceuticals), consumers of animal products and animal rights activists, each group having valid but differing points of view. In theory, the animal rights activists represent the third party rights of the animals and this is good. In practice, however, their perception of welfare may not equate to that of the animal.

There is a multiplicity of legislation relating to animal welfare but the major issues of ethics and practice are largely incorporated within three Acts of Parliament. These are:

(1) Unnecessary suffering: the Protection of Animals Act 1911.
(2) Quality of life: Agriculture, (Miscellaneous Provisions) Act 1968.
(3) Necessary suffering: Animals (Scientific Procedures) Act 1986.

The Protection of Animals Act (1911) is to welfare legislation rather as Plato is to philosophy, i.e. it says most of what needs to be said and in simple language. Its first definition of cruelty was clearly a response to the public opinion of the day, namely 'cruelly to beat, kick, ill-treat, over-ride, over-drive, over-load, torture, infuriate or terrify any animal', exemplified by being nasty to horses in the street. The second action said to constitute cruelty is much better defined because it is much simpler, namely 'to cause unnecessary suffering by doing or omitting to do any act'. This, in essence, covers all sins of commission and omission. Porter (1991) has summarized 11 pieces of UK legislation relating to the 1991 Act which deal with such specifics as Performing Animals (1925), Abandonment (1960), Administration of Poisons (1962), Anaesthetics (1964). All these relate to deliberate acts deemed to constitute unnecessary suffering and are reasonably straightforward provided, of course, that we can properly define 'unnecessary suffering'.

Ruth Harrison, in her seminal book, *Animal Machines* (1965), alerted public concern to the fact that the welfare of farm animals could not be ensured by legislation such as the 1911 Act and its descendants, designed simply to prevent conscious acts of cruelty. This concern for the quality of life experienced by farm animals led to a new generation of legislation, the Agricultural (Miscellaneous Provisions) Act 1968 and its descendants, the Welfare of Livestock Regulations 1978, 1982, 1987, 1990 (see Moss, 1993; Porter 1991). These are designed to regulate husbandry practices in part through legislation and in part through Codes of Practice which do not constitute regulations as such but can be used to define minimum welfare standards in the event of a prosecution under the 1968 Act. Similar legislation is emerging slowly from the Commission of the European Communities. Once again, this legislation has been drafted in response to public pressure. It is, however, inherently more difficult to create definitive legislation to guarantee quality of life than it is to prevent deliberate acts of cruelty. Most new legislation designed to improve quality of life for farm animals in intensive systems relates to minimum space requirements, a very limited concept of quality.

The third general category of legislation relating to the welfare of animals is that which permits cruelty in certain circumstances. The Cruelty to Animals Act 1876 'did not disallow' specified acts likely to cause pain when performed by licensed persons for scientific purposes. Its infinitely superior successor, the Animals (Scientific Procedures) Act 1986, not only expands the definition of welfare to include 'pain, suffering, distress or lasting harm' but also requires every such procedure with laboratory animals to be subjected to a cost:benefit analysis to determine whether the cost to the animal, however slight, can be justified in terms of the potential benefit to mankind or, of course, other animals. In essence, this Act defines and quantifies 'necessary suffering' in the context of laboratory animals. It has nothing to say about 'necessary suffering' in the vastly greater number of animals reared for food.

All aspects of animal welfare which require legislation fall into one of the three broad categories outlined above, namely:

(1) deliberate, unjustifiable acts of unnecessary cruelty;
(2) quality of life;
(3) the need to justify scientific, or otherwise 'unnatural' procedures.

The Protection of Animals Act (1911) can deal satisfactorily with most deliberate acts such as mutilations, and slaughter methods. The application of the law should be to minimize suffering in the light of new knowledge, but the principle is sound and does not need to be refined.

The Agriculture (Miscellaneous Provisions) Act 1968, its descendants and similar Directives from the Council of Europe for the protection of farm animals do not carry the near Biblical element of 'thou shalt not' implicit in the Protection of Animals Act 1911. They have, as indicated earlier, been drafted in response to pressure from the welfare-minded consumer lobby and are attempts to achieve a compromise between consumer demand for systems that are 'free' or 'natural' and producer demand for low cost, efficiency and low disease. Legislators have been faced by problems of defining the needs of farm animals for space, freedom, social contact and the opportunity to make a constructive contribution to the quality of their own lives. Given such complex questions, it is no surprise that legislation to date hardly merits being written in tablets of stone. UK legislation has achieved a ban on veal crates and the sow stall. Euro-legislation on the veal calf has sunk into a morass of Orwellian doublespeak, e.g. 'All calves must be provided with a diet adapted to their physiological and behavioural needs. This does not apply to the production of veal calves for white meat.' Attempts to improve the welfare of the laying hen are bogged down in wrangles over trivial changes in space allowances (e.g. 600 *v.* 450 cm^2 per bird) that do not attempt to consider the quality of space and, in the opinion of both sides of the argument (producers and welfarists), will have negligible effects on welfare one way or the other.

Although legislating for quality of life is very difficult, I believe that in the specific case of the laying hen, there is sufficient evidence to legislate for an improvement in minimum standards to provide a recognizable nesting area, a suitable perch and 900 cm^2 free space per bird. Such legislation would constitute an unequivocal improvement on the *status quo*, subject to the guarantee that the new law would remain unchanged for at least the next 10 years. I repeat what I wrote in Chapter 8: the farming industry can play to almost any set of rules, properly enforced throughout the European Community. What it cannot be asked to accept is constant reinvestment in capital equipment to accommodate constant shifts in our definition of acceptability.

I do not pretend that such legislation would be entirely satisfactory when considered merely in terms of its direct effect on the welfare of birds in cages. It cannot be, since all 'quality of life' legislation has to be a compromise. However, legislation that attempts to work for the common good by reconciling the differing aspirations of reasonable men does not have to be proscriptive, it merely needs to fine-tune market forces. The reason why the battery cage has become so dominant is that no other system can compete economically as a mass producer of eggs. My suggestion for improved minimum standards for the battery cage will not achieve optimal environmental standards for hens but it would impose a tax on the battery system and so encourage producers to improve welfare by alternative means. Expanding this argument, I suggest that the whole European approach to legislation for quality of life in farm animals is on the wrong track. Instead of agonizing at interminable length over trivial pieces of restrictive legislation almost totally confined to space requirements, it would be more constructive to consider legislating for incentives to improve welfare. Incentives imply cost, which means cost to the consumer. However, when 42% of European farm incomes are currently in the form of subsidy, governments cannot pretend that they cannot legislate by financial incentive to achieve the common good. If they control 42% of the income, they can do anything they like!

At the moment agricultural subsidies, for example those which encourage farmers not to grow food, are seen by the consumer as achieving only the good of the farming community. There has, as yet, been no attempt to use subsidy as a direct incentive to improved welfare. If politicians were to devise subsidies designed to encourage high welfare systems, (and did not define the rules too precisely), these subsidies would be more popular with all parties, welfare-minded consumers, farmers who wish to farm with pride and the animals themselves. The political party which enforced such legislation might also be rewarded with a few more votes.

It is generally recognized that new biology involving the physiological and genetic manipulation of farm animals will require new legislation to protect man, the environment and, not least, the animals themselves. The welfare implications of new biology must be defined not by the method used to manipulate the animal but by its consequences. Unacceptable 'tinkering' has been defined by the Farm Animal Welfare Council as 'the manipulation of body size, shape or reproductive capacity by breeding, nutrition, hormone therapy or gene insertion in such a way as to reduce mobility, increase the risk of pain, injury, metabolic disease, skeletal or obstetric problems, perinatal mortality or psychological distress'.

It is neither ethical nor practical to legislate to stifle research *a priori* on the grounds that something might just go wrong. FAWC (1987) prefaces its definition of unacceptable tinkering with the words, 'We accept that scientific investigation aims to be impartial and without prejudice so that it is impossible to pronounce *a priori* how any particular piece of new knowledge will affect farm animals'. During the period of scientific investigation of any application of new biology to animal production the animals are protected by the Animals (Scientific Procedures) Act 1986 which applies a cost:benefit analysis to all procedures weighing the cost to the animal in terms of suffering, however slight, against the likely benefit to society (or other animals). I can think of no ethical reason why farm animals should not receive the same degree of protection from the law as laboratory animals. If they did, procedures which required a Home Office licence while conducted to advance knowledge would need to be submitted to a cost:benefit analysis at least as rigorous before being pronounced acceptable for commercial exploitation.

A valid objection to the imposition of controls on the application of new science is that it holds up progress. This argument is only valid, of course, if the progress can be shown to be humane. I suggested in Chapters 9 and 12 that most welfare problems arising from the application of new biotechnology can be resolved (one way or the other) within two generations, or the length of time required for experimentation under the 1986 Act. Some

complex, low incidence conditions like mastitis and lameness in cattle treated
with BST, cannot be resolved without allowing the procedure to expand onto
a commercial scale. I suggest, therefore, that all new technologies to
manipulate animal production and reproduction developed initially under
Home Office Licence should be subject to a two-stage review process. If after
two or three generations the procedure appeared not to 'reduce mobility,
increase the risk of pain, injury, metabolic disease, skeletal or obstetric
problems, perinatal mortality or psychological distress', then it should be
given a provisional licence for commercial exploitation, subject to a properly
designed monitoring procedure for untoward effects in practice (such as an
increase in the incidence of mastitis) and reviewed after, say, five years, the
costs to be met by those promoting the procedure.

Education

Since the welfare of animals within our dominion will be determined by the
extent to which we both value and understand their welfare, it follows that we
can best serve the animals' interests by educating man towards a perception
of welfare that is as close as possible to that of the animals themselves. This
applies principally to man the consumer and the farm animals whom we treat
as a commodity (whatever we may claim to the contrary). There is, of course,
no standard consumer; the majority remain content to eat battery eggs and
broiler chickens, more so than beef or lamb, which indicates that while their
concern for animal welfare may be real it is not paramount.

The food industry has attempted to exploit the separation of the consumer
from the realities of animal production by creating a series of distorted
images which are either pitched at the level of the colouring book (pictures of
happy chickens on boxes of 'farm fresh eggs') or which attempt to suspend
belief that meat ever was part of a living animal. This really is not consumer
education but propaganda. Moreover, it does not take a Machiavelli to
deduce that propaganda is a dangerous instrument unless one holds the
monopoly. The animal industry is now under constant attack from expert
manipulators of the media who create equally distorted images of uncaring
profiteers ruthlessly exploiting suffering animals and laying waste to the
environment. The vulnerability of the consumer to both forms of image is, of
course, in direct proportion to their ignorance of the truth. I believe that it is
in the long-term interest of animal farmers to contribute to the proper
education of consumers by demonstrating quite openly where their meat and
milk is coming from and how it is produced. An excellent test of animal
welfare is to discover whether their owner can display his animals with pride
to any fair-minded observer. For many farmers and farming systems this is
so. However, the special pleading required to suggest that the welfare of
broiler fowl or laying hens is satisfactory, despite their appearance, is deeply
unconvincing to almost any unbiased observer.

Two common, reasonable objections to this suggestion are:

(1) Most consumers do not want to know where their food comes from and such frankness might put them off altogether.
(2) It is only the affluent few who can afford to pay for high welfare products and we have a moral responsibility to provide cheap food for the majority.

The first objection is valid only if farm animals are valued simply as a commodity. Once one accepts that their life itself has a value then nobody who rears, kills or eats them has the right to wash their hands of the relevant moral decisions. This is not a call to veganism. I repeat my example of the lady who gives her beef cattle 'pre-slaughter counselling', so ensuring that they remain calm and do not suffer right up to the point of non-existence. This is a beautiful example of the fundamental point that reverence for life is compatible with a realistic, dignified approach to death.

The second objection is less easy to dismiss. Clearly, food prices for all should not be distorted by welfare standards prescribed by a vocal, affluent, sentimental minority. Indeed I have already argued that attempts to use legislation to impose absolute standards, for example, on animal housing tend to be over-simplistic, open to abuse and as likely to impede as to advance animal welfare. On the other hand, the vast majority of people in the developed world who can afford to buy meat and milk eat more of it than they need. We do not really consume meat, milk and cheese in order to live but because they are among the great luxuries that determine the quality of our own lives. This should impose on us the obligation to ensure a fair deal for the animals involved in helping to improve our quality of life. I have suggested, not entirely flippantly, that a fair deal can be defined as follows: *for six months the farmer feeds the pig and for the next six months the pig feeds the farmer*. The purpose of consumer education is to create an increased awareness of the realities of different systems of animal production and to encourage buying habits based on a compassionate, but not sentimental, recognition of the rights of farm animals to a reasonable quality of life and a gentle death. The farming industry themselves are just beginning to break free from the dogma that livestock are a commodity to be produced as cheaply as possible, not least because this tenet of economic faith is collapsing when faced by a static market which is spoiled for choice and overfed to the point of neurosis. I suggest that it is in the combined interests of the farmer, the consumer, the land and the animals to redefine food of animal origin not as a commodity but according to quality, itself defined by source, system of production and, not least, quality of life for the animals. I further suggest that it is right.

I have given particular emphasis throughout this book to the welfare of farm animals, partly because of the huge number of animals involved, partly because they are so completely under our dominion and partly because we tend to value them only as commodities. The principles that should govern our approach to the farm animals can, however, be applied to our treatment of all those animals within our dominion. The use of animals in scientific procedures is now controlled by legislation which is designed not only to minimize suffering but also justify each procedure in terms of its likely benefit to mankind or other animals. However, I have suggested that the attempt to hide behind the anodyne phrase 'scientific procedures' is not only a distortion of the truth (some, not all, scientific procedures constitute deliberate cruelty), it has failed to lull public opinion. Like the farming industry, the scientific profession has, to date, been economical with the truth. It should be possible to justify all scientific procedures, like all farming systems to 'the reasonable man'. If not, it is reasonable to conclude that there may be something wrong with the procedure or the system.

The aim of education must be to instil in people a proper sense of value for the life of sentient animals. The word 'proper' implies a sense of balance, the Middle Way. The welfare of animals is important but not all-important. Man will, whatever some would wish, care for animals in direct proportion to their value to him. However, our sense of value is not always directed by self-interest. Mankind has the capacity for compassion, and once we have met our immediate needs, we can afford to be compassionate. When we can afford the costs of altruism we can enjoy the benefits. 'Until he extends the circle of his compassion to all living things, man will not himself find peace.'

Further Reading

Bateson, P. (1991) Assessment of pain in animals. *Animal Behaviour*, **42**, 827–40.

Blowey, R. (1993) *Cattle Lameness and Hoof Care*. Farming Press, Ipswich.

Brambell, F.W.R. (1965) Report of technical committee to enquire into the welfare of animals kept under intensive husbandry systems. (Cmnd. 2836) HM Stationery Office, London.

Carpenter, E. (1980) *Animals and Ethics*. Watkins, London.

Christian, J.J. (1971) Population density and reproductive efficiency. *Biology of Reproduction*, **4**, 248–294.

Cooper, J.J. & Nicol, Christine J. (1991) Stereotypic behaviour affects environmental preferences in bank voles, *Clethrionomys glareolus*. *Animal Behaviour*, **41**, 971–977.

Curtis, S.E. (1983) *Environmental Management in Animal Agriculture*. Iowa State University Press, Iowa, USA.

Dawkins, Marian (1980) *Animal Suffering, the Science of Animal Welfare*. Chapman and Hall, London.

Dawkins, Marian (1993) *Through Our Eyes Only? The Search for Animal Consciousness*. Freeman, Oxford.

Eddy, R.G., Davies, O. & David, C. (1991) An economic analysis of twin births in British dairy herds. *Veterinary Record*, **129**, 526–529.

Edney, A. (1989) Killing with kindness. *Veterinary Record*, **124**, 320-322.

European Community (1991) Council Directive laying down minimum standards for the protection of calves. No. L 340/28.

Eyton, Audrey (1991) *The Kind Food Guide*. Penguin Books, London.

Farm Animal Welfare Council (1992) *Report on the Welfare of Broiler Chickens*. MAFF, Tolworth.

Farm Animal Welfare Council (1993) *Second Report on Priorities for Research and Development in Farm Animal Welfare*. MAFF, Tolworth.

Farm Animal Welfare Council (1994) *Report on the Welfare of Sheep*. MAFF, Tolworth.

Fogle, B. (1981) *Interrelation between People and their Pets*. Thomas, Springfield, Illinois, USA.

Foley, C.W., Lasley, J.F., & Osweiler, G.D. (1979) *Abnormalities of Companion Animals*. Iowa State University Press, Iowa, USA.

Forbes, J.M. (1988) Metabolic aspects of the regulation of voluntary food intake and appetite. *Nutrition Research Reviews*, **1**, 145–168.

Fraser, A.F. & Broom, D.M. (1990) *Farm Animal Behaviour and Welfare*. 3rd Ed. Bailliere Tindall, London.

Galef, B.G., Mainardi, M. & Valsechhi, P. (1994) *Behavioural Aspects of Feeding*. Ettore Majoran International Life Series Vol. 12. Harwood Academic Publishers, London.

Gentle, M.J., Waddington, D., Hunter, L.N. & Jones, R.B. (1990) Behavioural evidence for persistent pain following partial beak amputation in chickens. *Applied Animal Behaviour Science*, **27**, 149–157.

Grandin, Temple (1994) *Livestock Handling and Transport.* CAB International, Wallingford.

Gray, J. (1987) *The Psychology of Fear and Stress.* Weidenfeld and Nicolson, London.

Griffin, D.R. (1981) *The Question of Animal Awareness.* Kaufmann, Los Altos, California.

Hecht, S.B. (1993) The logics of livestock and deforestation in Amazonia: directly unproductive but profitable investments and development. *Proc. VII World Congress on Animal Production.* Edmonton Alta, Canada 41–62.

Home Office (1986) *Guidance on the Operation of the Animals (Scientific Procedures) Act 1986.* HMSO, London.

Huntingford, Felicity and Turner, Angela (1987) *Animal Conflict.* Chapman & Hall, London.

Iggo, A. (1984) *Pain in Animals.* Universities Federation for Animal Welfare, Potters Bar, Hertfordshire.

Kempson, S.A., and Logue, D.N. (1993) Ultrastructural observations of hoof horn from dairy cows: changes in the white line during the first lactation. *Veterinary Record,* **132**, 524–527.

Kestin, S.C., Knowles, T.G., Tinch, A.E. & Gregory, N.G. (1992) Prevalence of leg weakness in broiler chickens and its relationship with genotype. *Veterinary Record,* **131**, 191–194.

Kestin, S.C. (1995) Welfare aspects of the slaughter of whales: Analysis and interpretation of 1992 and 1993 humane killing data. *Animal Welfare* **4**, 11–28.

Kirkwood, J.K. & Webster, A.J.F. (1984) Energy-budget strategies for growth in mammals and birds. *Animal Production,* **38**, 147–156.

Kirkwood, J.K. (1985) Patterns of growth in primates. *Journal of Zoology,* **205**, 123–136.

Kyriazakis, I. & Emmans, G.C. (1991) Diet selection in pigs: dietary choices made by pigs following a period of underfeeding with protein. *Animal Production,* **52**, 337–346.

Lawrence, A.B. & Rushen, J. (1993) *Stereotypic Animal Behaviour: Fundamentals and Applications to Welfare.* CAB International, Wallingford.

Ley, S.J., Livingstone, A. & Waterman, A.E. (1989) The effect of chronic clinical pain on thermal and mechanical thresholds in sheep. *Pain,* **39**, 353–357.

Linzey, A. (1976) *Animal Rights.* SCM Press, London.

Lorenz, K.Z. (1966) *On Aggression.* Methuen, London.

McFarland, David (1989) *Problems of Animal Behaviour.* Longman, Harlow.

MacInerny J. (1991) A socioeconomic perspective on animal welfare. *Outlook on Agriculture,* **20**, 51–56.

Meat and Livestock Commission Yearbooks: Pigs, Beef, Sheep. MLC, Milton Keynes.

Meat Manufacturing and Marketing (1993) New guidance on stunning and slaughter in pig abattoirs. October 1993, p 24–26.

Medawar, P.B. (1972) *The Hope of Progress.* Methuen, London.

Medway Report (1979) *Report of a Committee to Investigate Welfare Aspects of Shooting and Angling.* RSPCA.

Menzel, R. (1948) Observations on the pariah dog. In *The Book of the Dog.* Ed. B. Fitzgerald. Mouton, The Hague.

Ministry of Agriculture, Fisheries and Food. *Codes of Practice for the Welfare of Livestock.* Cattle, pigs, poultry etc., MAFF, Tolworth.

Moss, R. (1993) Welfare in national and international legislation. In *Livestock Health and Welfare*. Ed. R. Moss. Longman, Harlow.

Paton, W. (1992) *Man and Mouse*. 2nd edition. Oxford University Press.

Pimentel, D. & Pimentel, M. (1979) *Food, Energy and Society*. Arnold, London.

Poole, T. (1987) *The UFAW Handbook on the Care and Management of Laboratory Animals*. 6th ed. Longman, Harlow.

Porter, A.R.W. (1991) Animal Welfare. In *Legislation affecting the Veterinary Profession in the United Kingdom*. Royal College of Veterinary Surgeons, Belgrave Square, London.

Rifkin, J. (1993) *Beyond Beef. The Rise and Fall of the Cattle Culture*. Dutton Books, Washington, D.C.

Russel, W.M.S. & Burch, R.L. (1959) *The Principles of Humane Experimental Technique*. Methuen, London.

Ryder, R.D. (1975) *Victims of Science*. Davis-Pointer, London.

Schweitzer, A. (1933) *My Life and Thought: an Autobiography*. Trans. C.T. Campion. Allen and Unwin, London.

Scott, J.P. & Fredericson, E. (1951) The causes of fighting in mice and rats. *Physiological Zoology*.

Sherwin, C.M. (1994) *Modified Cages for Laying Hens*. Universities Federation for Animal Welfare, Potters Bar.

Singer, P. (1990) *Animal Liberation: A New Ethics for our Treatment of Animals*. Avon, New York.

Smith, Jane A. & Boyd, K.M. (1991) *Lives in the Balance. The Ethics of Using Animals in Biomedical Research*. Oxford University Press.

Stevenson, P. (1994) *A Far Cry from Noah*. Green Print, London.

Toates, F. (1986) *Motivational Systems*. Cambridge University Press, Cambridge.

Wathes, C.M. & Charles, D.R. (1994) *Livestock Housing*. CAB International, Wallingford.

Webster, A.J.F. (1981) Nutrition and the Thermal Environment. In *Nutritional Physiology of Farm Animals*. Eds. J.A.F. Rook & P.C. Thomas. Longman, London.

Webster, A.J.F. (1993) *Understanding the Dairy Cow*. 2nd ed. Blackwell Scientific Publications, Oxford.

Webster, A.J.F. (1992) Energy expenditure, studies with animals. In *The Contribution of Nutrition to Human and Animal Health*. Eds. E.M. Widdowson & J.C. Mathers. Cambridge University Press.

Webster, A.J.F. (1993) Energy partitioning, tissue growth and appetite control. *Proceedings Nutrition Society*, **52**, 69–76.

Webster, A.J.F., Saville, Claire and Welchman, D.B. (1986) *Improved Husbandry Systems for Veal Calves*. University of Bristol, Bristol.

Wells, M.J. (1978) *Octopus*. Chapman & Hall, London.

Winick, M. (1988) *Control of Appetite*. Wiley, New York.

Index

aborigines, 74
access system for veal calves, 188–91, 189
acclimatization, 70–74
adaptation, 70–74, 117–20
adrenal hormones, 117–19
agoraphobia (in hens), 12, 13
aggression, 79, 108, 109, 149
agonistic behaviour, 108
Agriculture (Miscellaneous Provisions) Act (1968), 259–60
alarm, 117–19, 118, 224
altruism, 107, 209, 257, 265
analgesics, 91, 92, 94
anger, 257
animal handling, 153–5, 158–60
animal mind, 23
animal rights, 6, 7
animal welfare research, 240–42, 257–9
Animals (Scientific Procedures) Act (1986), 88, 91, 182, 211, 229–34, 237, 244, 259–62
antagonistic behaviour, 79–81
anxiety, 28, 64, 84, 90, 104, 113, 206, 226, 235, 237, 253–4
apathy, 28
  learned apathy, 14, 31
appetite, 30, 40–45
ascites, 76

bar-chewing, 56, 57–9
barren environments, 64, 81–4, 146
battery cages for hens, 76, 78, 144, 157–8, 169, 261
beef production, 137, 138–40, 183–6
behavioural needs, 31, 33
biotechnology, 242–6
bird behaviour, 110, 123

blowfly strike, 88, 192
boredom, 201–2, 225, 255
bovine somatotropin (BST), 172, 175–6, 183, 242, 244–6, 263
Brambell Committee, 10, 63, 78, 156
breeding and welfare, cattle, 180–83
  dogs, 201, 210–13
British Union for the Abolition of Vivisection, 229
Buddhism, 14, 247–8, 257

cannibalism in poultry, 77, 108
castration, 192–3, 206–10
cat behaviour, 55, 206–8
cattle, 67, 72, 75, 167–91
  behaviour, 53, 63
  calves, 77, 169
  see also dairy cows
  veal calves, 58, 59, 65, 117, 186–91, 187, 189
circuses, 225–7
Clethrionomys glareolus, bank voles, 82
Codes of Welfare for Farm Animals, 65, 129
cognition, 7, 27–31, 258
Compassion in World Farming, 15, 194
competition, 108
cold stress, 28, 67, 68–70
colostrum, 179
comfort, 28, 31, 62, 74–78, 76
comfort behaviour, 79
companionship, 31, 107, 122–24, 205, 208–9, 255
conflict, 108, 121
conformation and lameness, 156, 173–5, 174

congenital abnormalities, 211–13, 212

cooperation, 121–23

Cordelia, 8

cost:benefit analysis in animal welfare, 249, 260–62

   livestock production, 130–34, 132, 242

   scientific procedures, 230–38, 235

'crazy chick disease', 49

crib-biting, 56, 59–61, 203–4

crowding stress, 119

Cruelty to Animals Act (1911), 230, 260

curiosity, 28, 64, 86, 253

dairy cows, 77, 167–83

   production, 137, 141, 142

   production diseases, 143

death and dying, 15, 104–6

debeaking, 93, 156

Declaration of Independence, 14–15

deer behaviour and welfare, 93, 110, 197, 219

deer hunting, 219–21

dehydration, 54, 101, 103

depression, 90, 101, 103, 113

displacement behaviour, 31, 34

dog behaviour, 46, 109, 110, 122–4, 169, 200, 204–10

'dog-sitting' in sows, 77, 149

domestication, 4–6, 45–7

dominance hierarchy, 79, 108, 111

donkey behaviour, 208

double-muscling, 184

Draize tests, 232, 245

dust-bathing, 76, 157

dyspnoea, 101

economics of livestock production, 130–34, 132

economic theory of motivation, 33

education, in animals, 62, 121, 144

   to improve animal welfare, 263–5

electronically controlled feeders, 149, 189

elephant behaviour, 105

embryo transfer, 181–3

energy cost of growth, 24–6, 25

environmental enrichment, 84–86

environmental requirements, 62–81, 62

Escherichia coli, 176

Eskimos, 4, 74

euthanasia, 213–15

evolution of mind, 24–27, 64, 255

exhaustion, 28, 36, 117, 118, 177, 236, 254

exploration, 64

factory farming, 69, 136, 146

Farm Animal Welfare Council, 10, 62, 79, 156, 163, 181, 184, 193, 211, 240, 243, 262

farrowing crates, 150–52, 151

farrowing of sows, 85

fear, 28, 30, 45, 64, 104, 112–16, 113, 160, 223–5, 235, 253–4

   fear of isolation, 122

   fear of novelty, 113, 114

   innate fears, 30, 114–15

   learned fears, 113, 114–15

feather pecking, 76, 79, 111

feelings, 19, 27–31, 28

fever, 100, 101

fighting, 79

fishing, 222–5

'five freedoms', 10–14, 12, 59, 62, 76, 117, 169, 101, 225, 236, 251–2

food selection, 47–53, 52

foraging, 45, 64

fox behaviour, 46, 200

fox hunting, 46, 219

frustration, 157, 201, 225, 255

gas stunning, 154–5, 160

general adaptation syndrome, 116–21, 118, 254

genetic engineering, 213, 228, 232, 242–6
Gloria, the artificial chicken, 159
goat behaviour, 46
grief, 255

habituation, 71, 74
heat exchanges, 65–70, 66, 67
heat stress, 28, 67, 68–70, 160
'higher feelings', 255
high-welfare foods, 129
hock burn, 75
homeothermy, 65–70, 67, 119
hopelessness, 14, 28, 35, 206
horses, 59–61, 60, 75
    horse behaviour, 124, 203–4, 208
housing, 62–86
hunger, 21, 28, 36, 39–53, 235, 253
    metabolic hunger, 39–45, 50, 171–2
    for specific nutrients, 47–53
hunting, 218–22
hygiene, 62, 74–8, 75, 76

impotence, 28
inappetence, 101, 102
infectious diseases, 101, 120
intensification and sustainability, 136–40
intensification of livestock systems, 130, 134–40

lactation, 142, 169–71
lameness, 93, 172–5, 173, 252
laminitis, 95, 102, 173
laparoscopy, 193
LD$_{50}$ tests, 232, 239–40
learned helplessness, 35, 81, 103, 113, 116, 238
legislation for improved welfare, 144, 259–63
    battery hens, 161–2, 261–2
    broiler chickens, 162–3
    control of biotechnology, 182–3, 244–5, 262
    incentives, use of subsidies, 162, 192, 261–2
    slaughter, 164–5
    sow stalls, 165–6
    transport, 164–5, 196
    veal calves, 188–90
leg weakness, in broilers, 156, 163
libido, 28
limbo, 36, 37, 252, 255
limits to productivity of animals, 142–6
longevity, 105, 255

'MacFarland's Egg', 36, 36–38, 47, 83, 121, 172, 205
magnesium deficiency, 53
malaise, 28, 44, 47, 54, 235, 237, 254
mastitis, 175–7
maturation and brain development, 24–7
maturation rates, 24–7, 25
metabolic body size, 140
metabolic diseases, 177
metabolizable energy requirement, 42, 140–42
mice, 3, 81, 119, 232, 233, 242
milking machines, 175–7, 177
MOET, 181, 185–6, 193, 244
moods, 27–31, 28, 57, 90
mood-altering drugs, 30
motivation, 31, 121, 241, 258
motivational priorities, 31, 32, 36
mutilations, 88, 192, 206

naloxone, 57
natural selection, 23, 107
nursery accommodation for pigs, 150–52
nutrient requirements, 42, 43

obstetric problems, 181–5, 213
opiates, 96, 115, 118, 241
oral satisfaction, 40, 45, 55–61, 147, 202–5

pain, 28, 29, 57, 75, 76, 89–99, 91, 92, 101, 153, 160, 236, 252–3
  chronic pain, 95–7, 102, 156, 174, 185, 214
  indices of pain, 91, 91–5
  pain in fish, 94, 223–5
  pain thresholds, 91, 94–6
  pharmacology of pain, 91, 92, 93–4
patenting of life forms, 242, 245
pets, 199–201
pigs, 66, 73, 75, 77, 146–55
  behaviour, 44, 59, 85
  breeding sows, 59, 77, 84, 146–52, 148, 165–6
  food selection, 52
  growing pigs, 152–3
  pig production, 137, 146–53
play, 64, 124, 202
pleasure, 28, 29, 37, 44, 121, 124, 250
poultry production, 155–60
  broilers, 51, 75, 76, 120, 137, 155–6, 162–4, 252
  laying hens, 10, 12, 73, 75, 76, 81, 137, 157–8
preference tests, 31
primates evolution, 25, 26
  behaviour, 82, 84, 105, 114, 123, 225–6
production disorders, 142, 171
Protection of Animals Act (1911), 87, 221, 255, 258–61

quality assurance marketing schemes, 129–30, 161–3, 264
Quantock system for veal calves, 186–8, 187

rabbit welfare, 75, 78, 93, 199
rat behaviour and welfare, 48–9, 53, 71–74, 75, 116, 245
  diet selection, 48–9
  Zucker rats, 49–52, 50
rebound behaviour, 31, 34, 80
rehydration, 101

relief of sickness, 100–4
rest, 28, 74–6
resting area, properties, 75
robot milking, 176, 177
round heart disease, 49
Royal College of Veterinary Surgeons, 88, 103
Royal Society for Prevention of Cruelty to Animals, 129, 194, 223, 226

salmon behaviour, 110
satiety, 28, 40
schizophrenia, 110
scientific procedures, 229–40, 231, 232
  refinement, reduction and replacement, 231–3, 238–40
security, 28, 31, 62, 74, 75, 76, 79, 121
sensuality, 28, 73
sentience, 23, 245, 249–50
sexual behaviour, 110, 121–22, 205–20
sheep production, 191–3
  behaviour, 67, 110, 114, 122
  welfare, 168, 183, 191–3, 239
shooting, 218–22
sickness, 99–104, 101
slaughter, 106, 154–5, 164, 197–8, 223
  casualty slaughter, 198
  ritual slaughter, 4, 106, 168
sodium appetite, 47, 53
sow stalls, 61, 147–50, 148
space requirement, 78–81, 144, 261
stable vices, 203–5
stalking, 218–20
stereotypic behaviour, 31, 35, 56, 255
  locomotor stereotypies, 82–4, 204
  oral stereotypies, 40, 55–61, 203–5
stress, 35–8, 70, 102, 116–121, 226, 254–5
  social stress, 119–120
  see also general adaptation syndrome

submission, 109
subsidies, 162, 192
suffering, 6–7, 19–20, 35–38, 36, 90,
        205, 229–33, 250–52, 256
supermarkets, 128
survival of the fittest, 24–7, 107
sweating, 68–73, 115

tail-biting in pigs, 111–12, 153
tail docking, 88, 112, 192
thermal comfort, 28, 62, 63, 65–70
thermal panting, 72
thermoneutral zone, 67, 68
thirst, 28–9, 40, 47, 54–5
tigers, 3, 46, 81, 226, 248
tongue rolling, sucking, 56, 58, 186
Tour de France, 141, 142
'toys', 86
toxicology testing, 238–9
transportation, 70, 72, 163–5, 194–6
    cattle, 117, 194–6
    pigs, 72
    poultry, 70, 114, 158–60
    sheep, 72, 194–6
triangulation, 241
turkeys, 156

twitching the horse, 96, 97

ulcerative colitis, 226
unnecessary suffering, 87–9, 131,
        221, 258–61
utilitarianism, 6, 214, 251

vegetarianism, 130
vigour, 28, 30
vivisection, 229, 237–9

weaning, 116, 152, 178–80
weaving, in horses, 56, 82, 202–4
Welfare of Animals at Slaughter Act
        (1991), 88
Welfare of Animals During
        Transport Order (1992), 197
welfare of farmers, 143–5
whaling, 224–5
wild animals, 45, 79, 216–27
wildlife parks, 225–7
windsucking, 56, 59–61, 60, 203
wolf behaviour, 200–1, 208
work rates of animals, 140–42, 142

zoos, 201, 225–7